HEALING HERBS ALREADY IN THE KITCHEN . . .

Rosemary

A simple cup of rosemary tea is as effective as aspirin for headaches and other inflammatory symptoms, including the relief of arthritic pains. Rosemary is also good for the hair and scalp . . .

Dill

Dillweed is effective in treating the symptoms of children's colicky stomachaches and pains. A dill tea is also good for adult stomachaches and insomnia caused by indigestion . . .

Anise

Coughs and colds respond to a tea of anise seed. A good tea for gas, indigestion, bloating, and nausea is made by combining a pinch each of powders of anise seed, ginger, cardamom, cinnamon, and an even smaller pinch of black pepper. Steep the spices in boiled hot water or scalded milk . . .

Books by Michael Tierra

The Natural Remedy Bible (*with John Lust*)
The Way of Herbs
The Way of Chinese Herbs

Published by POCKET BOOKS

THE WAY OF
HERBS

FULLY UPDATED—WITH THE LATEST DEVELOPMENTS IN HERBAL SCIENCE

MICHAEL TIERRA
L.Ac., O.M.D.

POCKET BOOKS
New York   London   Toronto   Sydney

POCKET BOOKS, a division of Simon & Schuster Inc.
1230 Avenue of the Americas, New York, NY 10020

ISBN-13: 978-0-671-02327-0
ISBN-10:   0-671-02327-6

First Pocket Books trade paperback printing August 1998

20

POCKET and colophon are registered trademarks of Simon & Schuster Inc.

Cover design by Joseph Perez
Front cover illustration by Amy Panzer

Text design by Stanley S. Drate/Folio Graphics Co. Inc.

Printed in the U.S.A.

Dedicated to my teachers:
Dr. Christopher,
Hari Das Baba,
Foon Lee Wong
Miriam Lee,
Efrem Korngold,
and Lesley Gunsaulus Tierra
for her loving support and encouragement.

A special thanks to Steven Foster for the
critical eye he applied to this edition.

CONTENTS

FOREWORD

When I first met Michael in 1980, he had just completed the first edition of *The Way of Herbs*. At that time, the Western herbal renaissance had begun and was being led by a handful of herbal masters and their next generation. Traditional Chinese medicine (TCM) was even younger in this country, having just been introduced in the West because of the interest of a few Americans. Ayurvedic medicine from India was only beginning to be introduced. Michael had studied all of these, along with Native American herbology from the Karok Indians in Northern California.

Through the study of these various ancient traditional systems of healing, Michael discovered the importance of a theoretical foundation for the application of natural medicines. This was especially emphasized while Michael was living and traveling in India, studying Ayurvedic medicine. He realized he didn't know how to use the local herbs of India. It struck him that an ancient theoretical foundation should be applicable to herbs known or unknown, no matter where they grew. Since his knowledge of Chinese medicine was greater than his knowledge of Ayurveda, he decided to apply the theoretical principles he had learned from Chinese herbalism to those of India. The effectiveness of the herbs was not only far greater when he did this, but he learned a great deal more about the herbs as well.

Realizing the true importance of energetics and how that influences the appropriate use and subsequent effectiveness of herbs, Michael's next step was to apply this same theoretical foundation to Western herbs. This step had never been taken before, except by some of the Native American tribes through their own energetic herbal systems, and through the now defunct Greek humoral system used hundreds of years ago. Michael experienced over and over—with patients and students— that when Western herbs were used without regard for their energies, the effectiveness of the herbal therapy was often compromised. When the principles of a theoretical foundation were applied, however, Western herbs took on a new dimension of meaning and use. Michael felt a strong call to revise our Western use of herbs at that time, to bring a systemized basis of herbal understanding back to the West.

A good example of the effectiveness of a system of principles of herb use involves the Native American herb, echinacea. Michael had already popularized the knowledge and use of this incredible natural antibiotic. He discussed its importance during lectures to students around the country in the seventies. Soon it caught on like wildfire, its usage and sales soaring not unlike the current explosion in the United States of St.-John's-wort for helping alleviate depression. Over time, it became known as a major immunity-potentiating herb.

Ironically, however, after about 10 years of popularity with vegetarians, the miraculous effectiveness of echinacea dropped among vegetarians. This is because echinacea has a cold energy and vegetarians tend to get illnesses of a cool nature. When echinacea was combined with an energetically appropriate herb for vegetarians, however, such as Siberian ginseng, its effectiveness for vegetarians was regained. Michael had a further reason to bring energetics to Western herbs.

He also saw the incredible importance of diet and its influence on illness and the effectiveness of Western herbs. Just as traditional medicinal systems throughout the world developed theoretical foundations for using herbs, they also did this with food. Michael began teaching the use of an energetically balanced diet along with herbs. He explained the therapeutic use of foods along with identification of the energetic imbalances in the body. This he included in the first edition of this book.

Since the original publication of *The Way of Herbs*, Western herbalism has expanded tremendously. Starting with the experience and knowledge that a few spread to their students throughout the country over two decades, the awareness of and use of Western herbs and alternative therapies have exploded into the mass market—down to the household level. Herbs and natural treatments, such as homeopathic remedies, are now sold in mainstream store chains. Increasing numbers of medical doctors are incorporating herbal and natural remedies into their medical practices. Special TV reports and newspaper articles frequently discuss specific herbal "miracle" cures. Acupuncture is now acknowledged and accepted as an effective medical therapy by the National Institutes of Health (NIH).

The formation in 1992 of the Office of Alternative Medicine under the auspices of the NIH during President Bill Clinton's administration has meant the allocation of special funds to investigate the validity of alternative medicine, which, it can be hoped, will include research on herbs and include the thousands of years of empirical evidence and extensive past research documented by many European and Asian countries. The continuing evidence of the safety of herbs, along with the paucity of their adverse effects as reported by poison control centers, supports this widespread acceptance of alternative medicine and herbs.

This fertile climate has helped to foster the introduction of potent herbs from around the world into American markets. Herbs long recognized for their therapeutic medicinal uses in Europe have found their way to store shelves and mainstream use. For instance, ginkgo leaf came on strong because of its usefulness in improving memory and eyesight and in forestalling Alzheimer's disease. Next, vitex (chaste tree berry), successfully employed for premenstrual syndrome, menopause, and other hormonally related complaints, burst onto the market. St.-John's-wort, now acknowledged in the West for its effective treatment of depression, has long been a European alternative to the antidepressant pharmaceuticals so overly prescribed in American society. There are many other potent herbs, less well known because of a lack of mainstream publicity, that are currently available.

Along with the expansion of herbal usage in America has come the explosion of the herbal industry. Herbal products are widely varied and sold in a myriad of forms. Entire multimillion-dollar companies have sprung up from grassroot beginnings in home kitchens. Herbal training and jobs have burgeoned, from herbal experts who serve as consultants to manufacturing companies and product distributors to teachers in schools and salespeople in stores. There is an increasing number of students—thousands—not just in the United States but around the world, enrolled in colleges, specialized schools, and correspondence courses.

The incredible growth and increasing sophistication of the herbal industry since the 1970s has both enhanced the knowledge and availability of alternative healing agents as well as created some problems and confusion. The false marketing of certain herbs through ignorance and desire for profit has tended at times to give the industry a bad name. Using ephedra (ma huang), for instance, for quick energy or weight loss is unwise, and marketing it as appropriate for either use is misleading.

Further, the current pharmaceutical process of standardization has created disagreement and misunderstanding. While its benefits guarantee a specified amount of the herb's active principles to be found in every batch produced, its problems are many. There is no agreement among companies as to which constituent should be standardized and to what degree. Thus, different companies extract and standardize different constituents and to varying potencies. This leads one to wonder about the effectiveness, importance, and need for the standardization process at all. Certainly, it needs to be guided by a governing body of trained herbalists.

On the other hand, the spreading use of concentrated extracts in herbs is a valuable addition to the industry. The real value in an herb, after all, is in its wholeness. Condensed extracts ensure the strength and effectiveness of the whole herb. It also keeps the dose manageable and the product affordable.

Over time, the tremendous growth of herbal medicine and its accompanying industry has created the need for professional recognition of herbalism and competent herbalists in America. Long ago, Michael recognized this need. He was both inspired by the national organization of herbalists in Australia when he taught there in the early 1980's, and encouraged by the professional herbal licensing bodies in the United Kingdom. At once, he saw the importance and necessity for such an organization in America. For many years, he discussed this need with other herbalists and students at herbal gatherings and schools. They began talking about it as well; then suddenly, the time was ripe and herbalists were ready.

In the early summer of 1989, the American Herbalists' Guild (AHG) was founded by some two dozen herbalists. Since then, its membership has grown to encompass professionals, students, and associate members. Its annual symposiums bring together herbalists from all parts of America and of differing backgrounds and expertise. Although not without its problems and drawbacks, the AHG has striven to recognize the competency of professional herbalists in all types of fields, from Native American and folk healers to Western medical and TCM herbalists.

Also recognizing the need for accrediting herbalists in Chinese Medicine, the NCCAOM (National Certification Commission for Acupuncture and Oriental Medicine) several years ago created a national examination and licensing for those demonstrating expertise in Chinese herbalism. While recognition from such organizations is vital and necessary at this time for all types of herbalists, it is not without controversy. These are only some of the issues facing herbalists at this time.

Because of the explosion of herbalism, natural medicine, and their accompanying industries, education in the use of herbs is of extreme importance. It is essential to keep the major herbal reference books updated so they reflect the latest directions in herbal medicine. It is time the many incredible and valuable herbs successfully employed in other countries became known and used. Although some have long been in mainstream use, others are just becoming known. Still others are important alternatives to many of our plants now endangered by overharvesting. *The Way of Herbs,* now a bible for herbalism, strives to keep abreast of this need and the growing knowledge of new herbs and available research.

In this revised edition of *The Way of Herbs,* several changes have been made. Thirty-two new herbs have been added and information on many of the existing ones appearing in the previous edition has been updated on the basis of the latest research and herbs most recently added to the modern Western pharmacopoeia. While many of these herbs have been used for centuries, others are being discovered in the West for the first time. Further, since the 1980s, dietary knowledge has evolved through Michael's research and experience with thousands of patients and students. In this new version of *The Way of Herbs,* he has updated the dietary information to reflect this wisdom.

Moreover, an entirely new chapter on the botanical treatment of cancer has been added. With one of every five people estimated to contract cancer during their lifetimes and with the shortcomings of conventional medicine in treating cancer, Michael feels it's extremely important for people to be aware of an effective and rational alternative treatment approach. Herbs and diet have brought relief to thousands of people with cancer, not only today, but in years gone by. That natural treatment has to make a comeback represents an example of the abandonment of a natural system of healing because it doesn't offer sufficient economic benefit to support multimillion-dollar pharmaceutical and medical industries.

Interestingly enough, alternative medicine is received more openly in such countries as China and Cuba, where profit is not the dominant concern. This is where supportive statistical research can be found, including human trials. Unfortunately, this research is not recognized in the Western world because it does not include double-blind studies.

Acknowledging the importance of healing sick people, researchers in these countries won't administer a valueless substance (the placebo of double-blind studies) just to authenticate the findings of a study. As a result, the proven health benefits of many herbs and natural remedies are denied to those in need in America.

Lastly, this revised edition includes material on the use of magnets. Since the early 1990's, Michael has found magnets to be extremely effective in alleviating pain. Used by one of three people in Japan, they are beginning to be employed in hospitals for pain relief and the healing of broken bones. They offer the most direct and immediate relief of pain and inflammation in a myriad of conditions and are easily combined with the use of herbs and diet.

The extensive growth and use of alternative medicine and natural remedies in America is making it possible for people to discover valuable alternatives for health, healing, and disease prevention. As global awareness of herbalism continues to expand, it is hoped that the reader become more informed about the myriad herbs available to us from around the world. May this revised edition further the wise use of herbalism by all those interested in herbs and natural healing.

LESLEY TIERRA, L.AC., DIPL. AC., DIPL. C.H., AHG
author of *Herbs of Life, Healing with Chinese Herbs,*
coauthor with Michael Tierra of *Chinese Traditional Herbal Medicine,* volume I
August, 1998

EDITOR'S PREFACE

Michael Tierra has been practicing herbal medicine and acupuncture in Santa Cruz, California for the past decade. He has an extensive background of study with traditional healers of America, India and China. From these diverse cultures, he has developed a unique approach to herbalism that is firmly rooted in practical experience. I have also been deeply involved in herbal medicine, but with a background in biochemistry, physiology and practical pharmacology. Much of my work has been with investigations of herb safety and efficacy from a scientific viewpoint. For years, Michael and I have been working and teaching in Santa Cruz, representing two very diverse aspects of herbal medicine. In that time, I have come to gain a deep respect for the traditional medical systems that gave rise to much of our current knowledge and Michael has gained a keen interest in the scientific explanations and clinical evaluations of herb action. It was therefore most appropriate and timely that we should join forces in producing this book. From the original manuscript Michael provided, we have developed a valuable synthesis of the many aspects of herbal knowledge that make up *The Way of Herbs*.

I am often asked the question: "Do herbs really work?" I answer both yes and no. The human race has been practicing medicine for many thousands of years and from all available reports, it has been reasonably successful. Herbal medicines have been a large part of all medical systems over the millennia, but they have been put to a very hard test by the severe conditions of a developing world. The greatest assault on health has come from the unsanitary conditions of city life and from bad diet. The unequal distribution of foods leaves some individuals without adequate nutrients while giving others deadly dietary excesses, especially in the form of highly processed foods. Where practiced, improved sanitation and proper diet have done more for health than any medicine that has ever been used. Few people seem to manage these conditions in their lives, and so medicines are required to perform a monumental task.

Herbal medicines have worked very well for those who have used them properly, and the literature is replete with success stories. Many remedies have been consistently recommended across cultures and time on the strength of their efficacy. In fact, most modern pharmaceuticals are based on chemical constituents that were at one time isolated from the traditionally used herbs (although a large number are now being derived from bacteria, fungi and animal sources as well). So I must say that herbs work.

Modern pharmaceuticals are directed against symptoms. They act swiftly and powerfully to remove the symptoms of disease. Compared to this type of action, it would seem that most of the herbs do not work. For in many cases, an herbal treatment will be gentler and more gradual in its action and it will rely primarily on allowing the body to heal itself by a slow, natural process. Using herbal therapy, the body will become stronger and the individual will take the time to learn something about the factors that led to the disease in the first place, thus giving the opportunity to prevent reoccurrence. The quick and powerful action of modern pharmaceuticals will bring superficial relief. Their primary action is to give temporary relief from the responsibility of taking proper care of one's health. These drugs, when relied on in this way, will lead to a more severe disease later. For you will have pushed aside the warning signals that you are doing something wrong. Herbs don't work that way.

However, too many people turning to alternative medicine try to cure themselves by using "a sprinkle of herbs in a cup of boiling water," thus drinking what they think of as an herbal tea. This will accomplish nothing. It is a great myth that drinking beverage teas will cure ailments and provide a healthy life. It is one thing to eliminate the bad habit of drinking coffee and black tea by replacing it with an herbal beverage, and another thing to treat an ailment with a potent medicinal tea or other herbal therapy. Herbal therapies will generally require a fairly large dose of herbs and an extended period of treatment. In fact, it is important to continue the treatment beyond the point where the symptoms have vanished, to bring strength to the deepest levels from which the ailment had sprung forth.

Many of the mild herbs need to be taken in the amount of one ounce per pint (two cups) of water in making a tea. This will yield about one and one-half cups of tea, which is to be taken a half cup each time, three times daily. Other herbs, with stronger action, are taken as alcohol extracts (tinctures) that are about four times as concentrated as a tea, or in capsules that are sometimes taken as frequently as every two hours, two capsules each time (sixteen per day). The herb tea bags found in a store will usually have only about one-fourteenth of an ounce of herbs; the bottles of prefilled capsules will often have the instructions "take one or two capsules daily." These instructions are generally not for therapeutic use of the herbs. (Small "homeopathic" doses are valuable only when the proper formulation is applied according to the principles of that medical system.) When treating acute diseases, the therapy will be applied for several days, and chronic ailments may be treated over a period of months.

It is not possible to overemphasize the value of a dietary change in treating an illness. It will be difficult to obtain success with herbal therapy or any therapy without proper attention to the role of diet. It is very important that upon becoming sick, one immediately eliminate hard-to-digest foods, using a simple but nutritious and balanced diet. Then the energy that goes to digesting foods and dealing with toxins in the diet is no longer diverted from the essential process of healing. Once the crisis of the acute ailment is over, it is necessary to progress through dietary changes to correct the imbalance that allowed the illness to appear and to strengthen the body against further disease.

In his practice, Michael gives considerable attention to the condition of the patient in terms of the Oriental concept of balance between Yin and Yang, and he has made extensive notes on the subject. Here, however, we have attempted to present this valuable aspect of diagnosis and treatment in a way easily accessible to our Western readers. The concept of Yin/Yang balance suggests a basis for many healthful dietary changes, as well as for determining the best herbal therapy. It is a major point of departure from the modern Western approach to health and disease. Michael also relies heavily on the use of Ayurvedic diagnosis and treatment, but this field of study is still quite difficult to present in a book such as this, so most of the references to these techniques have been reserved for a subsequent work. There both the Chinese and the Ayurvedic systems will be presented, and adequate space devoted to full explanations of both theory and practice. These traditional methods do not replace, but augment, modern medical diagnostic practices.

In the "Kitchen Medicines" and "Western Herbs" chapters we have tried to eliminate any information that would not be of immediate use to the reader. Those who wish more information may consult the sources described in the Bibliography. We have provided dosages and descriptions of methods of application, and the number of herbs has been restricted so as to minimize the common problem of information overload found in many herb books.

The chapter on "Obtaining and Storing Herbs" is based on my own experience, not only as an herbalist, but as a person who has worked with herb companies that produced the herb products you find in retail stores. I suggest that the reader take special note of the concern for the species of the plants and also the form in which they are purchased and stored.

If you will observe carefully the rules for "Making an Herbal Formula," you will find it easy to produce a very large number of useful and effective herbal preparations. The formulas presented are those that Michael feels are among his most valuable, and most of these clearly fit the general formulation technique. A few are less obviously derived from the rules set down, but they are nonetheless useful recipes and indicators of the range of herbal preparations. Some modifications have been made to allow the formulas to be produced from herbs available in stores or by mail order. If you are able to gather fresh herbs, these can be used and many substitutions can be made, so that local herbs will be generally adequate for the entire formula.

I have also added the chapter titled "Cautionary Notes on Herb Use." It will be important to read this section carefully and observe warnings presented there. I have done considerable research into the problems of herbal toxicology, but this field is poorly developed. The majority of concerns have briefly been presented in this chapter.

I am often asked if herbs are safe. To this, I again answer both yes and no. When herbs are used properly they are as safe as any natural food and they are far safer than other drugs. When used improperly, they can cause a number of unpleasant effects, and can even cause death. While there are many mild herbs that need to be used in fairly large doses, there are also some very potent herbs that must be used in relatively small doses. Herbs should not be used without an adequate knowledge of their traditional uses and application. When the body reacts negatively to any therapy, it is important to look carefully at the dose, and the appropriateness of the treatment. We have placed a number of cautionary notes throughout the text. When herbs are used properly, they are not only safe, but they are without side effects.

In collaborating with Michael in producing this book, I have taken special care to include much practical information for one not only to get started using herbs, but even to proceed towards the point of becoming a herbalist. You will find information here that has not been collected into any other single reference source. On the strength of this knowledge, you can move to familiarity with other herbs and techniques as necessary.

I have long been interested in providing an accessible education in herbal knowledge. Working with the Herb Trade Association and Dr. Paul Lee of the Academy of Herbal Medicine, I helped produce three major Symposia on herbs, which brought together university researchers, government officials, herb suppliers and herb users. The Symposia have led to an ongoing interaction between such groups to bring out the important knowledge of herbs from many vantage points. The Third International Symposium on Herbs eventually led to the establishment of the Institute for Traditional Medicine and Preventive Health Care. Established in 1979, the Institute carries on research and education with emphasis on herbal medicine. An advisory board of cooperating scientists from around the world has assisted our organization in its efforts. Active coordination of international research products is a major part of the emphasis of the Institute. Projects underway include: evaluation of ginseng in the prevention of heart disease; prevention and treatment of ailments of the female reproductive system; study of tobacco substitutes and herbs that can be smoked to alleviate the symptoms of asthma and bronchitis; the use of herbs with disinfectant, antiseptic and antibiotic activity. The Institute also has an agricultural research station in the Catskills, Cold Mountain Farm, where it is evaluating methods of production for a variety of important medicinal herbs, including American ginseng, goldenseal and lady's slipper.

Two research associates with the Institute are Calvin Cohen and Grace Marroquin. They have helped extensively with the preparation of this book by reviewing all the sections, making numerous valuable comments and suggestions and providing helpful insights. Both Grace and Cal have contributed their own herbal knowledge as well as experience in apprenticeship with Michael and myself. They are currently involved in carrying out clinical trials of herbal treatments.

Among our tasks in studying herbs has been the review of the literature to separate out vital information from that which is frivolous or outright incorrect. We have come to consider *The Way of Herbs* a unique book about herbs. Unlike most other herbals, it concentrates on important medicines that can be used again and again in a wide variety of treatments. The information about the herbs has been centered around the nature of the systems affected and the important properties of the herbs. Other aspects of the herbs, such as their history in medicine, growing region, appearance and minor uses, can all be learned from the other books mentioned in the Bibliography. We have deliberately focused on ways you yourself can learn to use the herbs.

I have included a few herbs in the "Herbs to Know" chapter that I have studied and used, but that Michael has not generally prescribed. These include kava kava, stoneroot and tienchi, herbs that are subjects of our research projects. In addition, I have provided a section on smoking herbs in the "Methods of Application" chapter. This is a method that Michael also uses, but it is of particular interest to me in terms of our research regarding asthma and bronchitis. As a result of Michael's very high regard for echinacea, which we hope has been adequately brought out in this book, our research group is in turn undertaking a detailed study of this herb as an antibiotic and blood purifier.

Rarely does an herb book provide any insight into the proper method of formulation and preparation of herbal therapies. *The Way of Herbs* provides the basic information necessary to use not only the herbs presented, but also any other herbs, in both the formulas presented and in formulas that you will design to fit your basic needs. This book contains the most comprehensive guide to date to the potential problems of herb use, from inadequate concern for the diet, to insufficient dosage, to excessive use. In addition, this book contains the most detailed instructions yet available for the methods of herbal application, both for the therapeutic techniques and for the production of useful herbal preparations in your home.

It has been very difficult to obtain good information on Chinese herbs despite the fact that their use is becoming very popular. From the thousands of herbs available in Chinatowns, Michael has picked the most widely used and highly valued to introduce to our readers. The herbs are well worth the trouble to track down and purchase, for they are superior tonics among the range of herbs available. This is the only book that details the use of these herbs in a context that the Western reader can readily understand.

The Way of Herbs thus brings together the most important aspects of several herbal traditions. It will be an invaluable contribution to every library of herb books and an essential manual for all who wish to practice herbal medicine effectively.

SUBHUTI DHARMANANDA, PH.D.
Institute for Traditional Medicine and
Preventive Health Care
Santa Cruz, California
June 1980

INTRODUCTION

THE HERBALIST'S PATH

It is a mistake to view herbology only as a science studying the therapeutic properties of plants. More than this, the path of the herbalist is a cultivated attitude towards nature and all of creation. I remember the time that I spent with the Karok Indians of northern California—whenever I presented one of them with an unfamiliar plant, the inevitable question was "What's it good for?" Certainly the Indians love nature as their home, but rather than merely holding an aesthetic viewpoint about it they combine a sincere appreciation for its beauty with a functional attitude based on the idea of "use, not abuse." This is also the attitude of the herbalist towards nature. It is in contrast to the lack of appreciation demonstrated by those who retreat to the wilderness to dump all of their repressed desires symbolized by the beer cans, pop bottles and other debris left in their wake. The view of the herbalist is also in contrast to the many pseudo-ecologists who make futile attempts to maintain natural environments as aesthetic monuments with no functional purpose, leaving signs saying "do not touch," "do not pick the plants," etc.

The herbalist, along with the American Indian, appreciates nature not only for its beauty but also for the valuable resource of wild foods and medicines that grow in these all-giving bowers. Thus the herbalist views nature as a positive force, and as a provider and teacher. Everything is seen as having a purpose that can only be revealed if we learn to be patient, and engage our senses both subtle and gross in allowing us to trust and understand the secrets this teacher can reveal. Nature communicates her secrets directly to us in terms of forms, colors, fragrances, sounds and flavors as well as by way of the more subtle information that comes to us through our intuitive imagination.

A certain perspective is necessary for this communication to occur. We must cultivate an attitude of respect for all living plants and animals and accept them as a gift. We must learn not to slight even the smallest

living thing, while maintaining an attitude of deep reverence and grati-
tude. This will enable us to better understand what benefit we can be
for each other's evolution. The way of the native Americans shows us a
reciprocity, a give-and-take attitude about nature. In northern California
no real cultivation of food was done; everything was found and gathered
in the wilds. However, the forests were periodically burned to keep
down the underbrush, keeping the ground clear for gathering acorns,
dynamizing the soil with fire and ash, encouraging the growth of edible
herbs and berries.

At first when we enter into an unfamiliar natural sanctuary, we may
only recognize one or two familiar plants. Rather than ignoring them or
taking them too lightly, we should see them as friends and diving mes-
sengers whose presence may allow us a welcome security and familiarity
until we learn about the many other unfamiliar plant-friends growing
in the area. Everything has a purpose and a use because everything has
qualities and properties. It is part of the human's divine purpose to
become more conscious and aware of the environment we all share.

While it may be our ultimate destiny to transcend nature, we must
first rediscover our rightful place in it. Those of us who have grown
up in cities have of necessity suffered from a separation from nature. I
remember living in a wilderness community during the late 1960's.
During the first few months, I mistakenly attempted to come to terms
with my relationship to the strange yet exotically attractive forest where
I lived by doing the only thing my previous conditioning would let me
conceive of—going out each day with my rifle in hand and playing the
role of the great white hunter. Thankfully I was so inept that any half-
way intelligent animal could hear or sense my approach from a long
distance, and I never bagged anything during that period. It was during
those days that, perhaps partially out of embarrassment from coming
back each day with nothing in hand, I became attracted to the wild
herbs of the forest and each day brought back various specimens to
identify.

At this time we harbored a number of black beret revolutionaries
who were seeking temporary refuge from the confusing and paranoid
vibes pervading cities and ghettoes. They evidently felt threatened by
the strangely peaceful forest, with its gentle quiet streams and new fallen
snow. Somehow they became very frightened of the raw quiet and deep
silence. They often imagined some terrifying animal, a projection of
their inner distrust and unfamiliarity with the environment, uneasily

expecting something to issue forth from that profound natural peace and eat them alive—or perhaps some governmental authority might be hiding behind a big Douglas fir tree, just waiting to get them. In any case, no matter where they went, it was an absurd picture seeing them strutting in their most downtown "macho" attitude, wearing their black beret and always carrying a pistol or a rifle. This was the only model they had for dealing with the unfamiliar.

It seems that after a while, when people realize that they are alone and nothing will eat them, they begin the often destructive process of letting down their societal inhibitions; then we find the tendency of country folk to spend their free time drinking, getting high and ultimately making themselves sick. Through such ignorance we miss the incredible lesson that nature has to teach us, the lesson of how to just *be*. Nothing to compete with (except perhaps the squirrels for the spring harvest of hazelnuts), no egoistic posturing for a job or a raise, no struggle with the Russians for the oil of the Middle East, no desperate search for approval or acceptance from societal peers or acquaintances. Nature offers us a rare freedom from the painful and stressful concerns of society.

The path of the herbalist is one path that can offer a vital link to the natural and interaction with nature's wilds. It gives us a point of view by which we can see ourselves as being connected with the entire process of life. It has been stated that in very ancient times everyone was born with knowledge of the use of herbs. Eventually, some of that was lost due to the development of extended societies leading to the development of future civilizations. During that transitional period people began to look to the wild animals and birds to guide them in understanding the healing power of herbs and plants. The American Indian, for instance, would watch the bear, who was considered to be the closest, physiologically, to the human, and learn what it would eat both for food and for medicine. Ayurvedic medicine has many herbs named after, certain animals, such as one called garuda bhuti, named after an eagle— probably because it was first found in eagles' nests. The Chinese still use precious nests of certain birds in a soup considered to be of great benefit as a whole-body tonic.

While such indications are often valuable, it was discovered that there were exceptions. One hermit yogi sádhu, for example, would eat only those foods that he saw monkeys eat. But one day he was discovered poisoned and dead because he had eaten one thing which, while not poisonous to monkeys, proved to be a deadly poison to humans. For this reason, certain principles, ideas and concepts had to be extracted from our previous experience with natural foods and medicines in order to safeguard and deepen our understanding. Humans begin to observe more closely the various colors, shapes, fragrances and tastes, along with the geographical location and season in relation to the healing and nutritional properties of plants. It was from these beginnings that the study of herbology evolved.

The first thing to emerge in the classification of herbs was a recognition of their cooling or heating properties. Thus it was noted that everything was encompassed by a cycle of polarity of night and day, sun and moon, wet and dry, male and female, hot and cold, full and empty, light and heavy, smooth and rough, etc. It was further observed that there was in fact a relationship between these obvious characteristic qualities and certain disease conditions of the body. An individual with a hot disease such as a high fever was treated with a cooling, detoxifying medicine such as a cool fruit or the tender leaves or petals of a flower such as hibiscus, elder, yarrow, red clover blossoms, mint, etc. Diseases characterized by coldness, weak digestion, poor circulation, etc., would be treated with deep rooted herbs and plants or barks of certain trees that would affect the deeper organs and secretions of the body, such as ginseng, dandelion, prickly ash bark, bayberry bark, burdock root, etc.

As ancient as this discovery was, this basic hot and cold relationship of plants and diseases is still a fundamental principle of all natural healing. Of course, there is much more to it than this, and as with any complex system, it is made complex by superimposing one clear and simple thing upon another over and over until it seems to defy our total comprehension. Thus the path of the herbalist may also encompass the laboratory with the identification and extraction of certain vital biochemical agents found in herbs.

There is an ever increasing danger of becoming far too out of touch with nature—not only external nature but, perhaps, our internal psychological nature as well. The herbalist must cultivate an attitude to maintain his or her balanced connection with the vital roots of existence. Such ritual practices as talking or praying to a plant, making an offering before picking or harvesting it or bringing the first-picked herbs to the people who live in that area, will help to raise and maintain one's consciousness at a level necessary for the proper practice of herbal healing. It must be understood that herbal healing involves a specially directed and trained imaginative and intuitive sense that cannot be taught mechanically but must rather be discovered and acquired with practice.

True "holistic" healing involves a healing of both mind and soul, and native shamans, curanderos and medicine men and women are always very aware of this fact. Using various tricks and performances to entice and help others to see themselves in a more positive way, they offer herbs as plant-sacraments providing a specific point of focus for all of their creative play. The herbs became what the Hindus called yantras or sacred objects, gross (more perceptible) manifestations of subtle healing energies.

The herbalist's perspective remains with him or her whenever he or she may travel. I often wondered how I would fare as an herbalist if I found myself in a foreign country where I could not identify a single plant. I almost found myself in such a place when I lived for a few weeks in a village in southern India. I barely recognized one herb, except gota kola, which grew everywhere as a common weed. Yet within two weeks, with a little personal effort (such as checking a few botanical books on the area but, most important, asking questions of the local folk), I learned the medicinal use of several plants, enough to prescribe them to the villagers for their various ills. They appreciated this for the same reasons as people everywhere appreciate being reminded of those simple and valuable things that can be found growing freely around them such as the common weeds.

In walking through wilderness trails and discovering wild plants and herbs, one should take the opportunity to notice the many conditions under which herbs and plants grow. An herb growing in one locale may be better suited for particular diseases than one growing under a different set of climatic conditions. For instance, we can find chaparral growing in veritable stands and fields in high desert places throughout the western United States. Recently I discovered a few chaparral plants growing on a high windy peak in Baja California under conditions quite different from any of the other chaparral I had ever previously gathered. Upon tasting a leaf of this specimen, I noted it was much less bitter than the common desert chaparral. Just as the climate and outward conditions of our life affect our characteristics and personality, so also do the growing conditions of a specific area affect the characteristics of the medicinal plants that can be found growing there. I decided that this particular "Baja" chaparral was especially good for diseases involving the liver because of the traditional relationship in Chinese medicine between the wind and the liver.

Other considerations I have noted for various reasons are as follows:

1. Herbs growing on the north side of a mountain are more tonifying and strengthening because of the increased power and stamina they must develop in order to survive in a more difficult growing area.

2. Herbs growing in lowlands or near water are more beneficial for urinary diseases.

3. Herbs growing in high, dry desert regions tend to be of more benefit to the spleen and pancreas because they would help the traditional function of the spleen-pancreas according to Chinese medicine, to transform moisture in the body.

4. Herbs growing in fertile, nitrogenous soil would be of more benefit for the digestion and assimilation. Also herbs whose job is to fix nitrogen in the soil, including the leguminous plants such as clover and alfalfa, would help in our metabolism of proteins and cell formation.

5. Herbs growing in cold, harsh weather tend to be more building and heating in contrast to herbs growing in hotter, more temperate climates, which would tend to be more eliminating. While both can be detoxifying in their respective ways, there is a subtle but important tendency manifested by herbs found growing in different geographical localities.

6. The tastes of herbs are important indicators of their properties. The sweet taste is nutritive; pungent is dispersing; salty taste influences water balance and digestion; sour is digestive and cooling; bitter is cooling and detoxifying. Many herbs have a number of tastes and therefore a number of properties.

7. As we walk, often a plant will greet us with a striking scent. It is a known fact that the sense of smell has a direct connection with the subconscious mind. It is one of the powers of aromatic herbs and plants to help us to get more consciously in touch with our subconscious process. Aromatic herbs such as mugwort, pennyroyal, bay, sandalwood, rose, sage, etc., can be used in special talismans and dream pillows to help the individual get more in touch with their dreams and psychological processes. Usually these aromatic herbs can be used internally in a variety of ways,

ranging from a sweating tea in fevers (the volatile oils of aromatic plants are eliminated through the pores of the skin), to antibiotic treatment of internal infections of the bladder, lungs, etc., to digestive, carminative herbs for better assimilation.

When you are gathering herbs, take time, make your peace with the environment and its life as well as with the living plants that pass their life cycle there. Avoid the tendency to plunder and pluck about unconsciously. Before taking an herb, offer a prayer of thanksgiving or a good thought of appreciation. Herbs have feelings not at all dissimilar in many respects to our own, and we and they can both be persuaded to give more of ourselves and our energy if we can be genuinely persuaded to feel good about the process. In any case, never take more than a third of the foliage of a plant. Never strip the bark around the entire circumference of a tree unless you deliberately intend to kill it. Bits and pieces can be taken from various parts of one tree and from various trees, and each tree can still heal itself over.

During various seasons, the vital energy of herb plants is found in different parts. In the spring it is in the newly formed leaves and buds; in the summer it is in the fruit and blossoms; in the fall and winter it is in the roots. These are the best times for gathering these various parts of medicinal herbs and plants. If there are only one or two specimens don't bother them. Always gather where there is an abundance—then you can be certain that the herbs you get are potent. When drying the herbs, carefully spread them out on a screen in a well-ventilated, partially shaded place. Turn them once each day so they will dry evenly, thus preventing decay and browning of the leaves.

In conclusion, we might direct our attention not only to the powerful beneficial aspects of medicinal plants, but also to their ability to poison and inflict harm. Poisonous herbs are used in minute "homeopathic" dosage, often one part in thousands, to effect profound cures of both acute and chronic illnesses. In any case, never eat a strange herb or plant of which you have no positive identification. There are methods of determining whether certain herbs are poisonous or not but all of these involve tasting them, and there is some question whether this is 100% effective; there is thus always the chance that you could have an unfavorable reaction.

The path of the herbalist is to open ourselves to nature in an innocent and pure way. She in turn will open her bounty and reward us with her many valuable secrets. May the earth bless you.

INTRODUCTION TO THE
REVISED EDITION

Since the first publication in 1980, I have received hundreds of letters and comments from individuals who have experienced personal benefit from the use of *The Way of Herbs*. Many have reported how they have successfully treated themselves for acute diseases ranging from the common cold, flu, and fever, to recurring bladder infections, skin diseases, hepatitis, and even to more serious diseases such as cancer. All of this attests to the efficacy of herbs as a safe alternative healing modality.

There were also many students who were able to gain a greater understanding of herbal medicine and to integrate the principles set forth in this book into a professional medical practice. This included not only holistic health practitioners but many professional medical doctors and nurses.

The success of *The Way of Herbs* is, I believe, due to the fact that the greater part of my information is based upon personal clinical experience. This in contrast to many similar books that seem to be based on nothing more than second- or third-hand information. Certainly, the integration of sound, balanced dietary principles is, and always will be, an important part of a successful herbal practice. I have, therefore, integrated the macrobiotic approach that classifies foods according to the same traditional principles as herbs. By macrobiotic, I do not mean a severely restricted diet consisting of only brown rice but a balanced traditional diet, combining many whole grains, beans, organic vegetables and fruits in a wholesome way.

Another important aspect of the success of *The Way of Herbs* has been the integration of all aspects of health and healing under ancient unifying principles first expounded by Yogic, Taoist and Buddhist sages and priests thousands of years ago. They first classified herbs energetically according to their nature and indications following the principle of bipolar opposites, hot-cold, acute-chronic, external-internal, Yin-Yang and the five flavors.

In this book I have added a considerable number of herbs to the materia medica, giving the book greater breadth and scope. I have also made several revisions and additions to the body of the text as well, adding more specific disease treatments.

In my opinion, the most important aspect of my contribution is the attempt to classify herbs energetically. I believe that without using herbs from this energetic perspective, we will be no different than those who use Western drug medicine, which tends to treat symptoms without addressing the underlying causes. Symptomatic medicine is undoubtedly useful in providing immediate relief of acute symptoms but it is the unique power of nature's herbs and foods when used according to traditional bipolar principles that can effect deeper levels of true healing. In fact, without considering the unifying principles of hot and cold, Yin and Yang, etc., to herbal therapy, we increase our potential for failure.

All of this has to do not only with the exact nature of the symptom or disease but also with the circumstance from which it arises in the body in the first place. Symptomatic medicine may temporarily destroy a particular germ or virus with a drug. However, if it is applied without attending to the overall imbalance of the system, problems may resurface or, worse, bury themselves deeper into the system to create more serious chronic conditions. All of this tends to result in increased attempts to beat the system into submission with higher concentrations of stronger drugs, thus risking further damage to the innate life force or immune system of the body.

It is my experience that if we have selected the correct treatment strategy, we need neither such high doses of chemical drugs nor even costly concentrated extracts of herbs to achieve positive results.

To many, a confusing aspect of all this is that any given imbalance can be expressed in a number of valid ways: emotionally, chemically or physically. Thus, it is possible for one to apply sound energetically balanced principles to the therapeutic use of drugs and chemicals as well.

Just the simple evaluation of the constitutional strength of the patient with regard to the proposed treatment can avoid most serious side effects, which inevitably lead to patient dissatisfaction. Still other levels of energetic reasoning can reveal the relationship between a particular food or life habit and a given disease. How much better it would be if doctors perhaps learned to recommend first a simple diet of whole grains and beans for a few days along with a harmless antiinflammatory herb such as echinacea root and perhaps a mild purgative such as rhubarb or cascara bark before routinely resorting to "blitzing" the entire system with an antibiotic that disturbs the delicate balance of the entire system.

It is through these simple practices, hardly a full-blown herbal or alternative-medicine practice, that increasing numbers of medical doctors are achieving a distinguished record as "holistic medical doctors." It is through such methods that alternative practitioners can help their fellow humans by treating the whole person.

Still another important aspect of the success of *The Way of Herbs* has been its demonstration of the therapeutic results of using food and herbs together. How many times I have seen individuals fail to achieve lasting positive results because they are energetically antidoting the properties of the herbs they are using with an inappropriate diet.

Simply put, there is no magical wand that with a wave will cure all diseases. However, if a disease is of a cold, deficient nature, we will achieve positive results by using a stronger diet of all cooked foods with herbal roots and tonics. If, on the other hand, the disease is of an excess, hot nature, we may use a lighter diet with lighter, more eliminative and detoxifying herbs. From this perspective, we can always perceive one's ignorance or lack of experience when one speaks of cures and remedies regardless of lifestyle or diet.

In this third revised edition, I have substantially increased the number of herbs in the materia medica, updating their energetic classifications with my current understanding as well as offering current scientific biochemical constituents. Since traditional herbalists generally find that herbs work better in compound formulas, especially for more chronic symptoms, I have offered a simple formulation for most of the herbs. I hope this will make the knowledge contained under the description of each herb more useful.

Thus, like a familiar ancient melody, *The Way of Herbs* winds paradoxically through the maze of contemporary scientific specialization: our exploration into the far reaches of outer space, the miracle of organ transplants, genetic engineering, the age of the computer. I hope *The Way of Healing* will continue to support and guide those who seek balance by choosing the path of nature.

MICHAEL TIERRA
January, 1990

THE WAY OF
HERBS

BALANCE: THE KEY TO HEALTH

A DEEPER UNDERSTANDING OF HEALTH AND DISEASE

Health is a reflection of the balance between the different aspects of ourselves (body, mind, soul) and our environment, our experiences, our associations and our food. There cannot be sickness in any of these categories without its being reflected to some degree in all of the others.

The cornerstone of all natural healing is summarized in the statement *"all healing comes from within and the body heals itself."* Before any true healing, as opposed to mere symptomatic relief, can occur, two important prerequisites must be met:

1. understanding the basic cause of our sickness on all levels, physical, emotional and spiritual;
2. being willing to surrender to our own deepest wisdom and implement whatever positive alternatives may appear to be helpful.

It is a mistake to reach for a remedy before taking the time to acknowledge the two foregoing conditions. Strong allopathic drugs with dangerous side effects may give quick symptomatic relief but are often the cause of weakness and diseases that may occur later. Even natural remedies such as herbs, vitamins and dietary changes may be inappropriate if they are not accompanied by a good healing attitude. We will develop a healthy attitude when we finally choose to see our problems from a larger perspective, as a process of readjustment or as valuable lessons to be learned.

I believe that there is an eternal force that drives us onward through countless changes, trials and errors. As a stream must follow its long course through the forest and mountains, flowing sometimes gently and smoothly while at other times encountering obstacles and rapids, so our life must flow through its various changes. We cannot hold ourselves back from experiencing those changes. *Such opposition is the primary cause of all sickness.*

The incessant yearning for an ideal may be said to propel us through these changes, including changes of health and disease. In this sense there are no accidents. Rather, we are moved by the silent force of evolution, which, more often than we suspect, foils our most careful plans and our expectations of staying the same. Life has evolved in adaptation to an ever-changing environment. As it attains the blossom of consciousness, it develops within each one of us the capacity to generate the changes and the lessons that will effect yet a higher adaptation and awareness.

It is essential to realize that every disease has a positive aspect. The ailment informs us of our resistance and of our imbalance and it provides a focal point for discovering all the negative energies we have cultivated. In the healing process, our lessons are learned and the body is brought naturally back to a reflection of total balance. If we fail to see the positive aspect of a disease, it will not be possible to get rid of the negative aspects.

We put ourselves in situations that cause illness, and thus create our sicknesses, for several reasons:

1. to grow and learn;
2. to help foster compassion in ourselves and others;
3. to repay old "karmic" debts that we may be carrying;
4. to provide an excuse for death to occur;
5. to get love and attention.

None of these reasons involves such matters as bad diet, accidents or self-neglect—all the usual diatribe offered in most well-intentioned discourses on natural healing. *The fact is that bad diet, accidents, self-neglect and other "causative factors" are themselves a reflection of the sickness we are experiencing.* They, along with the physical symptoms that must ultimately follow, are also only symptoms rather than the deep underlying causes.

A disease healed naturally leaves a person stronger. In the natural process of healing we come to understand our weaknesses and thus replace them with true strength. The highest form of ancient healing made no attempt to cure disease but rather sought to sustain the individual through the use of mild foods, herbs and spiritual disciplines as the individual healed himself, from within and completely, body, mind and soul. Any attempt to offer a remedy that would stop the natural process from occurring was considered an interference with the integrity of the individual's own self-generated healing process. As Lao Tzu put it in the *Tao Te Ching*, "A person will get well when he is tired of being sick."

The knowledge and the use of certain herbs and foods was a prerequisite among the ancient healers. Herbs, unlike the synthetic chemicals of most modern medicines, promote the natural functions of the body. They play an important part in the process of strengthening from within. Yet they are effective only if the other manifestations of the disease are also corrected, especially the diet. Enduring changes in the lifestyle, intended to remove unhealthy dietary practices and unnecessary stress, can only be made with the proper spiritual realization. Thus any treatment of an illness must take into account the needed spiritual growth of the individual. Disease gives us the opportunity to reach a higher consciousness. The process of healing is a reflection of our new awakening.

THEORY OF USING HERBS

The use of herbs can be a very simple healing art. In fact, it has long been known as the "Art of Simpling." Herbs were known as "simples" because a single herb could be used to treat a wide variety of maladies. I once helped a woman on a Canadian Indian reserve gather red alder bark, of which she would make large amounts of tea to drink instead of water. The tea cured her of her lower back pains and of a problem of frequent urination; it also helped normalize her blood pressure. On another occasion, I was preparing a tea of freshly picked mugwort and comfrey to be used as a wash to relieve someone's poison oak. This same herbal brew was subsequently used for someone who had a sprained ankle; on another who got a deep scratch from a frightened cat; and finally, for an individual who was suffering from a bad case of indigestion and who got relief by taking a few teaspoons of the tea. Sometimes older people and others suffer many sicknesses and feeling very weak come to me and say, "What herb should I take?" My favorite reply is "Any herb."

If one goes to the bookstore and looks through herb guides, it is not uncommon to come across encyclopedic works with the complexity of hundreds of herbs used in numerous special formulas. Herein lies a danger to anyone practicing herbalism: getting lost in this complexity and being separated from the basic and simple experience of involvement with a few herbs. There is, of course, a place for this complexity, for ultimately the complexity of the herbs must match the complexity of the individual. However, everyone can begin with the most important principles of Simpling.

Three Principles of Simpling

The first principle is to use the herbs that grow nearby. The type of illness that is contracted in a particular area is somewhat dependent on the environmental conditions. For example, people in northern climates tend to suffer conditions of bronchitis, while people in southern climates tend to suffer from parasitic infections. Similarly, the herbs that grow in that area take on the characteristics of their environment and are particularly useful for the treatment of those ailments associated with the climate and other conditions of the area. In any region, there are perhaps a dozen important herbs that can be used to treat most illnesses encountered there.

The second principle is the use of mild herbs. Mild herbs can be taken freely and will exert a general effect on all the body systems, aiding in the process of healing many different types of affliction. Thus almost any herb of mild action that grows in the area may be used.

The third principle is that these mild herbs must be used in large doses. Since the herb is very mild, only in a large dose will it have the power to overcome most illnesses.

Perhaps the most important lesson I have learned in my training as an herbalist has been to use large doses of these mild herbs. There is an important difference between beverage teas, which use only a small amount of the herb, and medicinal teas, which use much larger amounts. Too many people are drinking herb teas to cure their ailments thinking that a sprinkle of herbs in a cup of boiling water will do the trick. In general this is not the case. One may need to drink several cups of a much stronger tea for several days to effect a satisfactory cure.

Adding Complexity

The local herbs will effect a cure when properly used over an extended period of time by bringing the healing energy of the environment to the user. For a quicker change in one's condition, it may be necessary to reach out to other places to find herbs useful for this purpose.

The complexity of herb use comes when a person is:

1. unwilling to use the large doses of mild herbs;
2. impatient for relief of symptoms;
3. eating a diet derived primarily from foods of other climates, foods eaten out of season or processed foods;
4. unwilling to devote the time and energy to identify and gather the local herbs.

Unfortunately, most of us fit one or more of the above categories. In such cases, one must become familiar with a much larger variety of herbs and must be careful in adjusting the dose to account for their powerful effects. The herbs will be used in basic formulas that complement and balance their properties to make them applicable to the specific ailment and constitution of the user.

No matter which approach one uses, in order for an herbal treatment to be truly effective it is essential that the individual eliminate the factors causing the illness. The components of the lifestyle, especially the diet, have the greatest effect on the balance of the body.

Duration of Treatment

In general, for most acute ailments one will obtain favorable effects in just three days by using herbs and making the appropriate adjustments in the diet and other components of the lifestyle. Even so, one should continue the herbal therapy for one to two weeks after the symptoms are gone to insure a most complete healing and avoid reoccurrence of the ailment. Because the herbs have a beneficial and normalizing effect on the whole body, other physical conditions, which were not the main object of the therapy, will also be improved. If a positive experience from the therapy has not been obtained within about three days, it is necessary to change the herbs being used.

Herbs are also used in the treatment of chronic diseases of long standing. In this case, several herbs are compounded together into a balanced formula to be taken over a period of time at the rate of two or three cups of tea a day. It is important to understand that these chronic diseases have been developing over a long period of time and have probably involved a number of organic functions as well as a major adjustment on the emotional level. For these reasons, one may not get immediate results, although occasionally someone will report significant improvement even after only one week. One can generally expect to require about one month of treatment for every year the disease has been developing.

If one is undergoing such an extended period of herbal therapy, it must be understood that the body, as with everything else in nature, functions cyclically. That is, there is a period of maximum effectiveness in the use of herbs, and that effectiveness is benefited by regular breaks in the program. I adopt the "cycle of seven" as a standard. Of the seven days in each week, one day should regularly be reserved to fast and forgo the taking of herbs, thus giving the body a rest and preparing it to respond with renewed vigor after the fast.

The main problems that arise in the use of herbs are lack of commitment, lack of consistency, insufficient or extreme dosage, a formula that is not specific enough and last, but perhaps most important, a wrong diet.

Three Functions of Herbs

One must be able to coordinate the various herbal qualities as closely as possible with the nature of the individual being treated. Herbs have three general functions in the body and are compounded according to the state of the individual. The three functions are:

1. eliminating and detoxifying—using eliminative herbs that act as laxatives, diuretics, diaphoretics and blood purifiers (see the chapters on "Herbal Therapies" and "Herbal Properties" for definitions of these terms);
2. maintaining—using herbs that counteract the physical symptoms, allowing the body to heal itself;
3. building—using herbs that tone the organs.

The first stage in an herbal treatment is generally to eliminate, removing toxins that are both a physical cause and a result of the disease. However, this step causes some depletion of energy and should not be used for persons who are weak or who are suffering a long-term degenerative condition. Instead, one uses herbs to build up the system for those who are weak, such as those recuperating from disease, and those with recurring sickness. Whether eliminating or building, an herb that stimulates the overall process is included in the formula.

For persons suffering long-term degenerative diseases or very severe symptoms of an acute disease, the first step is to use herbs that will maintain the body through the crisis and stabilize the condition. Once this has been achieved, it is possible to proceed with the appropriate use of elimination and building.

Persons who have a diet rich in animal products and refined foods have a special need to eliminate toxins and have a characteristic condition for which leaf and flower herbs are most effective. Others who go to the opposite extreme and have a diet rich in raw vegetables and fruits also need to eliminate toxins, as they usually suffer from poor assimilation, and are best treated by the roots and barks of the herb plants (see the chapter on "Diagnosis and Treatment").

Herbs can also be regarded as special foods, and it is often of great benefit to take several herbal tonics to aid the major systems of the body. For convenience these are taken in pill or powder form or as a tincture (see the chapter on "Methods of Application"). These tonics bolster the organs of the body and are useful in preventive medicine as well as in the treatment of chronic diseases and congenital weakness. One may, for example, simultaneously take a kidney tonic, blood purifier, lower bowel tonic, glandular balance formula and an herb tea that is specific for a particular ailment. Such a combination may be taken in full doses of each tonic separately, or the formulas may be combined to form a single dose made up of smaller amounts of each component. The former is a full-potency treatment, while the latter is a maintenance dose that is usually satisfactory for long-term treatment and prevention. In this way, one may begin to match the complexity of the individual with a complex herbal program.

· 3 ·

HERBAL THERAPIES

There are a number of ways in which the body responds to herbal treatments, and these have traditionally been divided up to produce a basis for eight general methods of therapy. These methods are:

1. stimulation
2. tranquilization
3. blood purification
4. tonification
5. diuresis (control of fluid balance)
6. sweating
7. emesis (vomiting)
8. purging

Each therapeutic method is suitable for particular kinds of diseases, and it is often appropriate to combine several methods for the most effective treatment.

In applying therapy of any kind, one must regulate the treatment according to the energy of the body. Thus, while the use of certain herbs to eliminate toxins through purging or emesis can be very effective, they are not appropriate for one who is weak or of low energy since these methods will reduce the body energy further. *It is important, then, to follow the changing course of the disease each day and to decide which therapy is most appropriate for that condition.* Familiarity with these eight therapeutic methods will make it possible to choose an effective course of treatment to promote quick recovery.

Stimulation

The purpose of this therapeutic approach is to stimulate the vitality of the body to throw off the sickness. Herbal stimulants, when combined with other herbs, will promote their functions of eliminating, maintaining or building. Effective herbal stimulants include ginger, cayenne, garlic, black pepper and cloves. (A very useful stimulant formula, composition powder, is described in the chapter on "Making an Herbal Formula").

Stimulants increase the metabolism, drive the circulation, break up obstructions and warm the body. It is particularly useful to apply this therapy in the beginning acute stages of a disease. The body's underlying strength can then be stimulated to throw off the disease. The herbal stimulants can also restore vitality that has been reduced by chronic diseases.

Many ailments are attributable to blockages in the natural flow of blood, lymph, nutrients (digestion and assimilation), waste products (from food and metabolism) or nerve energy. Stimulants are an important means of breaking through these blockages, which are cold, inactive areas of the body. The increase in energy, circulation and warmth brings back the normal activity. Thus the dynamic balance of all aspects of the physiology may be restored.

Ailments characterized by reduced energy, causing one to feel slow and sluggish (as with colds and flus), are successfully treated by stimulant therapy, usually in combination with other therapies. In addition, prolonged, low-grade fevers may be treated with warming herbal stimulants such as black pepper and cayenne. In this paradoxical situation, the fever may be neutralized as the body is aided in its natural production of warmth, thus allowing the fever to subside.

Stimulants are also commonly used to overcome sluggish digestion. Many of the aromatic culinary herbs and spices are useful in treating indigestion and gas by stimulating the action of the stomach and small intestine.

Most people are familiar with the current campaign against the use of stimulants, particularly coffee and black tea. Despite the charges against the use of such beverages because of their stimulating properties (attributed to caffeine and related substances), the proper use of stimulant herbs is, according to herbal traditions, beneficial in treating a wide variety of conditions. The extensive use of stimulating beverages without regard to bodily needs will, on the other hand, be harmful. But most importantly, the major problem with coffee and, to a lesser extent, black tea is that they have a notable acidic effect, producing toxic conditions in the blood and digestive tract when taken in large amounts. This eventually contributes to the development of other ailments. Thus one should not confuse these overused beverage stimulants, which have a clearly detrimental effect, with other herbal stimulants, which, when properly administered, are very helpful in the treatment of certain diseases.

Stimulant therapy is not to be used when there is extreme weakness, as often occurs after severe and prolonged disease, since there is then no basic strength to stimulate to a better action. Stimulants, however, may be slowly added to help other herbs maintain the body through this critical time and build back the strength. Stimulants are also not used when the body is eliminating toxins through the skin in the form of eruptive skin diseases, since the use of stimulants will enhance that elimination process and make the disease symptoms appear worse. Minimize the use of stimulants in cases of nervousness and hypertension. Finally, stimulants, including hot, spicy foods, should be avoided when there is chronic imbalance in the colon. The stimulants will overwork this organ and may lead to problems with elimination and hemorrhoids.

Tranquilization

This therapy is used when there is great unrest, nervousness or irritation interfering with the process of overcoming the disease condition. There are three types of tranquilizers: demulcents, nervines and antispasmodics. These treatments may be taken intensively over a period of one or two days, as often as every hour.

Demulcent herbs and soothing foods will lubricate the joints, bones, gastrointestinal tract and even the irritating conflicts of our lives. Herbs such as slippery elm bark, marshmallow root and comfrey root, and foods such as warm milk and watery oat or barley cereals, are used to comfort and quiet a person while the process of healing carries on. Any mucilaginous substance will be effective; it may be taken along with warm milk and honey to promote its soothing effects.

Nervines are substances that feed the nervous system and balance its energy. These are also called nerve tonics. The nervine herbs include skullcap, catnip, wood betony, lady's slipper and valerian.

Antispasmodics calm the nervous tension in the muscles, including both the skeletal muscles and the smooth muscles of internal organs. These also help relieve pain due to tension or convulsion. Herbal antispasmodics include lobelia, valerian, kava kava, black cohosh, and dong quai.

In all cases, it is important to have adequate calcium in the diet since this strongly effects the function of the nervous system and muscles.

It is not uncommon to use tranquilization therapy along with stimulant therapy. The tranquilizers will not counteract the stimulants, but will buffer their effects.

Blood Purification

Most herbalists agree that if one can purify the blood and neutralize excess acidity, all diseases will eventually subside. For this reason, blood purifiers occupy a prominent place in herbal therapies.

The blood and lymph of the body carry a variety of toxic substances, most of these being acids. These substances include constituents taken in with food and drink, such as chemical preservatives, which the body cannot easily eliminate. Also included are natural wastes of the body, which may be produced in excess, or inadequately eliminated, when the body's organs are functioning improperly. In traditional Chinese medicine theory, the toxins of the blood are considered excess "heat," and toxin-producing infections are called hot diseases. The site of the body most responsible for the purity of blood is the small intestine, which must separate useful nutrients from the totality of substances ingested. Secondary organs affecting blood purity include the liver, kidney and colon.

There are several ways to purify the blood:

1. directly neutralize acids with the strong alkalinizing effect of some herbs (e.g., dandelion and slippery elm);
2. stimulate the vital organic functions of the body, especially the

liver and kidneys, lungs and colon (e.g., Oregon grape root, gold-enseal);

3. dry excess moisture and remove excess fat where toxins are re-tained (e.g., plantain, mullein, chickweed, gota kola);

4. eliminate excess "heat," especially from the small intestine (e.g., rhubarb root).

The best herb for blood and lymph purification is *Echinacea angustifolia,* sometimes called "prairie doctor" or "Kansas snakeroot." It contributes to some extent to all these ways of purifying the blood. Other useful blood purifiers include: burdock root, dandelion, red clover, sarsaparilla, sassafras and Oregon grape root.

The use of blood purifiers is particularly important for the treatment of infections. Not only does the herb help remove toxins produced by the infection, but it can also remove the excess moisture that provides the medium in which it grows. Furthermore, the infection may be totally eradicated because the herb will stimulate our natural defense mechanisms. For example, echinacea promotes the production of white blood cells which can then destroy the invading bacteria or virus.

Tonification

Herbs that can build the energy of the organ systems are used as tonics. They are commonly recommended for those who are weak and run down, having low vitality. Tonic therapy is used in the recovery from acute ailments and in building energy back for those suffering chronic diseases. It is also useful in maintaining a healthy condition and overcoming minor imbalances.

Tonics are nourishing to the organs. Some of the herbs act primarily to provide nutrients: vitamins, minerals and sugars. These are referred to as Yin tonics (see chapter on "Diagnosis and Treatment"), the most valuable being the seaweeds (kelp and Irish moss), alfalfa, comfrey and dandelion leaf. Others, in addition to providing some of these nutrients, act to balance and stimulate the energy of the organs, improving their ability to assimilate and utilize nutrients. These are the Yang tonics, the most valuable being the Chinese root tonic herbs (see chapter on "Western Herbs"), burdock, dandelion, parsley, Oregon grape root and goldenseal root.

Tonic herbs are used to counteract a deficiency (weakness or critical shortage) in the body. Usually if the body is deficient in one function, there will be deficiencies in all the other functions and in the vital substances (minerals and vitamins). When one is very weak and out of balance, the use of strong, stimulating Yang tonics is not advised, as these will drive the system further out of balance. Therefore, the milder acting, nutritive Yin tonics are first used. These are usually the fruit, flower and leaf herbs. Later a stimulating tonic can be added to improve the assimilation and use of the nutrients. These Yang tonics are usually roots and barks.

The science and art of tonic therapy for treatment of chronic diseases, recovery from acute crisis and prevention of all ailments is most highly developed in the Far East. Several of the most important Chinese tonic herbs have been included in the chapter "Western Herbs."

Diuresis (Control of Fluid Balance)

The body fluids are comprised mostly of water. Through the control of this vital element, we are able to restore and maintain health and well-being.

The amount of fluids in the body can change very quickly. Our emotions are strongly linked to the balance of fluids in our bodies and thus can also change very quickly. In fact, changes of emotion are frequently related to changes in the water balance. For example, women commonly experience emotional sensitivity just before their menstrual period. At this time, these women are experiencing an increase in retention of body fluids. As the fluids are released during the period, the emotions again fluctuate and are eventually returned to the normal equilibrium.

Having too much water retained in the body leads to feelings of weakness, paranoia and depression. Too little water in the body, on the other hand, may result in explosive anger and other forceful reactions. Water may be used to quiet the "fire" but too much water will "dampen one's spirits." Excessive water, especially when taken in with meals, will disrupt normal digestion by diluting the stomach's acids and enzymes. The internal organs may also become waterlogged; a common example of this is the occasional occurrence of hypoglycemia due to a waterlogged pancreas.

The primary method of reducing water in the system is through the use of diuretic herbs. Important diuretic herbs include: prince's pine, buchu leaves, horsetail, cleavers, corn silk, uva ursi leaves and juniper berries. The use of these herbs increases the flow of urine, decreases the blood pressure and helps purify the blood. Diuretics are also useful for weight loss by removing excess water, and for this purpose it is good to use the astringent diuretics such as cleavers and uva ursi.

To maintain a good water balance in the body it is important to regulate the intake of water. When thirsty, check the cause of the sensation. If it is due to spicy foods, it may be necessary to reduce the amount of spices in the food so as to reduce the intake of water. On the other hand, if one is thirsty following exercise, the thirst is a natural response to water loss. A large amount of fluid is taken in the water content of food. Persons suffering from excess water in the system should switch to less watery foods. The amount of fluids taken in with foods should also be limited for all persons, since excess water will interfere with digestion.

When undertaking a program of herbal treatments, one may need to consider the amount of water taken as tea, and if this is too much, use other methods of preparation such as tinctures.

Kidney weakness is also treated by the use of diuretics. The weakened kidneys may be further burdened by excessive water intake. A clear physical sign of waterlogged kidneys is bagginess or darkness under the eyes.

Sweating

Sweating is used to treat externally caused diseases such as cold, flu and fever. There are two methods of treatment: one with relaxing diaphoretic herb teas and the other with stimulating diaphoretic teas. Relaxing teas, such as those made with catnip or lemon balm, are used to treat ailments where the pores of the skin are closed and the energy has retreated from the surface. The volatile oils in the herbs exit through the pores of the skin, soothing and calming the body surface. The stimulating herbs provide heat, increase the circulation and promote sweating. They are used to treat weakness in the internal organs. Useful stimulant diaphoretics include teas made from boneset, elder flowers and peppermint, or a combination of cayenne, ginger, lemon and honey.

The herbs used for sweating are taken as warm teas. The same herbs, taken as cool teas, are useful as diuretics. Sweating occurs to some extent just by taking the tea, but is promoted by providing additional external heat to the body, such as taking a hot bath and then covering up with blankets, after taking two cups of the hot tea.

Emesis (Vomiting)

Emetic herbs induce vomiting and thus quickly empty the stomach of its contents. This may be a necessary treatment if one is feeling sick from eating too much food or a poor combination of foods. It is also recommended for treating poisoning by noncaustic substances that will not burn the esophagus when vomiting is induced.

Some people tend to create excess mucus as a result of certain foods they eat. The first line of treatment is to empty the stomach, where the mucus originates. Similarly, emetics can be used to treat colds that have resulted from overeating.

Ipecac, an herbal syrup found in most drugstores, is an excellent emetic. Lobelia can also be used. This is done by taking a full teaspoon of lobelia tincture (see chapter on "Methods of Application" for how to make a tincture) three times within an interval of about thirty minutes. In between taking teaspoons of lobelia tincture, one should drink as much peppermint tea as possible (about two quarts would be ideal) and tickle the back of the throat with the fingers to stimulate the emetic reaction.

Emesis greatly reduces the energy of the body and so should not be used by persons who are already very weak. The emetic treatment may be followed by a mild stimulating treatment, along with soothing, demulcent herbs, to recover the energy.

Purging

Purging, by the use of herbal laxatives, is valuable in treating ailments associated with the presence of excess secretions, buildup of toxins or weak elimination. Constipation is considered a serious problem because the retention of wastes in the body can lead to more serious diseases. Purgatives must not be overused, as they deplete the energy of the body, and thus they are only given occasionally to persons who are in relatively good health. Proper elimination is very dependent upon the diet; dietary factors should therefore be emphasized in the regulation of this important function.

Herbs work in a number of ways to promote elimination. Some, like cascara bark and rhubarb root, exert a laxative action by stimulating the secretion of bile into the small intestine and increasing the intestinal peristalsis (the natural rhythmic contractions by which the body moves the intestinal contents along). Others, such as licorice, slippery elm and various oils, are soothing lubricants that have a mild action and may be used to treat minor problems in adults or to treat children. Aloe vera combines both these kinds of actions and may be used for more advanced illnesses accompanied by poor elimination (see "Aloe vera" in the "Western Herbs" chapter). Bulk laxatives, such as psyllium seed, flax seed and chia seed, swell up with water and work by greatly increasing the bulk in the intestines. These herb seeds are also very nutritive. A combination of these laxative types, for example, with cascara, licorice, psyllium, flax and chia, provides a tonic laxative with nutrients, demulcent properties and stimulation.

· 4 ·

METHODS OF APPLICATION

In most parts of the world, healers achieve their cures with only a small variety of plants that are available in the region. Their success is due not only to their knowledge of these plants, but also to their ability to administer them in many different ways. One of the most commonly used preparations is the herbal tea, but there are many more methods of application, including:

1. bolus
2. douche
3. electuary
4. enema
5. fomentation
6. gelatin capsule
7. liniment
8. oil
9. pill
10. poultice and plaster
11. salve
12. smoking
13. syrup
14. tincture

The choice of method will depend on a number of factors; through familiarity with the nature of the different preparations, one will be able to choose the method that best fits the ailment, the individual and the herbs. For quickest results, and especially in treating severe acute ailments, it will usually be best to take the herbs while fasting or following a special cleansing diet (see "Therapeutic Diet" suggestions in the "Kitchen Medicines" chapter). The proper use of herbs and diet are certain to strengthen and heal your body if you reduce the intake of toxic or acid-forming foods, get plenty of rest and remove yourself from tension.

Medicinal Herb Teas

Herbs that have a relatively mild flavor and are to be taken internally are frequently taken as an herb tea. When purchasing herbs for making teas, the cut and sifted form is most useful because it is easily strained through any common tea strainer. Fresh herbs are first bruised by rubbing between the hands or using a mortar and pestle to break up the tissue structure and release the active principles. Herbs are prepared in nonmetallic containers such as glass, earthenware or enamel pots. Stainless steel has been found to be acceptable when these others are not available. Use distilled or spring water, rather than tap water, when possible.

There are two basic methods of preparing the tea infusion and decoction.

Infusion. If one is attempting to utilize the volatile oils in herbs such as the mints or eucalyptus, or the delicate plant parts such as flowers and soft leaves, the herbs are steeped in a tightly covered container with water that has just been brought to a rolling boil. This method is called an infusion. The herbs are not boiled at all, but are only steeped, allowing ten to twenty minutes in a tightly covered vessel. A "sun tea" is made by exposing the herbs in water to the sun for a few hours in a tightly covered glass bottle.

Decoction. To extract the deeper essences from coarser leaves, stems, barks and roots, the herbs are simmered for about one hour. This method is called a decoction. In many cases, the herbs are simmered uncovered and the volume of water is decreased by about half through evaporation. However, some of these coarser herbs contain important volatile oils, and these must be gently simmered or steeped in a covered pot (valerian, cinnamon and burdock roots, for example).

Combining Decoction and Infusion. Occasionally, a formula will combine roots and barks along with soft leaves and flowers. To make a tea, a decoction is first made with the coarser materials, then strained and poured over the delicate plant parts. This is then steeped, tightly covered, for ten to twenty minutes.

Amount to Use. Medicinal infusions and decoctions are very strong, and are not like the weak beverage teas familiar to most people. The beverage teas, such as those sold commercially in tea bags, are made using only about one-seventh ounce of herb per pint (two cups) of water. *The usual proportion in making a medicinal tea is one ounce of dried herb per pint of water.* The herb will absorb some of the water, so that after making the tea, perhaps only one and one-half cups of the tea will result from using one pint of water. In most cases, this will be the correct amount for one day, since the therapy usually requires taking one-half cup of the tea, three times daily. For convenience, perpare enough tea for three days of treatment all at once and keep it refrigerated in a tightly closed jar. Herb teas generally will not keep for more than three days in the refrigerator. They should be gently reheated in a covered pot.

If fresh herbs are to be used, the amount is doubled, since much of the weight of the fresh herb is water.

The standard dose of medicinal tea is one-half to one cup taken three times a day. Frequent small doses of two to three tablespoons (taken every half hour) are more effective than a few large doses when treating acute ailments.

In treating chronic ailments where the herbs are to be taken over a period of several weeks, it may be more convenient to use a tincture. Also, if one wishes to restrict the intake of fluids, the tincture will be more useful (see the information on "Diuresis" in the "Herbal Therapies" chapter). Herbs that are mucilaginous, such as slippery elm, comfrey root and marshmallow root, will give the tea a "slimy" quality. If this is disagreeable, the mucilaginous herbs may be put into gelatin capsules or pills and taken along with the tea.

Bolus

A bolus is a suppository made by adding powdered herbs to cocoa butter until it forms a thick, firm pie-dough consistency. This is placed in the refrigerator to harden and then allowed to warm to room temperature before use. It is rolled into strips about three-quarters of an inch thick and cut into segments one inch long. The bolus is inserted into the rectum to treat hemorrhoids or various cysts, or into the vagina to treat infections, irritations and tumors. The herbs used in the bolus may include astringents such as white oak bark or bayberry bark; demulcent healing herbs such as comfrey root or slippery elm; and antibiotic herbs such as garlic, chaparral or goldenseal. Goldenseal is particularly useful because it is a specific for treating mucous membranes and combines astringent, tissue healing and antibiotic effects.

The bolus is usually applied at night, and the cocoa butter will melt due to the body heat, releasing the herbs. Take precautions to protect clothing and bedding, and rinse away the residue the following morning.

Douche

A douche is generally used in the treatment of vaginal infections or for cleansing. I do not recommend that douches be used often because they disturb the balance of natural bacteria in the vagina. Repeated infections are usually a sign of a poor diet and general lowered resistance of the body.

The douche is made by preparing a strong tea using herbs such as goldenseal, plantain, uva ursi, comfrey, white oak bark or yellow dock. A small amount (one or two tablespoons per quart) of vinegar or yogurt may be added to promote acid balance. The douche is best applied in the bathtub or on the toilet, but never have the bag more than two feet above the hips. The herbal douche is slowly and gently inserted while still warm (body temperature) and retained for a period of ten to twenty minutes, if possible. If the liquid is forced in under too much pressure it may push the infection upward to the uterus. Don't douche if you are pregnant.

Electuary

An electuary is an old-fashioned way of giving unpalatable herbs to children who need them. A small amount of the herb is mixed with honey, maple syrup, peanut butter or other acceptable medium until a soft pasty mass is formed. Small children can even be persuaded to take cayenne in a little peanut butter coated with honey.

Enema

Enemas are administered for the treatment of nervousness, pain and conditions associated with excess toxins in the blood. One of the best herbal enemas is catnip tea. Others which are also very useful are those made from a combination of nervines, such as lobelia or skullcap, with astringents, such as yellow dock or bayberry bark. Use equal parts in making a strong tea for use as an enema.

Enemas are given cool (but not cold) if one is trying to remove old waste that has dried and hardened on the intestinal walls. A cool catnip enema is useful to reduce fever. Enemas are given warm for treating nervous conditions.

To prevent bowel irritation, it is good to mix two tablespoons of sesame oil and one tablespoon each of castor oil and honey to one quart of the warm water or tea to be used as the enema.

An enema is taken in first while lying on the left side, then on hands and knees, and finally while lying on the right side. This will help the solution to fill the lower intestines. The herbal fluid is to be retained for as long as possible and the procedure should be repeated during the course of an hour or until two quarts of water can be taken in and retained for a few minutes.

Fomentation

A fomentation is an external application of herbs that is used to treat superficial ailments, including swellings, pains, colds and flus. A fomentation can be used to stimulate the circulation of the blood or lymph in the area of the body to which it is applied. Herbs that are too strong to be taken internally may be used externally and the body will absorb a small amount slowly. A fomentation is also known as a compress.

A fomentation is prepared by making an herbal tea, dipping a moisture-absorbent towel or cloth into the tea and applying the towel over the affected area as hot as can be tolerated without burning. The towel is covered by dry flannel cloth and a heating pad or hot water bottle is placed on top of this. A plastic covering is used to protect bedding if applied overnight.

To stimulate circulation of blood and lymph, to relieve colic, to reduce internal inflammation and to restore warmth to cold joints, a ginger fomentation is recommended. Grate two ounces of fresh ginger root and squeeze out the ginger into a pint of hot water until the water turns yellow. Then apply the fomentation, having an alternate towel ready to apply as soon as one cools.

To help restore vitality to a part of the body that has been immobilized or weakened by a disease, the hot fomentation can be alternated with a shorter application of cold. Heat serves to relax the body and open the pores, while cold will stimulate the body and cause contraction. The alternation of hot and cold will revitalize the area.

The value of external herbal application is illustrated by the following experience. A member of my family was suffering from postoperative shock, showing extreme weakness and severe diarrhea. The condition was becoming critical since no nourishment was being assimilated and rapid dehydration was setting in as a result of the diarrhea. The doctors were quite concerned and didn't seem to know what to do. The hospital rules did not permit them to allow me to administer an herb tea that I thought would be of benefit. However, considering it harmless and probably of little effect, they did allow me to apply a hot fomentation of slippery elm tea over the abdomen with a heating pad to keep it warm throughout the night. The next morning, the diarrhea had lessened considerably; dehydration was almost completely stopped; and food was being digested properly. Improvement continued with no further applications of the fomentation being necessary.

Gelatin Capsules

Gelatin capsules provide a useful method of taking herbs when the herbs are:

1. to be taken in small amounts (one-half to three grams at a time);
2. bitter-tasting or mucilaginous;
3. to be taken regularly over a long period of time.

There are a variety of capsule sizes, but the most common are the small "0" (single 0) and the larger "00" (double 0) caps. The "00" capsules are generally used unless the capsules are to be taken by children or by someone who finds the larger capsules difficult to swallow. To facilitate washing down and dissolving the capsules, either take them with a meal or drink at least one half to one cup of water or herbal tea.

In many cases, it is necessary to purchase the herb already powdered in order to fill the capsules properly. The herb powdered in a blender or spice grinder may not be fine enough for this purpose. Place the powders in a small bowl and blend them well with a spoon. Separate the two parts of the capsule and press each through the powder to the side of the bowl so that some powder is forced into the capsule. Continue to do this until both ends are almost filled. Then carefully close the capsule. The amount of herb material that fills the capsule will depend on how finely it is powdered, how tightly it is packed and whether it is root, bark, leaf or flower.

Do not use very mild herbs that require large doses to be effective in the capsules. It will not be possible to get an adequate dose this way. Also, do not mix mild acting herbs, except those that are mucilaginous, with more potent herbs in a capsule, since the mild herbs will only dilute the potent herbs and will not be present in sufficient quantity to provide the desired effect.

The typical dose for herbs taken by capsule is two capsules, three times daily, though the actual dose will depend on the herb and the condition being treated. Some herbs, such as goldenseal, mandrake, poke and lobelia, should be taken in much smaller quantities, usually by incorporating them as constituents of a larger formula.

Gelatin capsules may be taken with meals, but if taken between meals *at least one-half cup water or herbal tea should be used to wash them down.*

Whenever a formula calls for using gelatin capsules, one may alternatively make pills, using twice as many pills as capsules to get about the same dose (see the section on "Pills" in this chapter).

Liniment

Liniments are herbal extracts that are rubbed into the skin for treating strained muscles and ligaments. They are also used for the relief of arthritis and some types of inflammation. Liniments usually include stimulating herbs, such as cayenne, and antispasmodic herbs, such as lobelia. Oils of aromatic herbs, such as eucalyptus, will penetrate into the muscles, increasing circulation and bringing relaxing warmth to the area.

Place four ounces of dried herbs or eight ounces of fresh bruised herbs into a bottle. Add one pint of vinegar, alcohol or massage oil and allow to extract. Shake the contents of the bottle once or twice a day. The extraction will require three days if the herbs are all powdered, but fourteen days if the herbs are whole or cut.

The vinegar acts as a natural astringent and also as a perservative. It may be used directly or diluted to 50% strength with water. Alcohol is an excellent extracting agent and preservative. One can use a grain alcohol such as vodka or gin, or, if only external use is intended, a rubbing alcohol. The application of the alcohol extract will be somewhat cooling, and the liquid will evaporate quickly, leaving the herbal principles in the skin. A massage oil can be mde by combining vegetable oils such as olive, sesame and almond. It is useful for extracting herbs with aromatic oils and for applications where one wishes to massage the area being treated. Oils are preserved by adding a small amount of Vitamin E, about 400 IU per cup.

Oils

When the major properties of an herb are associated with its essential oils, an oil extract will prove to be a useful method of preparing a concentrate from fresh herbs. Oils are prepared by macerating and pounding the fresh or dried herbs in a mortar and pestle. Olive oil or sesame oil is then added (one pint oil to two ounces of herb) and the mixture is allowed to stand in a warm place for three days. A quicker method is to gently heat the oil and herbs in a pan for at least one hour. Then the oil is strained and bottled. Yet another method is to extract the herbal properties with alcohol (see the section on "Tinctures" in this chapter), then add the oil and apply gentle heat to evaporate away the alcohol. A small amount of Vitamin E oil (about 400 IU per cup) will help preserve the quality of the preparation.

To obtain an oil made primarily of the essential plant oils, dip thin layers of cotton or cheesecloth in olive or sesame oil, wring out gently and cover each piece with a layer of herbs. Place these pieces of cloth on top of each other in a wide-mouthed jar, covered tightly, for three days and then squeeze out the oil from the cloths.

Oils are frequently made from spices, mints and other aromatic herbs.

Pills

Pills are used in the same way as gelatin capsules, but they have the advangate that they can be prepared entirely with herbs and the herbs need not be powered so finely. Coarse powders can be made from the dried and cut herb using a coffee and spice grinder. To the powdered herbs, add a small amount of slippery elm (or other mucilaginous herb powder), making up about 10% of the mixture. Slowly add water and mix it in with the herbs until a doughy consistency is reached. Alternatively, one can use a little gum arabic dissolved in boiling water as a good adhesive. Roll the dough into little balls about the size of a pea. The pills may be taken immediately, but to preserve them for later use dry them in the warm air or in an oven at low heat. Strict vegetarians prefer using the pills rather than gelatin capsules, since all available capsules are made from animal gelatin.

The pea-sized pills contain about half the dose of a gelatin capsule. Therefore when following a dosage schedule for gelatin capsules, use twice the number indicated when using pills as a substitute.

Poultice and Plaster

A poultice is a warm, moist mass of powdered or macerated herbs that is applied directly to the skin to relieve inflammation, blood poisoning, venomous bites and eruptions and to promote proper cleansing and healing of the affected area. Many poultices have the power to draw out infection, toxins and foreign bodies embedded in the skin; these usually include comfrey, plantain or marshmallow. To relieve pain and muscle spasm, herbs such as lobelia, lady's slipper, catnip, valerian, kava kava or echinacea are used. Usually a small amount of herbal stimulant, such as ginger or cayenne, is added to promote good circulation. The powdered herbs are moistened with hot water, herbal tea, a liniment or a tincture. Herbs that are not available in powder form may be added by using one of these other extraction methods and then adding it to the powder. A witch hazel extract, available at most drugstores, is useful for this purpose. In the wilds, a poultice can be made by chewing the fresh herbs, such as plantain, before applying them to the affected area.

A plaster is like a poultice, but the herbal materials are either placed between two thin pieces of linen or are combined in a thick base material and then applied to the skin. A classic mustard plaster is described in the "Medicines in the Spice Rack" section of the "Kitchen Medicines" chapter (see under "Mustard seed"). A very effective plaster for drawing out fever is made by squeezing out the water from tofu and then mashing the tofu together with 20% pastry flower and 5% grated fresh ginger root. This is applied directly to the skin for cooling the area. Tofu is a very useful base for many plasters.

Salve

A salve, or ointment, is a preparation that can be applied to the skin and remain in place due to its thick consistency. A salve can be made by first preparing an herbal oil, heating it and then adding melted beeswax sufficient to obtain the desired consistency (about one and one-half ounces per pint of oil). The quickest method is to extract the herbs in hot oil, allowing about two hours for roots and barks to extract in oil heated to just below the point where it will bubble. Keep the pot covered. Add leaves and flowers next, and continue to cook gently for another hour. Then add the melted wax and stir well. Alternatively mix one part of the powdered herbs into four parts of hot lard or other fat that is hard at room temperature. With either method, add a small amount of gum benzoin or tincture of benzoin to the salve to help preserve it (about one teaspoon of the tincture per quart of salve).

Smoking

For direct treatment of coughs and bronchial congestion, some herbs are smoked. This will provide immediate, but temporary, relief for the condition. Unlike tobacco, the herbs which are smoked for therapeutic purposes contain no nicotine or other addicting substances.

A small amount of the herb is smoked in a pipe, or a water pipe. The lungs are filled with smoke and then this is fully exhaled. Inhale the smoke about six to ten times for a single treatment.

The most commonly used herbs that are smoked are coltsfoot, rosemary, mullein, yerba santa and sarsaparilla. To aid in quitting smoking tobacco, lobelia, also known as Indian tobacco, is smoked. It contains lobeline, which is similar to nicotine but does not have the same set of effects. Thus it reduces the sensation of need for nicotine, but does not provide the effects that lead to addictive smoking.

There are a number of commercial herbal cigarettes available. Most of these contain herbs that are effective in treating bronchial problems, but they are also blended specifically for a particular flavor and therefore may not be as useful as an herbal formula you can develop for treatment. They are most useful in making a transition from smoking tobacco to stopping addictive smoking altogether.

In China, "Asthma Allaying Cigarettes" are commonly used in the treatment of asthma. They contain about a dozen herbs and have been extensively tested to reveal their efficacy in reducing lung congestion and aiding expectoration.

Datura stramonium, also known as jimsonweed and giant thorn apple, has been used extensively to treat asthma, often taken by smoking the leaves. However, this plant is extremely toxic and in large doses can not only cause severe neurological disturbances but may even be fatal. Therefore it is not recommended.

In India, a popular herbal cigarette is known as "Bidis." These contain herbs for coughs and congestion, but also include a small amount of datura. This has recently been recognized and has led to a reduced availability of the cigarettes in the United States.

Mugwort and catnip have been smoked for their calming effects to treat insomnia and restlessness. Damiana has been smoked for its aphrodisiac effects.

Peppermint is added to smoking blends for its cooling menthol. Licorice is added to provide a sweet flavor.

The smoking of herbs should only be an occasional practice, done with proper concern for the ability of the lungs to remove smoke particles and tars that are an inevitable result of burning plant materials.

Syrups

A syrup is often used in treating coughs and sore throats because it will coat the area and keep the herbs in direct contact. Add about two ounces of herb to a quart of water and gently boil down to one pint. Strain, and while warm, add one or two ounces of honey and/or glycerine. Licorice and wild cherry bark are two herbs commonly used both as flavors and as therapeutic agents in making syrups. Other herbs commonly used in cough syrups are thyme, comfrey root, anise seed, fennel seed, Irish moss and small amounts of lobelia. The syrups are used in doses of one-half to one teaspoon, as needed.

Tinctures

Tinctures are highly concentrated herbal extracts that can be kept for long periods of time because the alcohol is a good preservative. The final concentration of alcohol in the tincture should not be less than about 30%. Tinctures are particularly useful for herbs that do not taste good or are to be taken over an extended period of time, and they may be used externally as a liniment. Some herbs, such as black cohosh and chaparral, contain substances not readily extracted by water and thus should be taken in pills, capsules or tinctures rather than teas. Alcohol will generally extract all important ingredients from an herb.

To make a tincture, combine four ounces of powdered or cut herb with one pint of alcohol such as vodka, brandy, gin or rum. Shake daily, allowing the herbs to extract for about two weeks. Let the herbs settle and pour off the tincture, straining out the powder through a fine cloth or filter. It is best to put up one's tincture on the new moon and strain it off on the full moon so that the drawing power of the waxing moon will help extract the herbal properties.

The amount of tincture to be taken in a single dose varies from a few drops to two tablespoons. This amount of alcohol is quite small and for most people should not present a problem. However, if for any reason, such as a previous history of alcoholism, one chooses not to take any alcohol whatsoever, then the required amount of tincture can be stirred into a quarter or half cup of boiling water in order to evaporate the alcohol. If one is specifically extracting herbs for their alkaloid content, then an acidic extract can be made substituting apple-cider vinegar for alcohol.

Tinctures are usually made with the more potent herbs that are generally not taken as herbal teas. If a tincture is to be made with milder herbs, the dose will have to be increased to one or two tablespoons, about the equivalent of one-half cup of the tea.

Do not confuse tinctures with the commercially available "fluid extract." The fluid extract is made by techniques that utilize multiple solvent extraction, resulting in a very concentrated product. These are up to ten times as potent as the tincture and thus are usually taken in quantities of only six to eight drops (the equivalent of a teaspoon of tincture).

Page 353 of this book provides weights and measures for the preparation of herbal formulas.

Herbal Wines

The method of making herbal wines probably predates that of tinctures. The major difference is that the fresh or dried herbs themselves are used to help produce the alcoholic medium that will preserve their therapeutic essence. While it is a slower and somewhat more involved process than making tinctures, it has the advantages of being cheaper (not having to buy the alcohol), more organic and for me a lot more satisfying experience. Another decided advantage is that it provides a way to economically preserve and render therapeutically effective an overabundant harvest of garden-fresh herbs. Also, alcohol-based medicines are particularly good for digestive problems, poor circulation, and can be used externally as a liniment. So far I have made naturally fermented wines with comfrey, valerian, yarrow, lavender (delicious!), and angelica, to name only a few.

The basic method is to decoct hard roots and barks or infuse aromatic leaves and flowers using at least one half to one pound of the substance to a gallon of water. Allow this to cool to less than 100°C, and dissolve three pounds of honey or raw sugar to each gallon of liquid. Add one teaspoon of live baker's or wine yeast to each gallon and allow to stand in a warm place (around 70°C to 80°C) for two to three weeks, keeping the container loosely covered to protect the brew from extraneous wild yeasts. The first stage is completed when it stops fermenting. It should then be carefully strained through a cloth and bottled again with a loosely fitting lid until you are sure that it will not begin to ferment again. The dosage varies depending upon the herb used from a teaspoon to a small wineglass.

· 5 ·

HERBAL PROPERTIES

The remarkable aspect of herbs is their combination of several different healing properties. Thus each herb will have a combination of specific effects on particular systems of the body, and also some very general effects. By carefully matching the herbal properties with the symptoms being treated, it is possible to confront the entire scope of the disease at once, achieving a cure quickly and with the minimum possible dosage.

Every herb contains hundreds of biochemical constituents that may have an effect on the body. These constituents lend themselves to descriptions according to their physiological effects, or properties. Thus the tannins in many herb plants give rise to the properties "astringent" and "hemostatic," and the aromatic essential oils give rise to such properties as "diaphoretic," "stimulant" and "carminative."

Through the centuries of herbal practice, more than a hundred terms have arisen to describe these properties. Yet there are about three dozen terms that are adequate to describe most herbal effects, after one has eliminated equivalent terms and rarely mentioned properties. These have been included in this chapter to familiarize you with the most frequently considered herbal properties. Many of the same properties have already been referred to in the chapter on "Methods of Application" and will repeatedly be used in the description of the important "Western Herbs."

Alteratives: Also known as blood purifiers. These are agents that gradually and favorably alter the condition of the body. They are used in treating toxicity of the blood, infections, arthritis, cancer and skin eruptions. Alteratives also help the body to assimilate nutrients and eliminate waste products of metabolism. The choice of alterative depends upon matching the accompanying properties of the herb with the specific nature of the condition being treated. Hence red clover is used to treat cancer because of its effects on protein assimilation; echinacea is used to neutralize acid conditions in the blood associated with a stagnation of lymphatic fluids; sarsaparilla may be used when diuretic properties are needed, as with infections; cascara sagrada is used when a laxative is required, as with toxic conditions resulting from constipation; dandelion root combines hepatic tonic properties and diuretic properties, and is particularly useful for treating chronic problems of blood toxicity; elder flowers have diaphoretic properties, and are thus used to purify the blood during treatment of colds and flus. In addition to the herbs mentioned above, other alteratives include: alfalfa, aloe vera, angelica, burdock root, comfrey, goldenseal, gota kola, marshmallow, nettles, Oregon grape root, plantain, sassafras, uva ursi, chrysanthemum, dong quai, ginseng, ho shou wu, lycii, peony and rehmannia.

Analgesics: Herbs that are taken to relieve pain without causing loss of consciousness. Some analgesics are also antispasmodics, relieving pain by reducing cramping in muscles; these include cramp bark and dong quai, which are used to reduce menstrual cramps and associated pain. Others, such as cloves and kava kava, affect the nerves directly, reducing the pain signals to the brain. These may be applied for toothaches for relief. Other analgesics include: lobelia, catnip, camomile, wild yam, skullcap and valerian.

Antacids: Herbs that are able to neutralize excess acids in the stomach and intestines. In most cases, these also have demulcent properties to protect the stomach lining. Dandelion, fennel, slippery elm, Irish moss and kelp function as antacids.

Antiabortives: Herbs that help to inhibit abortive tendencies. These are taken in small quantities during early pregnancy, and include: false unicorn root, lobelia, red raspberry and cramp bark. The herbs will not interfere with the natural process of miscarriage when the fetus is damaged or improperly secured.

Antiasthmatics: Herbs that relieve the symptoms of asthma. Some, like lobelia, are strong antispasmodics that dilate the bronchioles. Others, like yerba santa, help break up the mucus. Some herbs may be smoked for quick relief. These include coltsfoot and mullein, which may also be taken as teas. Other antiasthmatics include: wild yam, comfrey, elecampane and wild cherry bark.

Antibiotics: Substances that inhibit the growth of, or destroy, bacteria, viruses or amoebas. While many herbal antibiotics have direct germ killing effects, they have as a primary action the stimulation of the body's own immune response. Excessive use of antibiotics will eventually destroy the beneficial bacteria of the intestines. In fighting stubborn infections it is a good idea to maintain favorable intestinal flora by eating miso, tamari or fresh yogurt. Important antibiotic herbs include: buchu, chaparral, echinacea, goldenseal, myrrh, juniper berries, thyme and garlic.

Anticatarrhals: Substances that eliminate or counteract the formation of mucus. A treatment for catarrh should also include the use of herbs that aid elimination through sweat (diaphoretics), urine (diuretics) and feces (laxatives). Anticatarrhal herbs include: black pepper, cayenne, ginger, sage, cinnamon, anise, gota kola, mullein, comfrey, wild cherry bark and yerba santa.

Antipyretics: Cooling herbs used to reduce or prevent fevers. Substances with strong cooling properties are called refrigerants. Cooling may refer to neutralizing harmful acids in the blood (excess heat) as well as reducing body temperature. Antipyretics include: alfalfa, boneset, basil, gota kola, skullcap, chickweed and the seaweeds.

Antiseptics: Substances that can be applied to the skin to prevent the growth of bacteria. This includes the astringents. Other antiseptics include: goldenseal, calendula, chaparral, myrrh and the oils of thyme, garlic, pine, juniper berries and sage.

Antispasmodics: Herbs that prevent or relax muscle spasms. They may be applied either internally or externally for relief. One of the most important antispasmodics is lobelia, which has been called the "thinking herb" because it has been used successfully whenever there was any uncertainty as to the method of treatment. Antispasmodics are included in most herb formulas to relax the body and allow it to use its full energy for healing. Other antispasmodics include: dong quai, black cohosh, blue cohosh, skullcap, valerian, kava kava, raspberry leaves and rue.

Aphrodisiacs: Substances used to improve sexual potency and power. Aphrodisiacs include: damiana, false unicorn, ginseng, angelica, astragalus, kava kava and burdock.

Astringents: Substances that have a constricting or binding effect. They are commonly used to check hemorrhages and secretions, and to treat swollen tonsils and hemorrhoids. The main herbal astringents contain tannins, which are found in most plants, especially in tree barks. Important astringents include: bayberry bark, white oak bark, yellow dock, uva ursi, calendula, myrrh, horsetail, juniper berries, prince's pine, stoneroot, squawvine and witch hazel.

Carminatives: Herbs and spices taken to relieve gas and griping (severe pains in the bowels). Examples of carminatives include: anise, caraway, fennel, cumin, dill, ginger, peppermint and calamus.

Cholagogues: Substances used to promote the flow and discharge of bile into the small intestine. These will also be laxatives, as the bile will stimulate elimination. Aloe vera, barberry, Oregon grape root, culver's root, mandrake, goldenseal, wild yam and licorice are cholagogues.

Demulcents: Soothing substances, usually mucilage, taken internally to protect damaged or inflamed tissues. Usually a demulcent herb will be used along with diuretics to protect the kidney and urinary tract, especially when kidney stones and gravel are present. Important demulcents include: marshmallow, comfrey, Irish moss, slippery elm, chickweed, licorice, psyllium, flax, chia seeds, aloe vera, burdock and fenugreek.

Diaphoretics: Herbs used to induce sweating. To administer diaphoretics effectively, the stomach and bowels should be emptied by fasting and using an enema. However, laxatives should not be taken before using these herbs. Sweating teas should be hot; when given cold they act as diuretics. One must distinguish between relaxing diaphoretics and stimulating diaphoretics (see the "Herbal Therapies" chapter). Relaxing diaphoretics include lemon balm and catnip. Stimulating diaphoretics are generally taken along with other stimulants, such as ginger or cayenne, and include: elder flowers, yarrow flowers, boneset, hyssop, peppermint and blessed thistle.

Diuretics: Herbs that increase the flow of urine. Diuretics are used to treat water retention, obesity, lymphatic swellings, nerve inflammations such as lumbago and sciatica, infections of the urinary tract, skin eruptions and kidney stones. Whenever a diuretic is given, a lesser amount of a demulcent herb is also given to buffer the effect of the diuretic on the kidneys (especially when the diuretic contains irritating properties) and to protect the tissues from the movement of kidney stones. Diuretics include: agrimony, horsetail, parsley, uva ursi, cleavers, buchu, juniper, marshmallow, plantain, nettles, burdock, dandelion, hawthorn and pai shu.

Emetics: Substances that induce vomiting and cause the stomach to empty (see the "Herbal Therapies" chapter). In small quantities these will not cause emesis, but will have other important effects on the body. Lobelia, black mustard seed, ipecac, bayberry, elecampane and blessed thistle are emetics.

Emmenagogues: Herbs that promote menstruation, usually causing it to occur earlier, and sometimes with increased flow. These have been used in the past to induce abortions, but extreme caution is advised. All of these, when taken in sufficient quantity to cause abortion, have other strong effects on the body. None of these should be taken when a woman wants to be pregnant. They are now commonly used to help regulate the menstrual cycle. Herbs with strong emmenagogue properties include: pennyroyal, juniper berries, myrrh, black cohosh, rue, angelica and wild ginger.

Emollients: Substances that are softening, soothing and protective to the skin. These include: oils of almond, apricot kernel, wheat germ, sesame, olive, linseed and flaxseed, and herbs such as marshmallow, comfrey root, slippery elm and chickweed.

Expectorants: Herbs that will assist in expelling mucus from the lungs and throat. Expectorants include: wild cherry bark, coltsfoot, yerba santa, lobelia, mullein, elecampane, horehound and anise. Also, to loosen mucus, inhale steam from boiled water with eucalyptus, bay leaves and sage.

Galactogogues: Substances that increase the secretion of milk. Anise seed, blessed thistle, cumin, fennel and vervain are galactogogues.

Hemostatics: Substances that arrest hemorrhaging. These include astringents and herbs that affect the coagulation of blood. Bayberry, blackberry, cayenne, cranesbill, mullein, goldenseal, horsetail, uva ursi, white oak bark, yellow dock, witch hazel and tienchi are hemostatics.

Laxatives: Substances that promote bowel movements. (See the section on "Purging" in the "Herbal Therapies" chapter for details.) A strong laxative that causes increased intestinal peristalsis is called a purgative in many texts.

Lithotriptics: Herbs that help to dissolve and eliminate urinary and biliary stones and gravel. For the kidney and bladder stones, use gravel root, cleavers, parsley, dandelion, nettle, uva ursi and horsetail. For the gallbladder, use wild cherry bark, Oregon grape root and cascara sagrada.

Nervines: Herbs that calm nervous tension and nourish the nervous system. See *Tonics*.

Oxytocics: Substances that stimulate uterine contractions to assist and induce labor, thus hastening childbirth. Oxytocics include: angelica, black cohosh, blue cohosh, juniper berries, raspberry, rue, squawvine, uva ursi and wild ginger.

Parasiticides: Substances that destroy parasites in the digestive tract or on the skin. Garlic, rue, thyme oil, cinnamon oil and chaparral are parasiticides.

Purgatives: See *Laxatives*.

Rubefacients: Substances that increase the flow of blood at the surface of the skin and produce redness where they are applied. Their function is to draw inflammation and congestions from deeper areas. They are useful for the treatment of arthritis, rheumatism and other joint problems and for sprains. Rubefacients include: mustard seed oil, cayenne, black pepper, pine oil, thyme oil, eucalyptus, cinnamon and cubeb oil.

Sedatives: Herbs that strongly quiet the nervous system. These will include antispasmodics and nervines. Useful sedatives include: valerian, hops, camomile, kava kava, passionflower, wood betony, catnip and skullcap.

Sialagogues: Substances that stimulate the flow of saliva and thus aid in the digestion of starches. Echinacea, black pepper, cayenne, ginger, licorice and yerba santa are sialagogues.

Stimulants: Herbs that increase the energy of the body, drive the circulation, break up obstruction and warm the body (see the "Herbal Therapies" chapter). Stimulants include: anise, cayenne, black pepper, cinnamon, echinacea, ginseng, sarsaparilla, dandelion, elecampane, angelica, ginger, yarrow, rosemary, garlic, onion, juniper berries, sage, pennyroyal, bayberry bark and astragalus.

Stomachics: See *Tonics*.

Tonics: Herbs that promote the functions of the systems of the body. Most tonics have general effects on the whole body, but also have a marked effect on a specific system.

Vulneraries: Herbs that encourage the healing of wounds by promoting cell growth and repair. Aloe vera, cayenne, comfrey, fenugreek, garlic, calendula, rosemary, thyme, marshmallow and slippery elm act as vulneraries.

NERVE TONICS (nervines)	HEART TONICS (cardiac tonics)	STOMACH TONICS (stomachics, bitters)	URINARY TONICS (diuretics)
skullcap	hawthorn	agrimony	rehmannia
lobelia	lily of the valley	gentian	fu ling
valerian	ginseng	barberry	parsley
lady's slipper	motherwort	don sen	gravel root
fu ling	rehmannia	elecampane	

LIVER TONICS (hepatics)	BILIARY TONICS (stimulates bile)	SEXUAL TONICS (aids sexual functions)
dandelion	Oregon grape root	damiana
sassafras	goldenseal	ginseng
stoneroot	rhubarb	dong quai
cascara	parsley	burdock
mandrake	wild yam	licorice

·6·

DIAGNOSIS AND TREATMENT

It is much more important to know what sort of patient has a disease than what sort of disease a patient has.

—Sir William Osler

Until the advent of modern medicine, diagnosis and treatment were based upon four things:

1. a general theory of health and disease;
2. an intuitive appraisal of the patient's condition and the nature of curative agents;
3. directing the patient toward making those changes necessary to promote self-healing;
4. experience.

More recently the theory of health has been all but lost, and only pathology is studied; intuition is often replaced by distant analysis; the role of "healing" is placed on the drug or on some kind of physical intervention (surgery, radiation, antibiotics, etc.); and experience has been replaced by a continuous onslaught of new synthetic drugs and physical techniques that nature never counted on in the evolution of the human body.

There are a number of traditional medical systems that provide a pathway to better interaction between patient and healer and to the active participation of the patient in healing his/her disease. These many traditions differ primarily in the particulars of the theory of health and

38

disease and in the curative agents available to them. All rely on the idea of balance in health, and disease as a reflection of imbalance. All rely on an intuitive approach to diagnosis and treatment.

Diagnosis in these traditional systems takes on a very different meaning in that the ability to recognize the underlying cause of a disease is already an integral part of the treatment. As was mentioned earlier, an ailment provides a focal point for discovering all the negative energies and direct and immediate knowledge of how to stop feeding the disease process. This knowledge, seeking more for the cause than the symptom, is the first step in healing oneself.

The Chinese system of diagnosis and treatment is a commonsense approach to healing with over 5000 years of proven efficacy. The general concepts of balance are similar to those used throughout the Orient, in East Indian Ayurvedic medicine, and even by the native Americans.

The most important concept to understand about the system involves the ability to diagnose imbalances using the theory of Yin and Yang.

The Yin/Yang theory is a teaching method and does not define anything absolute. It shows the way to develop an intuitive approach to diagnoses and treatment. Thus it is important to avoid getting too attached to the symbols Yin and Yang for they are only tools.

Yin and Yang represent the two essential opposites that make up all opposites. They find their physiological roots in the complementary action of the adrenal glands. The adrenal cortex controls the more Yin, parasympathetic nervous system dealing with body maintenance, including digestion, circulation, elimination, anti-inflammation and reproduction. The adrenal-medulla controls the sympathetic nervous system which is involved in the anti-stress or "fight or flight" response, the immune system, protection and stimulation of primary bodily response. Thus, the Ancient Chinese texts say that the root of Yin and Yang in our bodies is in the kidneys, meaning the small adrenal glands which are attached to the kidneys.

Treatment is based upon counterbalancing Yin-cold-deficient-chronic diseases with Yang-warm-full foods and herbs and Yang-hot-excess-acute disease with Yin-cool-empty foods and herbs.

The most important pairs of opposites to evaluate are as follows:

YIN	YANG
cold	*hot*
internal-chronic	*external-acute*
wet	*dry*
weak	*excess*

In the process of diagnosis, one looks for Yin-like or Yang-like conditions in both the basic constitution of the person and in the nature of the ailment. The chart of Yin conditions and Yang conditions shows examples of characteristics you might find present.

There are seven basic laws governing Yin/Yang theory and twelve theorems:

Laws Governing Yin and Yang

1. All things are the differentiated apparatus of one infinity.
2. Everything changes.
3. All antagonisms are complementary.
4. No two things are identical.
5. Every condition has its opposite.
6. The extreme of any condition will produce signs of its opposite.
7. Whatever has a beginning has an end.

YIN CONDITIONS

COLD: poor circulation; cold hands and feet; subnormal fevers; muscle cramps and spasms; desire for warmth

DEFICIENT: anemia; vitamin, mineral or protein deficiencies; underweight; paleness; clear urine; low vitality; timidity; shallow, weak breath; fatigue and tiredness

DEEP: involves internal organs; sensitive emotional states; tolerates or prefers deep massage

WET: history of eating raw fruits and vegetables; frequent urination; watery stools containing undigested foods; thin, clear mucus

OTHER DIAGNOSTIC   pulse feels slow, deficient, weak, sunken or deep; tongue
FEATURES: appears pale, lightly coated

YANG CONDITIONS

HOT: inflammatory; high fevers; burning sensation; irritability;
                    desire for cool things; hot hands and feet

EXCESS: rapid breathing; loud, coarse speech; forceful; high blood
                    pressure; insomnia; overweight; red face; cloudy urine

SUPERFICIAL: acute ailments; ailments due to exposure to cold, damp wind;
                    aversion to deep massage or pressure on the abdomen

DRY: constipation, dry mouth; mucus is thick (white, yellow or tinged
                    with blood); history of eating meat

OTHER DIAGNOSTIC   pulse feels rapid, forceful, full; tongue is heavily furred, coated
FEATURES: white, yellow, red or purple

Theorems of Yin and Yang

1. Infinity divides itself into Yin and Yang.
2. Yin and Yang result from the infinite movement of the universe.
3. Yin is centripetal and Yang is centrifugal; together, they produce all energy and phenomena.
4. Yin attracts Yang and Yang attracts Yin.
5. Yin repels Yin and Yang repels Yang.
6. The force of attraction and repulsion between the two phenomena is proportional to the difference in their Yin-Yang constitution.
7. All phenomena are ephemeral and are constantly changing their Yin and Yang constitution.
8. Nothing is solely Yin or Yang; everything involves polarity.
9. Nothing is neutral; either Yin or Yang is always more abundant.
10. Yin and Yang are relative: large Yin attracts small Yin; large Yang attracts small Yang.
11. At the extremity of their manifestation, Yin produces Yang and Yang produces Yin.
12. All physical forms are Yin at the center and Yang at the surface.

To illustrate these opposites, the chart of Qualities of Yin and Yang shows examples of the differing attributes.

QUALITIES OF YIN AND YANG

QUALITY	YIN	YANG
Tendency	to condense	to develop
Position	inward	outward
Structure	space	time
Direction	descending to earth	rising to heaven
Color	dark, purple, blue	bright, red
Temperature	cold	hot
Weight	heavy	light
Catalyst	water	fire
Light	dark	light
Construction	interior	exterior (surface)
Work	psychological	physical
Attitude	gentle, negative, introspective, intuitive	active, positive, outgoing, aggressive
Biological Classification	vegetable	animal
Energy	feminine	masculine
Nerves	parasympathetic	sympathetic
Taste	sour, bitter	acrid, pungent, sweet, mild

Since one rarely ever sees purely Yin or Yang conditions but rather a combination of both, we must follow the principle of considering the primary manifestation of symptoms first and the Yin-Yang constitution of the individual second. Generally, for acute ailments, consider the most serious symptoms; for chronic ailments, consider the basic constitution and behavior of the individual.

In general, an individual with a Yang-type constitution and diet (high in red meat and rich foods) will tend to have Yang diseases while a person with a Yin-type constitution (little or no meat, foods lacking in whole protein) will tend to have Yin diseases.

This is, however, not always the case, and a severe excess of Yin or Yang character can cause what are called "false Yin" or "false Yang" symptoms. As an example, one who is thin, weak, complains of coldness and eats a primarily vegetarian diet would be considered to have a

Yin constitution. But, in extreme imbalance, this person may suffer from a disease that has Yang characteristics such as high fever, red nose and cheeks, thick yellowish discharge from the lungs. These are called false Yang symptoms and should be treated by providing herbs specific for congestion and fever (treating the acute symptoms) along with a diet to bring the Yin condition back to balance (treating the chronic deficiency).

The method of treating an imbalance of Yin and Yang constitution is to provide a diet and herbal therapy that provides more of the Yin or Yang nature that is lacking. Hence those with a Yin constitution are given a diet and herbs with a somewhat more Yang character than they usually use, and those with a Yang constitution are given a diet and herbs with a more Yin character. It is important to avoid using herbs and foods that are too extreme in their Yin-Yang nature as it is almost impossible to obtain a good balance that way. Rather, one should use substances that are themselves close to balance, thus the therapeutic diet emphasizes the use of 50% whole grains on a daily basis.

The following chart indicates the relative Yin-Yang qualities of common foods and herbs. Since Yin and Yang are relative, fruits would be classified as being more Yin than vegetables but within the realm of fruits there would be those that have more Yang or Yin qualities than others.

Qualities of foods and herbs that represent the Yin character include those that have a cool energy, with moist, light, "empty sweet" (simple carbohydrates and sugars such as juicy fruits, honey and sugar), sour, or bitter tastes. Examples would include most herbal laxatives, anti-inflammatory herbs and blood purifiers, citrus fruits, leafy vegetables and herbs. These generally aid in the Yin-cooling processes of the body.

Qualities of foods and herbs that represent the Yang character include those that have a warm energy with a dry, heavy nature, concentrated proteins and nutrients, pungent, salty, or "full" sweet (complex carbohydrates and full proteins) tastes. All flesh foods are more Yang than vegetable foods, and lean red meat is generally more Yang than fatty light-colored meat. The more Yang parts of a plant are the deep roots, requiring a long time to mature, harder leaves, barks, and stems. These generally aid in the Yang-warming processes of the body involved with maintaining and stimulating the immune system and circulation.

Foods and herbs that are more Yin in quality can be balanced by preparing them in such a way as to accentuate their Yang qualities and vice versa.

The basic ways to "Yinnize" foods and herbs are as follows: Add more liquid, use cool or raw, add empty sweets such as sugar, honey or fruit.

To "Yangize" foods and herbs add heat, age, pressure or salt. Thus cooking, pickling in salt and using a pressure cooker are ways to balance Yin foods by making them more Yang. Eating cold or raw foods, juices, fruits, or taking more liquid is a way to counterbalance Yang foods such as red meat. For this reason, Oriental vegetables are practically always cooked and meat is most often served in soup.

The Tastes of Herbs and Foods

One might inquire how the ancients, lacking direct knowledge of biochemistry, determined the nutritive and therapeutic properties of foods and herbs. All herbs and foods were classified according to energy and taste. Herbs and foods that are more Yang were considered to have a warm energy, while herbs and foods that are more Yin had a cool energy. Generally, if something had a stimulating quality in some way, it was considered Yang; and if it had a soothing or calming energy, it was considered Yin.

There are five recognizable tastes used in Chinese herbology. They are as follows:

1. Sweet—Soothing, nutritive, tonifies the stomach and spleen, subclassified in terms of empty and full. Herbs with a warm-sweet nature—such as ginseng, astragalus, tienchi—are considered Yang. Herbs with a cool sweet nature—such as fruits and berries—are considered Yin.
2. Salt—Stabilizes and regulates body fluids. This refers to all kinds of salts, some of which are purging. Has a direct effect upon the kidneys and bladder. Example: seaweeds.
3. Sour—Tends to be cooling at first and stimulates enzymatic process of digestion and metabolism. Has a direct effect upon the liver and gallbladder. Examples: lemon, hawthorn berry, rose hips.
4. Bitter—Cooling and detoxifying. The bitter taste usually indicates the presence of alkaloids having a tendency to neutralize harmful body acids. Herbs and foods with this taste are considered to have a direct effect upon the heart, circulation, small intestines. Examples: cascara, Oregon grape, gentian, rhubarb root.

5. Pungent or Acrid—Stimulates the removal of stagnation and obstructions of both energy and blood. The spicy taste also counteracts the formation of mucus (unless taken in excess). Again, there are acrid-cool herbs, such as peppermint and various culinary spices, and acrid-warm herbs, such as cinnamon, peppers, and aconite.

In Ayurvedic medicine, herbs are said to have both a primary taste and effect, and secondary taste and effect. Generally anything that is salty or sweet tasting will have a secondary sweet or sedating taste. This includes nutritional substances such as seaweeds, grains, meat and vegetables. Foods and herbs with sour, pungent or bitter tastes will have a secondary taste, being pungent or stimulating. Sometimes the primary taste is of greater importance and sometimes the secondary taste is. The way to control this is by using a small amount if you want only the primary taste and effects, and a larger amount if you want the secondary taste and effects.

In applying the energetic understanding of foods and herbs, one must not neglect the valuable insights of the Western scientific system in explaining the action of a medicine. Thus the biochemical constituents are even more important in appreciating certain peculiar characteristics of herbs than the energy and tastes themselves. In ancient medicine, the unknown property indicated by the biochemical constituents of certain plants or medicine was considered to be the even more potent "magical" property. However, the great value of the energy and tastes principle is that it allows the practitioner to have a unifying commonsense principle by which to organize and sort out complex and subtle information regarding the patient's overall health, diagnosis, and treatment.

Foods

MORE YIN		BALANCED			MORE YANG			
WATERY FRUITS	SMALL FRUITS	LEAVES	ROOTS	SEEDS	DAIRY	FISH	POULTRY	RED MEAT
orange	cherry	spinach	carrot	rice	cheese	cod	chicken	pork

Herb Tonics

MORE YIN			BALANCED	MORE YANG		
SMALL FRUITS	FLOWERS	LEAVES	NEUTRAL ROOTS AND BARKS	BITTER ROOTS AND BARKS	LONG ROOTS	PROCESSED ROOTS
hawthorn	camomile	comfrey	echinacea	rhubarb	dandelion	rehmannia
juniper	honeysuckle	alfalfa	eleuthero	gentian	burdock	red ginseng
lycii	elder	skullcap	slippery elm	cascara	ginseng	aconite (Ch)

· 7 ·

A BALANCED DIET

A good and proper diet in disease is worth a hundred
medicines and no amount of medication can do good
to a patient who does not observe a strict regimen of
diet.

—CHARAKA SAMHITA (ca. 300 A.D.)

Diet is the essential key to all successful healing. Without a proper
balanced diet, the effectiveness of herbal treatment is very limited.
With the appropriate eliminative or balanced diet, herbal treatment will
prove itself to be effective where no medicine will work and will often
be faster than the quick but temporary relief offered by Western drugs.

The nutritional philosophy I have found to be the best and easiest
centers around the use of whole grains, properly cooked foods and
small amounts of fresh vegetables and fruits when they are in season.
This basic dietary approach is the foundation of traditional ethnic diets
of people around the world and is summarized by the principles of Yin/
Yang described in the previous chapter.

To construct a simple balanced diet, the intake of foods can be divided into three categories:

PRIMARY FOODS: Whole grains—20%–30% of the diet
Protein, including animal protein, tofu, tempeh,
and beans—20%–30% of the diet (Beans are
also high in carbohydrates and should be
consumed in smaller portions; vegetable sources
of protein, such as tofu and tempeh, are not as

high in carbohydrates but need to be consumed in larger volume to equal a corresponding amount of animal protein.)

SECONDARY FOODS: Fresh seasonal vegetables (mostly lightly cooked)—30%–40%

TERTIARY FOODS: Dairy, eggs, and fruits—5%–10% of the diet; fats and oils, including olive, sesame oils, and ghee—2%

PRIMARY FOODS

The primary foods consist of whole grains, neither grains that are refined or milled nor flour products. This is important because whole grains are rich in dietary fiber, which slows their absorption and prevents the overstimulation of the pancreas. In this way, there is a timed release of energy over a longer period of time and less tendency to store the carbohydrates of whole grains as fat.

If one's digestion is weak, which occurs because of overconsumption of refined carbohydrates or a weakening of digestive metabolism either constitutionally or from age, it may be necessary to consume milled or partially milled grains. It is common for contemporary Asian people to emphasize the use of white rice, for instance, over whole brown rice, despite the fact that Japanese folk healing advocates the use of brown rice, azuki beans, and miso for practically all diseases. This is more appropriate with animal protein when it is consumed to supplement the nutrition of the refined grains.

For Western people, where excess is a more common characteristic, white rice and indeed all refined grains and flour products (even when made with whole-grain flour) is a stagnant and deadening energy that can cause abnormal weight gain. Some Chinese practitioners even say that it is preferable to eat white rice so long as one has first-class animal protein with it. This may be true for those with weaker digestion, but digestion, being a capacity like any other muscle or body faculty, becomes weaker if it is not appropriately and regularly challenged. In the final analysis, one should always eat according to what one can digest and assimilate. Foods that are either too easy or too hard to digest can cause physical weakness.

If one is trying to lose or gain control of body weight, one should cut out or significantly limit all refined grains and foods made from milled flour. This being said, however, it is the combination of yeast with flour, as in bread or other baked goods, or fat with flour products, as in chips or pie crusts, that is the most problematical. The occasional use of low-fat, unleavened, freshly milled whole-grain flour products, as in many traditional cultures, offers an easier-to-follow alternative to a health diet.

In traditional societies, such as those in China, India, Japan, and Central America, whole grains and beans constitute a therapeutic diet as a primary treatment for disease or as the ideal diet to accompany the use of herbal therapy. The traditional Japanese diet for the folk treatment of most disease is a diet of miso and brown rice. In China, congee or rice porridge is taken alone or cooked with herbs as a regular morning breakfast and for convalescence. Congee is usually made with white rice to facilitate digestion; 1 part by volume of white rice is slowly cooked with 10 parts water over a course of 6–8 hours. Sometimes vegetables, small amounts of beans, other grains, meat, and medicinal herbs are also added. Congee, also called jook in Cantonese, is a traditional Chinese breakfast because it is easily digested. In India, a similar dish called kicharee (see page 55) consisting of a stew of rice and mung beans with ghee and certain spices is recommended to accompany healing of all diseases.

Considering the endurance of the empirical experience of these ancient societies regarding the value of grains, it is arrogantly premature to rush to contrary conclusions based on relatively recent hypotheses. If indeed whole grains are the "staff of life" as the Good Book maintains, then regularly refining—meaning to remove some vital nutrients from one's predominant food without replacing it from other sources—ultimately leads to deficiencies.

These primary foods are an essential part of a healing treatment. When American doctors and scientists went to the jungles of Mexico to study the herbal medicines used by the highly reputed curanderos (healers), they verified that many diseases they had considered difficult or impossible to cure were being successfully treated. Upon applying the same treatments here, they were unable to achieve good results and eventually abandoned the treatments. However, when one doctor returned to watch more carefully and determine the basis of the curanderos' effectiveness, he discovered that the patients, without any prompting on the part of the healer, would go on a restricted diet, eating cornmeal and beans. In fact, the young Indian children were fed only corn, whole grains and beans up to the age of eight years to prevent spoiling their tastes and so that in the event of sickness it would be easy for them to go on this restricted diet. This, he reasoned, was certainly the factor that was missed when the herbal medicines were tried elsewhere.

SECONDARY FOODS

The secondary foods are fresh, local, seasonal vegetables, which provide important vitamin and mineral nutrients. These foods, however, are somewhat Yin (those eaten raw or cold being more Yin, and those cooked being more balanced) and stimulate the process of elimination. Elimination is an important process, since the proper removal of waste and toxins, either ingested or produced through normal metabolism, is essential for health. Excessive use of these foods will lead to overelimination, leaving the body weak and cold, often with excess water. Therefore these foods should make up only 30–40% of the diet. In therapy, where elimination of toxins is called for and where the individual has been eating too much meat and processed foods, vegetables such as fresh salads are useful in the detoxification needed to begin healing. The most valuable vegetables are the seaweeds, such as hiziki, dulse, kelp, wakame, arame and Irish moss. These are very high in essential minerals and vitamins.

TERTIARY FOODS

The third level of foods are those we may eliminate entirely or should consume in smaller portions. These include the extremes of Yin foods (fruits) and Yang foods (red meat) or such congesting foods as milk.

Fruits are the most seasonal of foods. They represent the end cycle of a plant before a seed is formed. As such, from a macrobiotic holistic point of view, they are best consumed according to their natural cycle in each season. Of all foods, fruits are most capable of altering the chemistry of our blood to help us better adjust to the seasons and climates where we live. In this, they are particularly appealing in the warmer climates where they tend to ripen because they provide a more cooling, alkaline-forming energy to counteract hotter climates.

Most fruits have the advantage of being light and easy to digest, which makes them appealing in hot weather when our appetite is naturally lower. However, even in tropical countries where there is an abundance of fruit, such as in southern India or on tropical islands, the people know to avoid the temptation of overeating fruit. Its high sugar content tends to overstimulate the pancreas to secrete insulin, which actually causes lethargy from low blood sugar.

Fruits imported from warmer climates and overconsumed by people living in colder northern areas cause imbalance. It is important to appreciate the fact that fruits in general are Yin and therefore cooling and eliminative in nature. We should become more sensitive to recognize when a Yin cooling energy is not appropriate.

Fruit juice is a refined food that has a strong eliminative and weakening energy. It can be useful for special short-term therapeutic diets or fasts, but long-term overconsumption of fruit juice overloads the system with sugar, causing metabolic imbalance that further contributes to abnormal cravings that can lead to disease. It is a mistake for parents to substitute fruit juice for sugar sodas for very young children, believing that it may be healthy. When our children are at preschool age, we have the unique opportunity and responsibility to condition their appetite so that they ideally prefer simple foods. In most cases, this is what small children naturally prefer. However, the tendency is for parents to pass down their own dietary imbalances by introducing strong foods sweetened with sugar or to give flavored drinks other than water when children are thirsty. When hungry, small children are inclined to appreciate such simple foods as rice porridge, certain vegetables, warm dairy products (such as warm goat's milk), a little fish or poultry, and seasonal fruits. As parents, we should avoid the tendency to want to gain children's favor by introducing them to highly sweetened desserts and foods, ultimately spoiling their taste for life.

Protein and High-Protein Diets

Meat, eggs, and dairy are considered first-class, high-protein foods. Protein has two important functions: (1) to repair damage to tissues and cells as they normally break down, and (2) to stimulate and maintain bodily metabolism. Often, I have found that if vegetarians are not careful enough with maintaining their protein balance, they experience greater difficulty in healing injuries and broken bones. A higher metabolism means a more Yang quality and therefore stimulation to the various organ systems.

For some, especially those who have problems with nondiabetic hyperinsulinism caused by over consumption of carbohydrates, there may be problems associated with abnormal weight gain. The stimulation of insulin causes the burning of blood sugars, which if not fully consumed will be stored in the body as fat. For these people, higher protein consumption stimulates the release of glucagon from the liver, which commands the body to burn its stored fat deposits.

From this, we see that prolonged excessive consumption of carbohydrates and highly saturated fats along with insufficient protein consumption compromises key hormonal and metabolic processes that leads to, among other things, an imbalance of cholesterol and fat. This is directly related to cardiovascular disease, blood sugar imbalances, and either abnormal weight gain or weight loss, depending on one's innate constitutional predisposition. Many suffer from this because of the excessive consumption of overly refined carbohydrates, such as white sugar and refined-flour products. Among vegetarians, especially in the West, the tendency to consume insufficient protein in combination with the resultant overconsumption of carbohydrates over a prolonged number of months and years is an insidious health problem. Because of this, I have modified the ratio of protein to carbohydrate in the present edition of this book.

Fats and Oils

A certain amount of quality unsaturated fats and oils is important to one's health, not to mention that they add to the delectability of foods. It is the combination of a high-carbohydrate diet with fats and oils that causes overweight conditions and arteriosclerosis. In fact, when one lowers carbohydrate consumption and increases protein consumption, foods not only taste better, but appetite is satiated, carbohydrate cravings are lessened, and protein production is supported; the use of unsaturated fats and oils, such as olive oil, sesame oil, and clarified butter (ghee), in moderation actually assists in the burning of stored fat. It has been found that a certain amount of fat is essential for the absorption of vitamins A, D, E and K. Even The American Heart Association recommends getting between 15 to 30 percent of our calories from that wonderful substance that makes food so delicious.

One oft-quoted study conducted at the University of London involved putting patients on a low-calorie (1,000 calories) but high-fat (90% of their total calories) diet. Patients on this high-fat diet lost significant weight in a relatively short period of time. When the same patients were put on a high-carbohydrate, low-fat diet, there was virtually no weight loss.

Other Factors in a Healthy Diet

A balanced diet will also be a low-cost diet. Grains, beans and local vegetables in season are the cheapest food items. Exotic fruits and vegetables imported from distant climates will throw us off balance at a high price. There are also specific items to avoid: white sugar, denatured flour and artificial stimulants. These drain the energy of the body and make the assimilation of nutrients from whole foods more difficult. Thus the best diet is one that bypasses the recent technological changes in food supply and relies on nature for its health-giving qualities.

A healthful diet is not determined solely by the foods eaten. While many people claim to have a "good diet" simply because they eat natural foods, nonetheless, they may suffer a number of ailments resulting from poor food combinations, inadequate protein levels, and erratic eating habits. Such habits destabilize blood sugar levels and natural body rhythms whose regularity are essential to optimum health.

The following dietary schedule has proven very beneficial as an adjunct to herbal therapies and as a goal for daily health maintenance. In the morning, when the body and air temperatures are low (a Yin condition), eat a warming, cooked meal (Yang). Because this meal must fuel your body for its most active time, it should contain *substantial* amounts of proteins, carbohydrates, and other essential nutritional components. At lunch time, when the body and air temperatures are highest (Yang condition), eat a cooling meal with raw foods (Yin), such as salads. But, be sure to also include an adequate amount of protein to regulate blood sugar and provide metabolic components for the afternoon. At supper time, when the body and air temperatures are cooling (Yin), again eat a cooked meal (Yang). This meal should be relatively light, since the night is a time of less vigorous activity and because the organs of digestion should be allowed to rest during sleep. Yet, the meal should not be so light that you have a desire for a "midnight snack." Preferably, all eating should be completed at least three hours before bedtime.

For any dietary program to be successful in maintaining health, an adequate level of exercise is essential. Periods of vigorous exercise as well as moderate exercise will ensure natural hunger at mealtimes. A strong appetite for nutritious and balanced meals is a sign of good metabolism. The meals you take must be large enough to prevent any need for between-meal snacks. Cravings for snacks, especially carbohydrates, indicate poor control of blood sugar possibly due to inadequate protein levels in the meals or the use of caffeinated beverages.

A vegetarian diet can be very healthful, but it is difficult to get enough protein for optimum health unless attention is given to carefully combining sources of essential amino acids. A consistently low-protein diet will eventually lead to a number of deficiency conditions such as: emotional instability, low body weight, thinning hair, allergic sensitivity, bronchial and nasal congestion (production of copious amounts of clear mucus), hemorrhoids, tiredness, and cold extremities. Obesity can still be a problem even with a low protein diet if carbohydrates and fats take the place of protein in satisfying hunger. It is common for a person switching from a standard American diet to a vegetarian diet to feel much better for several months. However, if protein levels are inadequate, the conditions described above will begin to appear after one to two years.

Your body will signal direct warnings of poor eating habits primarily through indigestion and flatulence. Check for potential problems such as:

1. eating too fast and not chewing adequately
2. poor food combining
3. excess water taken with meals
4. excessive use of raw foods
5. overeating

If these activities persist over a long time, all the organs of digestion—stomach, intestines, liver, kidneys, pancreas—will be weakened and this will cause imbalances throughout the body.

Concentrated foods such as wheat grass, bee pollen, spirulina, and yeast can be very helpful as nutritional supplements, but should not be regarded as primary foods making up your dietary needs. These foods spare you the efforts to plan and prepare wholesome meals, but they do not provide the full range of food components essential to a good diet. Time spent in properly preparing and calmly eating balanced meals is your surest investment in health.

THERAPEUTIC DIET

At the first sign of acute disease one should abstain from all solid foods. In general, the diet should be wholesome, light, warm, easily digested and mostly liquid during the acute crisis. One should avoid heavy, hard-to-digest foods such as meat, cheese and bread. It is also important to avoid excess use of fruits and raw vegetables. Light soups and the appropriate herb teas should be taken. For those who need to eliminate toxins from a meat diet, some warm fruit juice can be taken.

Kicharee

As one's condition improves, more solid foods can be added to the diet in the form of steamed vegetables and soupy grains. Miso soup and kicharee are also helpful foods. Kicharee is made by mixing one-half cup cooked mung beans or lentils with one-half cup steamed brown rice and sautéing in sesame oil or clarified butter (ghee) for five minutes with a pinch of cumin seed, one-third teaspoon turmeric and one teaspoon ground coriander. Then add four cups of water and simmer for twenty to twenty-five minutes. If desired this can be topped with a small amount of yogurt. Kicharee is well balanced and high in easily assimilated protein. It also has blood purifying properties.

Ghee

Ghee is clarified butter, a delicious and fragrant oil that is semi-liquid at room temperature. It is very useful in cooking and makes an excellent base for herbal salves and oils. To make ghee, melt two pounds of unsalted butter in a saucepan until it reaches a slow, rolling boil. Remove from the heat and carefully skim off the foam with a spoon. Return the pot to the heat and repeat this procedure twice more, removing as much of the foam as possible and discarding it. Allow the pan to cool two minutes and then remove a thin film that forms. Let the butter cool down somewhat, and then, while still liquid, pour through a fine-meshed tea strainer, but stop pouring when the heavier solids at the bottom of the pan move to the strainer. Collect the ghee in a glass bottle, cool completely and cover. The whole process takes about twenty minutes. Two pounds of butter will yield about one pound of ghee. It can be stored without refrigeration for six months.

Four-Day Cleansing Fast

Fasting is done for a number of reasons; among them are:

1. as a way of becoming more sensitive to the body;
2. for a curative effect, especially with chronic ailments;
3. to lose excess weight or excess water;
4. to clean out accumulated wastes;
5. to free the blockages of energy flow in the body;
6. for longevity;
7. as a way of developing calmness, control and will power.

A four day cleansing fast is adequate to satisfy these concerns for most people. The method of fasting will depend on the nature of the usual diet and the constitution of the individual. For persons whose diet is high in meat and for those with a predominantly Yang constitution, the cleansing through "expansion" is most suitable. This relies on stimulating the process of elimination, especially through the bowels. For persons whose diet is predominantly vegetarian and for those with a Yin constitution, the cleansing through "contraction" is used. This method relies primarily on removing water from the system.

Expansion. The first three days of the fast are begun each morning with an herbal enema using a tea of raspberry, comfrey or catnip leaf. Then one or two eight ounce glasses of prune juice can be taken to stimulate elimination and to help draw the toxins down into the bowels. Every two hours throughout the day, drink a glass of fresh apple juice. To stimulate the secretion of bile and elimination of toxins, one should take a tablespoon of olive oil with one-half teaspoon of cayenne (one "00" capsule) two to four times per day. Persons who are overweight but who are not weakened may also use the weight loss formula (see the "Treatments for Specific Ailments" chapter).

On the fourth day, one begins to break the fast, and after the enema and prune juice, a lunch of some lightly cooked (steamed or baked) fruits or vegetables can be taken. Soupy grains may then be added, and a balanced normal diet can be resumed on the fifth day.

Contraction. Begin each day of the fast with an herbal enema using a tea of raspberry, comfrey or catnip leaf. Eat a small bowl of brown rice three times a day with no additional liquids. For a more effective fast, eat only one bowl of rice a day, taking a tablespoon whenever there is strong hunger, chewing it very well. No other foods or drinks are to be taken during the four day fast. However, this method of fasting may cause a mild constipation and if this occurs a small bowl of stewed prunes may be taken once each day.

To break the fast, on the fifth day, take only lightly cooked fruits and vegetables, and soupy grains. Resume a normal balanced diet, high in grains, on the sixth day.

This diet is very good for eliminating excess moisture, reducing coldness of the body and restoring the ability to assimilate nutrients. It will also help remove the sensation of excessive thirst for those who normally experience that condition.

Alternating Expansion and Contraction. Either method of fasting may precipitate a minor healing crisis. If one does not obtain significant changes in condition or experience a healing crisis, it may be useful to use the opposite cleansing method. Sometimes it is necessary to alternate between expansion and contraction to encourage the body to dump its toxic wastes.

Healing Crisis

The healing crisis is recognized in all systems of natural healing. The Chinese refer to this as the "law of cure." It is not uncommon with effective therapy that one seems to get worse before getting better. When the body is engaged in the elimination of toxins accumulated over the years, one may experience aches, pains and symptoms of diseases, from the most recent to those of childhood. This is because the toxins are being liberated from their storage places and are now actively affecting the body with full force. This is the healing crisis.

If you experience discomfort or marked weakness during the four day fast or as a result of taking the herbs and recommended diet, you should strengthen your determination to go through with it. Strength and improved well-being will return when the process of elimination has been sufficiently accomplished. The cleansing fast can be repeated after one month to help complete the process.

THERAPEUTIC FOOD RECIPES

Rice

Rice is the most balanced, perfect food, and in many countries, such as China, India and Japan, the word for rice is synonymous with the word for "food." It is considered to be the specific grain for strengthening the lungs. Brown rice, though somewhat harder to digest, strengthens the body and constitution and is the basic peasant food of people living in rugged mountainous regions and in the traditional Zen temples of Japan. Processed white rice is only a poor substitute for the healing properties of brown rice, although it is lighter and easier to digest.

Generally, white rice is more acceptable if one prepares it with a little meat at the same meal. In India there are many varieties of rice available; one such variety, Basmati, is considered the "epicurean" rice with the most delicious flavor. It is a naturally grown white rice, lighter and easier to digest than brown rice but more suitable for warm rather than cold climates.

During winter, one should select short-grain brown rice because it is more Yang in nature and therefore more warming. During the hot summer months, one can use long-grain brown rice as it is more Yin and cooling. Whenever possible, one should always select foods that are locally grown as organically as possible. This helps adjust the blood to the climate and environment of the area.

By adding more water to rice, it becomes a little more Yin and possibly easier to digest for someone with a weak Yin digestion. By pressure-cooking rice and other foods, one can use less water and the food will have a more Yang nature. Generally for vegetarians, pressure-cooked rice is preferable.

Boiled Rice

Wash the rice. Use 1 cup of rice to 2 or 3 cups of water. Add ¼ teaspoon of salt and cover. When the water starts to boil, lower the flame and simmer for 45 minutes to 1 hour.

Pressure-Cooked Rice

Cook 1 cup of rice with 1¼ to 1½ cups of water. Add ¼ teaspoon of salt. When the pressure regulator begins to indicate proper pressure, lower the flame to a simmering point. Let cook for 45 minutes. If the rice is too wet or uncooked, the flame was too low. If it is too mushy and wet, then possibly too much water was used.

For lighter, easier to digest rice, add 3 cups of water to 1 cup of rice in the pressure cooker, cooking it for 1 hour and then leaving it in the pot for another 2 hours.

Generally I make up a pot of rice to be stored in the refrigerator and heated up as needed for the entire week. Be sure to use only a stainless steel pressure cooker or good quality enamel pot. Aluminum and other kinds of metals can release toxic ions into the food and herbs and thus harm or alter their properties.

Rice can be served in a variety of ways: steamed as is; fried with a little ghee or sesame oil (about 1 teaspoon); with onions, chopped mushrooms, and so forth; combined with 10% aduki beans for a good protein balance; with pureed steamed spinach or other greens that are mixed into the cooked rice to make "green rice"; in soup; with the addition of spices such as thyme, basil, tamari soya sauce, or sesame salt (Gomashio).

For those who are very weak, it might be best to begin by serving rice cream.

Special Rice Cream

Use 1 cup of rice, 10 cups of water, and a pinch of sea salt. Wash the rice, drain and dry roast it in a pan, stirring constantly until it is golden brown. Add water and bring to a boil. Cook for 3–4 hours over low heat. Take a cotton cloth and wrap the rice in it to form a bag. With your fingers, squeeze the rice through this bag. You should be able to press out 3 to 3⅔ cups of rice cream. The remaining bran can be used in bread and muffins. Serve as is or with a bit of sesame salt, ghee or a teaspoon of honey.

Rice cream, along with pureed steamed vegetables and pureed mung beans, can be a basic diet for anyone in a severely weakened condition who finds eating other forms of whole grains, beans and vegetables difficult.

Other Grains

While rice is the most balanced grain in terms of Yin and Yang properties, other grains should also be considered. Certain grains such as millet and buckwheat are more warming and hence suitable for the cold winter season. Millet is particularly beneficial, along with aduki beans and sweet winter squash, for spleen-pancreas malfunction such as hypoglycemia. Buckwheat, which is actually the seed of an herb rather than a grain, is very Yang and stimulating to circulation. It is served as kasha in the winter to help keep the body warm.

Whole wheat berries are among the most nutritious grains in terms of protein content. They are almost too rich and therefore usually served partially sprouted by soaking them for a day or so before cooking.

Bulghur (cracked wheat) is about the fastest whole grain one can prepare since it is already precooked. Wheat is believed to have a particular effect upon the liver, which is why those with a weak liver may have difficulty digesting it and may exhibit allergic reactions. Actually, it is just what they need to heal their liver, but it should be made milder by sprouting before cooking and by eating only small amounts. Wheat served in this way is very calming to the nerves.

Buckwheat Cream

There are two ways to make buckwheat cream: by using buckwheat flour or by using whole buckwheat groats that are then ground in a flour mill. 1) Heat 1 teaspoon of corn oil in a skillet without burning it. Keeping the flame low, add the flour, stirring constantly and rapidly with a wooden spoon so that the flour will not burn. After the flour is brown, allow it to cool. Add 4 cups of water and heat over a high flame, stirring until it reaches the boiling point. Lower the flame and simmer for another 15–20 minutes, stirring and checking it occasionally. Keep it covered while cooking. Add salt to taste during the last 5 minutes of cooking. 2) Soft Kasha is made by toasting the whole buckwheat groats, then adding 1 cup to 5 cups of water and simmering, covered, for 25–30 minutes. This is a powerful food for stimulating Yang energy and bodily warmth.

Corn is the native grain of North and South America and is quite cooling and Yin in its properties. It is very beneficial to use during the summer months. A simple and favorite way to prepare it is to take the entire ear of corn and roast it in the oven, leaving the outer husk on until it is eaten.

Oats and barley are more Yin grains, having a greater moisture content and a softer texture. They are each used as oatmeal cereal for breakfast or in barley soup.

One of the most important things to remember about eating whole grains is the almost lost art of chewing. The fast pace of modern life, along with its stress, has caused us to forget to chew our food properly. One-quarter of digestion occurs in the mouth, where acid foods are neutralized by the alkaline secretion of saliva. One should develop the habit of chewing each mouthful at least fifteen to thirty times or more. The other three-quarters of digestion occurs in the stomach and small intestines.

Vitamins, Proteins, and Other Nutrients

The notion that deficiencies of a certain vitamin or nutrient should be remedied by concentrated doses or supplements is both false and possibly very dangerous. If our diet is properly balanced, we have no need for supplements. We forget that most deficiencies are caused by a breakdown of physical metabolism rather than a particular nutrient missing from the food we eat. If our diet is in balance, our body has the capacity to produce enough of the necessary vitamins needed to maintain health. Steaming or cooking food may destroy a small amount of the vitamins, but the process of cooking enhances our bodies' ability to assimilate what is there. Thus, Oriental nutrition teaches that for weak bodies, longer cooking is necessary, while for strong bodies shorter cooking is needed.

More important than vitamins in our diet are assimilable minerals. Minerals are the more Yang nutritional components whereas vitamins are the lighter, more Yin components. Mineral deficiencies are most severe in people who have eaten a primarily imbalanced "vegetarian" diet high in fruits, juices, liquids and raw salads. To supplement possible trace mineral deficiencies, one need only add a small amount of a sea vegetable such as kelp, dulse, nori, kombu, wakame, arame or hiziki to the daily diet.

There are many ways to do this, from taking six kelp or dulse tablets daily, to learning how to cook the other sea vegetables in soups and other food combinations.

Sea Vegetables

Kombu Soup Stock

Break a sheet of prewashed kombu seaweed into 4 or 5 pieces and soak in water for 10 minutes until tender. Cut into 1-inch squares. Boil the water in which the kombu has been soaked. Add kombu and another 6 cups of water and simmer for 15 to 20 minutes. Serve as is or store in a jar to use as soup stock. It will keep refrigerated for weeks. Kombu seaweed is very good for mild elimination of toxins, and it is often cooked with aduki beans as a particularly good combination. The moist slippery nature of kombu counterbalances the dry nature of aduki beans and therefore makes them even more digestible.

Wakame is very high in calcium and is used in miso soup, which will be discussed later. Nori seaweed is very high in protein and is sold in thin, dried sheets. It is frequently used as the outer wrapping of sushi. Stuffed with brown rice, beans, carrots, onions and toasted sesame seeds, this sandwich-roll is very useful to take for lunches.

Agar-agar seaweed is tasteless and can be used as a gel to create an interestingly textured food called vegetable aspic with water and vegetables, or a kind of "jello" when added to fruit juices. The high mineral combination of agar will counterbalance the Yin-eliminating aspects of the fruit juice, making it a pleasant, cooling dessert. Heat 1 quart of juice and dissolve 1 tablespoon of agar flakes. Chill to form a gelatin consistency. This method is also useful for thickening fruit preserves and jellies.

Protein, Beans and Meat

Protein toxemia is probably one of the major causes of cancer and other degenerative diseases in America and is largely due to eating excess animal protein combined with environmental and food toxins. Fortunately, economics is helping to limit this problem for the majority of people. However, vegetable sources of protein are, as in the case of the soya bean, even more abundant than meat and more efficiently metabolized with little or no harmful toxic by-products.

Chinese and Ayurvedic nutritions consider meat to be the most powerfully nutritious food. Because animal cell structure is closest to our own, meat transmutes itself very efficiently in our own body cells. This is both a virtue and a possible danger. The amount of meat we eat should be very small as there is an eminent danger of excess. Eating an excess of vegetable proteins like grains and beans is not nearly as important. The toxins of meat are particularly harmful to our bodies' immune systems; furthermore, the drugs and hormones given to animals tend to be stored in our own bodies in much the same way they were stored in the body of the animal.

Traditional standards of Chinese nutrition allow for not more than two to four ounces of meat to be ingested on a daily basis. Usually it is cooked in a soup broth along with herbs such as ginger or garlic to offset its possible toxic reaction. Organic meat is the best to use.

Beans are the best protein supplement when combined with whole grains. Beans are basically Yin because they are high in oil and fat and have an expanding energy, producing gas when eaten in excess. Certain beans are considered to be more therapeutically valuable for certain conditions than others.

Ideally, all beans should be soaked up to twenty-four hours before cooking. This step, along with throwing out the soak water, adding a piece of kombu seaweed, a pinch of salt, and later some suitable herbal condiments such as cumin seed or asafoetida will help to make most beans more digestible.

The Aduki (or Azuki) bean is a small red bean which has the least Yin qualities and is considered to be most like a grain. It is the preferred bean for healing and therapy, especially for kidney-adrenal malfunction. Cooked as a soup with a freshwater fish, such as trout, the broth is taken to eliminate excess fluid from the body.

The green mung bean is the easiest to digest and can be used to lower high blood pressure, demonstrating its cooling nature. For high blood pressure, a simple home remedy is to put two or three tablespoons of mung beans in a cup of boiling water in the morning. Allow it to stand until cool enough to drink, leaving the mung beans at the bottom of the cup. Repeat afternoon and evening by adding boiling water to the remaining mung beans. In the evening, drink the broth and eat the beans.

The black bean is very sweet and nourishes the Yin. It is often included in desserts and confections in the East. It is very good for the reproductive organs, increasing sensitivity in women. A folk remedy is to dry roast pre-cooked black beans and black sesame seeds. These should be done separately since the black bean will take longer. Using equal parts, grind the two into a flour. Take one teaspoon in warm water three times a day before meals.

The soya bean is highest in protein content having a 34.3% protein in contrast to beef which has only 20.0% protein. However, the soya bean is very hard to digest and needs not only twenty-four hours to soak but several hours in cooking to soften them and make them digest-ible. For this reason, they are seldom eaten by themselves, but are sub-jected to a number of ways of fermentation and processing to utilize their protein efficiently.

Miso

Fermented soya exists in the form of miso paste. This is sold in natu-ral food stores and is used as a delicious stock for soups that are tradi-tionally served with a few sprigs of freshly chopped scallions before a Japanese meal. Miso soup can be made as a simple broth, or with barley, wakame or kombu seaweed, carrots, onions, or buckwheat noodles. As a preliminary digestive aid to a main dish or a simple, easily digested meal in itself, miso is high in lactic acid and helps prevent poisoning of the intestines. It benefits the culture of favorable intestinal bacteria and the resulting production of B vitamins.

Anyone with a frail constitution should have miso soup at least once each day, preferably in the morning. This will neutralize the buildup of dangerous fermented acids in the intestines which gradually poison the cells of the body. A cup of miso soup supplies an abundance of valuable minerals, fat and four grams of protein. The protein content can be increased with the addition of small pieces of chopped tofu (soya bean cheese) cooked in the broth.

Miso contains a number of valuable bacteria such as lactobacilli which aid digestion by helping to break down carbohydrates, protein and the cellulose found in practically all vegetable food, including brown rice, carrots, barley and many others. Without these favorable bacteria, we cannot even digest healthy food properly.

Furthermore, miso soup, as well as whole grains and seaweeds, seems to detoxify radiation poisoning and is a specific for environmen-tal radiation poisoning and exposure to X rays. For these and many other reasons, miso soup is one of the most important therapeutic foods we have and is recommended for anyone who is trying to recover his health.

Miso Soup

2 sliced onions
2 sliced carrots
1/4 small cabbage

1 tablespoon sesame oil

4 cups of water

6 rounded teaspoons of Mugi miso (or other varieties)

*2 scallions, finely chopped to be added fresh just before serving
    (optional)*

Sauté the vegetables in oil, beginning with the onions. Other seasonal vegetables can be substituted as desired. Add boiling water to the pot in which the vegetables have been sautéed. Simmer for about 30 minutes. Dissolve the miso in a cup of hot water and add this mixture 5 minutes before the end of cooking. Try not to boil the miso as this will destroy the favorable bacteria and spoil the taste of the soup. This can be served with barley, buckwheat noodles, wakame or kombu seaweed, and small pieces of chopped tofu.

Another way of utilizing the nutritional power of the soya bean is by adding tamari soya sauce to vegetables and rice. A convenient method used in Chinese villages is to pickle well-cooked soya beans in tamari sauce, adding enough tamari to cover the beans. Three or four tablespoons of these pickled soya beans are added to every bowl of whole grain. In this form the beans can be stored almost indefinitely and will always provide a balanced protein necessary when one eats little or no meat.

Tofu and Tempeh

Tofu and tempeh can be used as meat substitutes and are delicious in whole-grain-bread sandwiches. The basic cooking method is to lightly sprinkle a little tamari sauce on a slice of tofu or tempeh and allow it to marinate for a while before sautéing in a little sesame oil or ghee. One can deck up a delicious vegetarian tofu or tempeh "burger" to rival or surpass those made with fatty meat. Tofu and tempeh also make delicious protein additions to grain and vegetable dishes. Just sauté in sesame oil or ghee.

Vegetables

Vegetables are important as the "balanced" Yin part of a balanced diet. They are more Yin than whole grains and beans but not as extreme as fruits and juices. Because a diet low in meat is basically a Yin diet, it

is necessary to add Yang heat to the vegetables to facilitate their digestion and assimilation. Raw vegetables are necessary if one is eating a lot
of meat because the "Yinness" of the vegetables will help to eliminate
the Yang toxins of the meat. However, too many cold, raw vegetables
and fruits in a diet lacking cooked foods and meat will depress metabolic function, lower resistance and immunity to infections, and cause
a general state of extremely nervous mental energy. Over and over again
I have encountered people whose health has been ruined by following
a dietary program of raw vegetables over a prolonged period, weakening
their circulation and digestive power sometimes to the point of no return.

I must emphasize that the principle of eating only well-cooked foods
for the very sick and weak and lightly steamed or sautéed vegetables for
those who are already healthy is crucial to balanced healing and nutrition. For those who are very debilitated, steamed vegetables are pureed
by either pounding them in a mortar and pestle or running them
through a blender.

Foods and vegetables that are high in potassium are useful for those
who eat a high-sodium diet of red meat and salt, but for those following
a more balanced grain-based diet, these foods should rarely be eaten.
The same is true of tomatoes and eggplants which, along with potatoes,
are part of the nightshade order. Most of these species, except for okra,
should not be eaten in excess. They are very high in potassium and
have a decided cool energy, tending to depress metabolic processes.

Vegetables that take a longer time to mature, such as carrots, kale,
cabbage and winter squash, are more warming and Yang than those
that mature more quickly, such as red radish, spinach, mushrooms and
summer squash (zucchini). Someone eating a Yin, primarily vegetable
diet based on whole grains and beans should emphasize those foods
and methods of preparation which are more Yang, while those who eat
meat in excess and are attempting to withdraw from this dangerous
habit should include more Yin-type raw vegetables for a limited period
of time to eliminate the Yang toxins of meat. (See Chapter 6, "Diagnosis
and Treatment," for methods of "Yinnizing" or "Yangizing" foods and
herbs.)

Pressed Salad

Finely chop lettuce or watercress leaves and wrap in a cotton cloth
to form a bag. Dip this into salted rapidly boiling water for 1 minute.

Drain and set on a plate with a weight on it to press out the remaining water from the greens. Let this stand and cool for some time. Remove the greens and serve with a light sauce made of 2 tablespoons of tamari sauce, 2 tablespoons of tahini (sesame butter) and 2 tablespoons of umeboshi plum juice or lemon juice. This is a most welcome dish that can be served in the heat of summer. It is also a way of making salad more Yang. The basic sauce, which can be blended with a little water to dilute it if desired, makes a healthful and delicious addition to any simple steamed vegetables.

Sesame Salt (Gomashio)

The sesame seed is very high in calcium and oil. Sesame salt is easily and quickly made in your kitchen and is a specific medicine for those who suffer from heat disease.

Use whole unbleached sesame seeds. Wash and rinse the seeds and toast in a cast-iron or stainless-steel pan. Stir constantly with a wooden spoon to prevent scorching. The color will change to a light brown. Remove from the fire and put in a suribachi, which is a ridged mortar and pestle usually available in Japanese grocery or import stores. Then separately roast sea salt. When the salt is sufficiently roasted, you may detect the smell of chlorine gas being released, usually occurring in the first few minutes. Chlorine, a very unstable Yin element, is removed from the sea salt to purify it. Then grind the salt and sesame seeds together in the suribachi, rotating the pestle counterclockwise while holding the suribachi between the legs. Combine in a ratio of 8 parts sesame seed to 1 part salt. The gomashio is finished when most of the seeds are crushed. A goodly amount of this sesame salt can be made and kept in a bowl on the table as a condiment to whole grains and vegetables.

Method for Aiding the Digestion of Fruit

Many people have trouble digesting raw fruit mostly because the fruit is too Yin, which aggravates their constitutional Yin imbalance. The result for many is bloating, hypoglycemic reactions, fatigue, and an aggravation of candidalike symptoms. For some, this can be alleviated by eating a piece of the peel of such fruits as citrus, or a few seeds of an apple or the shelled kernel of such fruits as apricot or peach (in large amounts, a cupful or more, these are actually poisonous). This may be especially important for vegetarians, whose diet tends to be more Yin. The more Yin part of a fruit is the fleshy, juicy part; the drier, more Yang part, which contains important digestive enzymes, is contained in the peel and seed. People who eat more Yang flesh foods are usually better able to tolerate fruit and juices without having to eat some of the peel or seed.

Another example of this is the eating of melons. Melons are watery and can promote mucus; the seeds of the watermelon, however, are actually used as a diuretic to remove excess water. Thus, to eat and chew some of the seeds while eating the fruit will help to antidote the more extreme Yin effects of eating the fruit alone.

Kuzu

Kuzu is starch that has been extracted from the root of the kudzu plant (*Pueraria thunbergiana*). It is cultivated and grows wild in Japan and in the southern states. We have not yet learned to appreciate the powerful healing properties of this plant, and it is considered the botanical scourge of the South, where it grows rapidly and envelops everything in its path.

The starch is used in much the same way as arrowroot, as a thickener in soups, desserts and beverages. Kuzu powder is a concentrated starch, high in minerals and calcium, excellent in teas and soups for colds, flus, and digestive and intestinal disturbances of many kinds. Those who have trouble digesting grains should try tamari-kuzu root sauce on steamed vegetables. This will gradually develop their digestive capacity to normal. It is both delicious and very beneficial to health.

Simply dissolve 1 to 1½ tablespoons of kuzu powder in 2 tablespoons of *cold* water (it will lump otherwise) and add to sautéed vegetables in a pan along with a little tamari soya sauce. This simple sauce—which can be varied by adding grated ginger root, garlic, lemon rind, miso, and honey and vinegar (to make sweet and sour)—forms the basis for the exquisitely delicious sauces enjoyed in both Chinese and Japanese restaurants. Usually those restaurants use arrowroot, which is a poor substitute, but in your own home I recommend seeking out and using kuzu root.

There are many other uses for this wonderful healing substance.

Check the bibliography at the end of this book for other books on ways to use kuzu root as food and medicine.

Umeboshi Plum (Pickled Salt Plum)

This substance is called the "king of alkalinizers." It literally seeks out and eliminates or neutralizes toxic Yin acids in the body, relieving indigestion, fullness and bloat from overeating, headache, hangover, morning sickness, colds, flu, aching pains in the joints and many other symptoms of acidosis.

By taking a basically Yin substance such as a plum and pickling and aging it in salt, thus "Yangizing" it, we are able to attract and neutralize Yin toxins in the body. The umeboshi plum is added to many sauces and substances which might otherwise cause acid Yin fermentation in the body. By adding a small amount of the ume plum, the toxic principle is prevented from occurring.

Rice Balls for Traveling

Take precooked brown rice, either plain or with some aduki beans, and add small slivers of carrots and other vegetables. Roll into a ball with a sliver of umeboshi plum in the center. Wrap with a sheet of nori seaweed. The umeboshi will prevent spoilage for days, making these rice balls particularly useful for traveling or for lunches.

Sample Diet

Following is a possible outline of a basic diet for one day:

BREAKFAST: whole grain cereal, rice cream, buckwheat cream, or miso soup. If desired, the cereal can be sweetened with raisins, chopped apple, dried fruits, walnuts or sautéed nuts; onions and mushrooms can be used with tamari sauce.

LUNCH: Sushi rolls, brown rice balls, or tempeh or tofu burger with pressed salad. If a warm lunch is possible, one can have kicharee soup, with pressed salad in the summer.

DINNER: miso soup, whole grain dish, steamed or sautéed vegetables with tofu slices and kuzu-tamari sauce, baked apple for dessert or agar-apple juice "jello."

HEALTHFUL BEVERAGES: roasted dandelion root tea, camomile tea, chrysanthemum tea, hibiscus tea, Bancha twig tea, mu tea, umeboshio tea, yanoh (a roasted whole grain and bean beverage).

· 8 ·

KITCHEN MEDICINES
HERBS AS SOURCES OF VITAMINS AND MINERALS

Most of us suffer from deficiencies in some vitamins and minerals. These deficiencies are not resolved by taking expensive food supplements, most of which are rapidly eliminated through the urine and wasted. This is because the deficiency is due to imbalance and poor assimilation or rapid elimination of these important nutrients. (Persons with diets consisting primarily of fruits and vegetables will excessively eliminate minerals and vitamins from the system, despite the high intake accompanying these foods. Persons with a diet rich in meats will fail to absorb the necessary nutrients from the food because the digestive and absorptive functions become separated with this kind of diet.) Adding large doses of purified vitamins and minerals will generally fail to overcome these problems.

The key to total nutrition is a balanced diet. Herbs are useful as a part of the balanced diet and also as an aid in remedying a long-term nutritional deficiency. This is done in two ways:

1. the tonic herbs improve the assimilation of vital nutrients by the organs (sometimes referred to as a "Yang tonic");
2. the nutritive herbs provide substantial amounts of balanced minerals and vitamins in a form that is easy to assimilate (sometimes referred to as "Yin tonics").

The most important herbs for providing nutrients are the seaweeds (kelp, Irish moss, etc.), the docks (yellow dock) and dandelion. The most important herbs for providing vitamins are parsley leaves, dandelion leaves and alfalfa.

Herbal Seasoning for Vitamins and Minerals

Combine one part each of the culinary herbs (garlic, parsley, watercress, sweet basil, oregano, marjoram and thyme), using whatever is readily available. Add one part each of kelp powder, dulse powder, nettles, comfrey, rose hips and capsicum. Then add one-quarter part each dandelion root powder and burdock root powder. Make a small amount of the blend and then adjust to taste.

Mineral Formula

A formula to supply easily assimilated minerals such as iron, calcium, silicon, magnesium, potassium, sulfur, iodine, zinc, magnesium and trace minerals. Good for all deficient and anemic conditions. Take:

Parsley root and leaf	Horsetail
Yellow dock	Comfrey root
Nettles	Watercress
Irish moss	Kelp

Simmer slowly *equal* parts of these herbs, four ounces to a quart of water. Continue to simmer until volume of liquid is reduced by half. Strain, keep the liquid and cover the herbs with water once more; simmer again for ten minutes. Strain again and combine the two liquids. Cook this down until the volume is reduced by half. Add an equal amount of blackstrap molasses. Dosage: take one tablespoon, three to four times daily.

MEDICINES IN THE SPICE RACK

A convenient place to discover the medicinal value of herbs is the kitchen spice shelf. The common culinary herbs and spices so often added to foods for flavor also have considerable medicinal use and it is likely that they were originally added to foods for these reasons as well.

Most herbal spices are carminatives (preventing and relieving gas), stimulants and aids to digestion. Many of them are also used to relieve nervousness, spasms and coldness. They are often regarded as "crisis medicine," being useful for the first acute stages of disease. Thus the kitchen spice shelf can be thought of as a safe and natural alternative to the synthetic drugs found in the medicine cabinet. Spices can be used to treat problems ranging from bleeding, diarrhea and headache to heart attacks and acute infections.

ANISE (PIMPINELLA ANISUM)

Anise is very useful for breaking up mucus and is thus used for hard dry coughs where expectoration is difficult. A tea is made by adding a cup of boiled water to three teaspoonsful of crushed seeds, steeping for twenty minutes, and sweetening with a little honey. The tea may be used to stimulate the production of mother's milk. The seeds may also be smoked or added to a cough syrup formula (see the "Methods of Application" chapter).

It is also used as a stimulant and carminative to treat flatulence and colic, taken as a tea. Added to laxative formulas, it will reduce griping (cramping of the bowels).

BASIL (OCIMUM BASILICUM)

Sweet basil is good to use as a tea for indigestion, fevers, colds, flu, kidney and bladder troubles, headaches, cramps, nausea, vomiting, constipation and nervous conditions. Its medicinal properties include carminative, antipyretic, stimulant, alterative, diuretic and nervine. A tea made of one ounce basil leaves to a pint of water simmered for twenty minutes with three powdered black peppercorns per cup will be effective for most fevers.

BAY (LAURUS NOBILIS)

The bay tree was dedicated by the ancient Greeks to Apollo and Aesculapius, the god of medicine. Bay was considered capable of increasing and maintaining health and happiness. One or two bay leaves added to soup and beans improves the flavor and also helps prevent gas and indigestion. They are too strong to be used in large amounts internally, but externally the leaves can be applied as a poultice on the chest with a cloth covering to relieve bronchitis and coughs. Oil of bay, which is made by heating the leaves in a little olive oil, can be applied with great benefit to rheumatic and arthritic aches and pains as well as to swellings and sprains.

BLACK PEPPER (PIPER NIGRUM)

Black pepper is an excellent remedy one can take at the first sign of most diseases. Yogis consider black pepper to be one of nature's most perfect foods and useful not only to cure disease but also as a preventive, taking a dose of seven peppercorns ground (one-eighth teaspoon powder) and mixed with honey each morning. The mixture of pepper and honey is useful to overcome cold mucous diseases and sore throats. When treating acute diseases it may be used three to four times a day.

CARAWAY (CARUM CARVI)

Caraway is an excellent aid to digestion. It is taken for indigestion, gas, colic and nervous conditions. An ounce of the crushed seeds is used in making a pint of the infusion, using boiled water and steeping twenty minutes, or letting the seeds stand in cold water overnight. The tea is then taken in frequent doses of two tablespoons until relief is obtained. Caraway is a mild stimulant and may be added to herb formulas for digestion and laxative formulas to prevent griping.

CARDAMOM (ELETTARIA CARDAMOMUM)

Cardamom is a carminative and stimulant commonly mixed with other spices to treat indigestion and gas. It warms the body and is good for diarrhea, colic and headaches. It is an important ingredient in Chai tea, an Indian spice tea valued for its warm, stimulating effects. To make this tea, grate one ounce of fresh ginger, add seven peppercorns, a cinnamon stick, five cloves and fifteen cardamom seeds and heat in one pint of water, simmering for ten minutes. Then add one-half cup of milk and simmer for another ten minutes. Add a sprinkle of nutmeg and a few drops of vanilla extract. Drink one cup of the tea, sweetened with honey, twice per day or as needed for warmth.

CAYENNE (CAPSICUM ANUUM)

The genus Capsicum includes red and green chilies, cayenne, paprika and bell peppers. Cayenne originated in Central and South America where it was extensively used by the natives for many diseases, including diarrhea and cramps.

Cayenne is a stimulant, astringent, carminative and antispasmodic, and is considered a superior crisis herb, useful as a first aid remedy for most conditions. Taken as a daily tonic, one-quarter teaspoon three times daily, it is of benefit for the heart and circulation, preventing heart attack, strokes, colds, flu, diminished vitality, headaches, indigestion, depression and arthritis.

Since cayenne is so hot, the idea that it will not be harmful is sometimes difficult for a beginning user to believe. However, I have used it hundreds of times as often as one teaspoon every fifteen minutes during a crisis and there has never been any problem. On the contrary, it helped to effect a speedy recovery from whatever disease was occurring. Cayenne is not irritating when uncooked.

Cayenne powder or tincture can be rubbed on toothaches, swellings and inflammations. A remedy for arthritis is to rub a little cayenne tincture over the inflamed joint and wrap a red flannel around it to remain throughout the night. The pain is usually relieved by morning.

For hemorrhage internally or externally, cayenne can be relied on to stop the bleeding by virtue of the fact that it normalizes the circulation. For the same reason, it is very well suited for those who have either high or low blood pressure.

When a little cayenne is combined with plantain and applied as a poultice, it has remarkable powers to draw out any foreign object embedded in the flesh.

CINNAMON (CINNAMOMUM ZEYLANICUM)

Cinnamon is stimulating, astringent, demulcent and carminative. It warms the system and is useful to add to balance cooling foods such as fruits, milk and desserts. Medicinally it is used to warm the organs to treat chronic diarrhea, cramps, heart and abdominal pains, coughing, wheezing and lower back pain. It is effectively used as a tincture given every fifteen minutes or so to stop bleeding from the uterus. Simmered in milk and taken with a little honey, cinnamon is very effective for indigestion, gas, diarrhea and dysentery.

CLOVES (SYZYGIUM AROMATICUM)

Cloves are stimulating aromatic buds of the clove tree and are effective in warming the body, increasing circulation, improving digestion and treating flatulence, vomiting and nausea. They will also help the action of other medicines. Allspice (*Pimenta officinalis*) has a very similar action and may be substituted. Add cloves or allspice to any herbal formula requiring a stimulant (see the chapter on "Making an Herbal Formula"). Oil of cloves gives quick relief for toothaches, and cloves may simply be chewed for this purpose.

CORIANDER (*CORIANDRUM SATIVUM*)

The coriander seeds are added to hot stimulating foods to impart a balanced coolness. It is diuretic, alterative and carminative. Steeped in tea, it is useful to relieve fevers (a small amount of black pepper may be added to stimulate its action). Use two teaspoons of crushed seeds in a cup of boiled water and steep twenty minutes. Coriander is added to laxative formulas to help prevent griping.

CUMIN (*CUMINUM CYMINUM*)

Cumin is an essential ingredient in making curries. It is one of the best spices to use to prevent and relieve gas (carminative). As such it is particularly useful to cook beans and fried foods with cumin. It is also a stimulant and antispasmodic useful in formulas calling for both qualities (see the chapter on "Making an Herbal Formula"). Cumin is of benefit to the heart and uterus and is given to women after childbirth to increase breast milk (galactogogue). The seeds may be used to make a tea (one teaspoon crushed seeds to a cup of boiled water) but because of the strong flavor, the powdered seeds may be taken in gelatin capsules, two capsules at mealtime in the evening. Externally, cumin can be used in liniments for stimulating circulation and bringing warmth to the area (see the "Methods of Application" chapter).

FENNEL (*FOENICULUM VULGARE*)

Fennel is a very valuable seed spice combining several herbal properties. It is antispasmodic, carminative, diuretic, expectorant and stimulant. A tea is made using one teaspoon of crushed seeds in a cup of boiled water, steeped twenty minutes. This is used to treat colic, cramps and gas and to expel mucus. The cooled tea can also be used externally as an eyewash. Fennel is useful in herb formulas containing strong laxatives to prevent griping. For chronic coughs, fennel may be used in making cough syrups (see the "Methods of Application" chapter).

FENUGREEK (TRIGONELLA FOENUMGRAECUM)

Fenugreek is one of the oldest recorded medicinal plants and one of the most versatile of the seed spices. The seeds are tonic, astringent, demulcent, emollient and expectorant. Fenugreek is useful for all mucous conditions and lung congestion. A decoction is made using one ounce of the crushed seeds with seven crushed black peppercorns in a pint of water to relieve congestion and eliminate excess mucus. The decoction of fenugreek alone is useful for ulcers and inflamed conditions of the stomach and intestines. It is also used in the treatment of both diabetes and gout. Fenugreek is considered to be an aphrodiasiac and rejuvenator. Eventually, it is used to make an emollient poultice applied to boils and carbuncles.

GARLIC (ALLIUM SATIVUM)

Garlic is a world-renowned cure-all highly espoused as a home remedy in practically every culture. It has the properties of being an alterative, stimulant, diaphoretic, expectorant, antispasmodic, antibiotic, nervine, carminative and vulnerary, to mention some of the more outstanding characteristics.

It is used in the treatment of all lung ailments, for high and low blood pressure, against parasites and infections, for headaches and for nervous disorders. Onions have similar characteristics and are often used in combination with garlic.

To preserve the beneficial effects of garlic it should not be boiled. The fresh juice is the most effective preparation. For nervous spasms, cramps and seizures, crush one clove of garlic in a glass of hot milk. For high blood pressure, take one clove of garlic each morning.

Prepare oil of garlic by placing eight ounces of peeled minced garlic in a wide-mouthed jar with enough olive oil to cover. Close tightly and shake a few times each day; allow to stand in a warm place for three days. Press and strain it through an unbleached muslin or cotton cloth and store in a cool place.

For colds, flus, fevers and infectious diseases take one teaspoon of the oil every hour. For earaches, insert a few drops in the ear with a wad of cotton. For aches, sprains and minor skin disorders rub the oil directly on the affected area.

Prepare syrup of garlic by placing one pound of peeled minced garlic in a wide-mouthed two quart jar and almost fill the jar with equal parts of apple cider vinegar and distilled water. Cover and let stand in a warm place for four days, shaking a few times a day. Add one cup of glycerine and let it stand another day. Strain and, with pressure, filter the mixture through a muslin or linen cloth. Add one cup of honey and stir until thoroughly mixed. Store in a cool place.

For coughs, colds, sore throats, bronchial congestion, high or low blood pressure, heart weakness and nervous disorders, take one tablespoon of the syrup three times a day before meals.

GINGER (ZINGIBER OFFICINALE)

Ginger is one of the most versatile herbal stimulants. It is of great benefit to the stomach, intestines and circulation. Ginger may be taken alone or with other herbs to enhance their effectiveness. Ginger tea, made by grating one ounce of fresh ginger and simmering ten minutes in a pint of water, is used for indigestion, cramps and nausea. Taken with honey and lemon it is an excellent treatment for colds and flus and acts as a stimulating diaphoretic. Ginger root should always be added to meat dishes to help the intestines detoxify the meat.

Externally, ginger is applied as a fomentation for the treatment of pain, inflammations and stiff joints. Simmer five ounces of grated ginger root in two quarts of water for ten minutes. Strain and soak a cloth in the water to apply to the affected area. Keep changing the cloth to keep a constant warm temperature on the skin. The skin should become red as the circulation increases.

Squeeze out the juice of fresh grated ginger and combine with equal parts of olive or sesame oil to produce an oil that can be massaged into the skin for relief of muscle pain. The oil can also be applied to the head for dandruff and a few drops on a wad of cotton inserted into the ear is good for treating earaches.

In all formulas calling for ginger, either the fresh or the dried root may be used unless otherwise specified. The amount used, by weight, is the same.

MARJORAM (ORIGANUM MAJORANA)

Marjoram is an antispasmodic, diaphoretic, carminative, tonic, expectorant, stimulant and emmenagogue. The tea, made with one-half ounce marjoram steeped in a pint of boiled water, is used for upset stomach, headache, colic and a variety of nervous complaints. It can be used for cramps and nausea associated with menstruation and for severe cases of abdominal cramps. It is also considered helpful for seasickness. Oil of marjoram can be used externally to relieve aches and pains and can be applied for this purpose to toothaches. It is added to the bath to promote a calming effect and to relieve insomnia. Marjoram is applied as a fomentation to painful swellings and rheumatic joints and in liniments to stimulate the circulation (see the chapter on "Methods of Application").

MUSTARD SEED (BRASSICA NIGRA)

Mustard seed is rubefacient, stimulant, diuretic, alterative and, in large doses, emetic. Internally, a teaspoonful of crushed seeds in warm water acts as a mild laxative and blood purifier, but a tablespoonful acts as a quick emetic.

Externally, the oil is used to stimulate local circulation. A mustard plaster is made by mixing powdered mustard with cold water to make a thick paste. The paste is spread on a cotton cloth. Another thin cloth is placed on the skin and the mustard cloth placed over it. The plaster should remain on until the skin begins to redden and a burning sensation is felt. The plaster is removed and the remaining mustard is washed from the skin. The mustard plaster is used for aches, sprains, spasms and cold areas needing circulation. It should not be used on tender, sensitive areas and if it seems too strong, the mustard powder may be diluted with a little rye flour. After removing the plaster, the skin may be powdered with rice or other flour and the area wrapped with dry cotton.

NUTMEG (MYRISTICA FRAGRANS)

A small amount of nutmeg, about the size of a pea, can be taken once daily over a long period to relieve chronic nervous disorders and heart problems. It may be added to milk and baked fruits and desserts to help digestion and relieve nausea. Large doses can be poisonous and may cause miscarriage.

ROSEMARY (ROSMARINUS OFFICINALIS)

Rosemary is of great benefit in treating headaches and may be used as a substitute for aspirin. It is astringent, diaphoretic and stimulant. It is useful for indigestion, colic, nausea, gas and fevers. It is high in easily assimilable calcium and thus is of benefit to the entire nervous system. A tea is made by adding one-half ounce of rosemary to a pint of boiled water and steeping for ten minutes in a covered vessel. Rosemary is also good for the hair and scalp; use a cooled strong tea as a rinse after shampoo. Rosemary is smoked with coltsfoot leaves to treat asthma and mucous congestion of the lungs and throat.

SAGE (SALVIA OFFICINALIS)

Sage is antispasmodic and astringent and is of particular benefit in slowing the secretions of fluids. Thus it is used for excessive perspiration, night sweats, clear vaginal discharge and to stop the flow of milk. It is also useful for diarrhea, dysentery, the early stages of cold and flu, sinus congestion, bladder infections and inflammatory conditions. A tea is made using one-quarter ounce of the herb in a pint of boiled water, steeping in a closed vessel for ten minutes. It should not be used for more than one week at a time, but during this period the tea may be taken up to three times per day. When combined with rosemary, peppermint and wood betony, it is effective for headaches. A half cup of the infusion, made from equal parts of these herbs (one ounce per pint of water), is taken every two hours until relief is obtained. Sage tea is also used as a gargle for sore throats and ulcerations of the mouth.

THYME (THYMUS VULGARIS)

Thyme is important as a parasiticide for intestinal worms. It is also antispasmodic, carminative, diaphoretic, expectorant and antiseptic. It is frequently used as a tea for bronchial problems such as acute bronchitis, whooping cough and laryngitis. An ounce of the herb is steeped in one pint of boiled water and then strained and sweetened with honey. It is also of benefit for the treatment of diarrhea, chronic gastritis and lack of appetite. It should not be used in large amounts, one ounce being adequate for a daily dose taken as tea. Externally, its antiseptic properties make it a useful mouthwash and cleansing wash for the skin. It will destroy fungal infections such as athlete's foot and skin parasites such as scabies, crabs and lice. For these purposes, a tincture made from four ounces thyme to a pint of alcohol, or the essential oil, is used.

TURMERIC (*CURCUMA LONGA*)

This root imparts its characteristic golden color to curry powder and to most Indian dishes. It is used as a blood purifier, stimulant and vulnerary. It can be applied both internally and externally to heal wounds, relieve pains in the limbs, break up congestion and as a restorative after the loss of blood at the birth of a child. It is of benefit to the circulation and it helps to regulate the menstrual cycle. Turmeric is also used for reducing fevers and for nosebleed. A teaspoon of turmeric powder is added along with a teaspoon of almond oil to a cup of warm milk. One to two cups are taken daily. This is particularly helpful in stretching the ligaments and to cure menstrual cramps.

· 9 ·

WESTERN HERBS

Acorns

Quercus species

PARTS USED: Fruit of the acorn tree

ENERGY AND FLAVORS: Sweet, mildly bland and slightly bitter depending upon how well they have been leached

SYSTEMS AFFECTED: Nutritive systems, lungs

BIOCHEMICAL CONSTITUENTS: Tannins, flavonoids, sugar, starch, albumin and fats

PROPERTIES: Nutritive tonic, demulcent, astringent

DOSE: Freely as desired

USED FOR: Nutrition

NOTES: Acorns are an ideal food for those with wasting, degenerative diseases such as TB and AIDS. One conjures nineteeth-century memories of George Sand serving the consumptive Frederick Chopin his regular daily acorn coffee and various homeopathic remedies. In fact, throughout the nineteenth century when tuberculosis was not an uncommon disease, the highly nutritious acorn porridge was one of the most commonly prescribed foods.

Acorns must be properly leached. First, the acorn is shelled and ground; the meal is then tied in a bag upon which cool water is allowed to wash the excess tannins for several hours. The meal can be dried and pan-toasted for use as a food or beverage. Some of the tannins probably remain, making this a near-perfect food for diarrhea. The acorn was a staple of the California Native Americans and is still eaten as a food by traditional people in many parts of the world.

Agrimony
Agrimonia eupatoria
COMMON NAMES: Sticklewort, Cocklebur
FAMILY: Rosaceae
PARTS USED: Aboveground portion
ENERGY AND FLAVORS: Slightly bitter, astringent, warm
BIOCHEMICAL CONSTITUENTS: Tannins, bitter glycosides, coumarins, flavonoids, nicotinic acid amide, silicic acid, polysaccharides, vitamins B and K, iron and essential oil
DOSE: 6–15 grams taken in a mild decoction or 10–30 drops of the alcoholic extract
USED FOR: Hemorrhage, irritable bladder, kidney pains (agrimony with marshmallow root), pulmonary and bronchial phlegm
NOTES: Agrimony is commonly used as an astringent and hemostatic to inhibit bleeding, restore tone to the stomach and intestines, and counteract flaccidity. It is indicated for any symptoms associated with bleeding, including blood in the urine and in the stools. It has also been shown to have antiviral properties.

A good antihemorrhagic combination is equal parts agrimony, cinnamon bark and yarrow.

To stop bleeding, the Chinese use the ashes of burnt hair or mugwort. The burnt ash of agrimony taken internally, as well as applied externally, is also more effective than using the unburnt herb to inhibit bleeding.

Ointments and boluses are made to shrink bleeding hemorrhoids.

Besides its antihemorrhagic and astringent effects, agrimony is specific for irritable bladder and renal pain caused by kidney and bladder inflammation.

In all cases where there is flaccidity and/or abdominal secretions with inflammation, agrimony can be employed. This may include bronchial or pulmonary cough, leucorrhea, dysmenorrhea, colitis, proctitis, ileocolitis and ulcerative stomatitis. The Eclectics also found it effective for erysipelas. Traditional Chinese Medicine regards it as one of the most important herbs for cancer.

Alfalfa

Medicago sativa

COMMON NAMES: Alfalfa, Lucerne

FAMILY: Leguminosae

PARTS USED: Aboveground portions

ENERGY AND FLAVORS: Sweet, neutral to cool energy

SYSTEMS AFFECTED: Stomach and blood

BIOCHEMICAL CONSTITUENTS: Leaves contain betacarotene, vitamins C, D, E and the coagulating vitamin K; it also contains various mineral salts including calcium, potassium, iron and phosphorus

PROPERTIES: Nutritive tonic, restorative (Yin) tonic, antipyretic, alterative, antianemic, antihemorrhagic, diuretic

DOSE: One cup of the infusion taken three times daily

USED FOR: Wasting, improving digestion and assimilation, weight gain, increase in strength and vitality, cystitis, prostate inflammation, lower-back pains, acidosis and rheumatic aches and pains, lowering fevers, increasing mother's milk, insomnia, to regulate the bowels

NOTES: Alfalfa, in Arabic, means "father." Perhaps this refers to its function as a superlative restorative tonic. It treats all chronic and acute digestive weaknesses, aiding the assimilation of protein, carbohydrates, iron and calcium, as well as various essential trace minerals. Thus alfalfa can be given two or three times daily as a substitute for tea whenever there is a need to increase flesh and generally to build and regenerate normal strength and vitality. In this, its indications are not at all dissimilar to its immune-potentiating Chinese relative *Astragalus membranaceus*. Alfalfa serves as an ideal cooling Yin tonic suitable for various acute and chronic inflammatory symptoms associated with degeneration and aging.

Alfalfa is indicated for chronic and acute cystitis, burning urine, prostatitis, peptic ulcers, as well as various arthritic and rheumatic complaints, including lower backache. It also increases mother's milk. It is slow and deep acting so it should be taken regularly on a daily basis for treating chronic disorders.

Aloe Vera

Aloe vera

COMMON NAME: Aloe vera gel

FAMILY: Aloeaceae

PARTS USED: Mucilaginous gel found inside the leaves and the dried powder of the leaf

ENERGY AND FLAVORS: Cold, bitter

SYSTEMS AFFECTED: Liver, heart, spleen

BIOCHEMICAL CONSTITUENTS: Contains two aloins, polysaccharides including glucomannans, anthraquinones, glycoproteins, sterols, saponins and organic acids

PROPERTIES: The gel is vulnerary, "Yin tonic"; the dried powder is cholagogic, laxative

DOSE: Of the gel and liquid, take two tablespoons three times daily in juice; of the powder, take one-half to one teaspoon

USED FOR: Maintaining beauty, counteracting wrinkles, female hormone regulation

DRIED POWDER USED FOR: Hepatitis, liver problems, constipation

NOTES: Aloe is called "kumari" in Sanskrit, which means "goddess." This refers to its common daily usage by East Indian women to maintain beauty and counteract symptoms of aging. Ayurvedic medicine considers aloe gel to be estrogenic, which accounts for its vitalizing and tonic properties for women.

In the West, aloe vera gel is considered one of the most effective healing agents for the treatment of burns and injuries. A diluted liquid is taken daily for its lightening enzyme-promoting activity.

Again, it figures prominently in gynecology since a teaspoon of aloe alone or in combination with turmeric root taken daily for at least three months regulates liver function and counteracts symptoms of premenstrual syndrome.

The dried powder of aloe is considered one of the best herbal laxatives and benefits the liver.

Amaranth

Amaranthus hybridus, var. *erythrostachys*

COMMON NAMES: Love lies bleeding, Red cockscomb

FAMILY: Amaranthaceae

PARTS USED: Aboveground portion, the seeds are used as food

ENERGY AND FLAVORS: Sweet flavor, neutral to cool energy

SYSTEMS AFFECTED: Digestive system, kidneys, blood

BIOCHEMICAL CONSTITUENTS: None listed

PROPERTIES: Astringent, nutrient, hemostatic, diuretic, alterative

DOSE: 6 to 30 grams or normal decoction

USED FOR: Bleeding, menorrhagia, diarrhea, dysentery, food

NOTES: Amaranth is a mild astringent used in strong decoction for menorrhagia and diarrhea (thus its common folk name "love lies bleeding"). It is also taken internally for ulcerated throat, stomach and intestines, as well as for symptoms of diarrhea and dysentery. The decoction is also used as a douche for leucorrhea.

My main use for this common wayside weed is as an acid-neutralizing green vegetable. Since a diet high in grains, beans, meat and dairy products naturally tends to be more acidic, most green vegetables, being alkalinizing, such as amaranth greens, should regularly be included in the diet to help neutralize the acidity of these foods. Thus, the fresh leaves of amaranth, commonly known as pigweed in Western countries because it is fed to pigs, is sold in most Asian marketplaces as a common vegetable. It has a flavor not unlike that of spinach, and it is similarly high in minerals such as iron, as well as being a rich source of vitamins A and C. Thus by adding such greens to our diet, based on traditional acidic grains, beans and proteinaceous foods, we experience easy digestibility and lightness.

The seeds of a Central American species, once used as a staple food by the Aztecs, have now been introduced into the health food industry.

Angelica

Angelica archangelica

FAMILY: Umbelliferae

PARTS USED: Primarily the root

ENERGY AND FLAVORS: Spicy, bitter, warm

SYSTEMS AFFECTED: Lungs, stomach, intestines, blood

BIOCHEMICAL CONSTITUENTS: Volatile oil, miscellaneous sugars, acids, flavonoids and sterols

PROPERTIES: Carminative, stimulant, emmenagogue, diaphoretic, expectorant

DOSE: 3 to 9 grams or normal tea infusion; of the tincture, use 10 to 30 drops three times daily

USED FOR: Coldness, rheumatic complaints, digestive weakness and gas, menstrual irregularities, alcohol addiction, coughs and colds

NOTES: Angelica is specific for lack of appetite, flatulence, dyspepsia, and weak digestion. It is also used as an expectorant in colds, coughs, and all upper-respiratory complaints. Because of its warming and stimulating properties, it is a warming circulatory stimulant, effective for all rheumatic complaints, including gout. Angelica root has definite emmenagogic properties and can be used to relieve cramps, delayed or stopped menstruation, and menopausal problems. The context for its use for the above are hypotonic conditions associated with coldness. Angelica's emmenagogic properties also mean that angelica should generally be avoided during pregnancy, especially during the first term. Angelica should also be avoided by diabetics as it has a tendency to increase blood sugar.

Angelica combines well with other emmenagogic herbs. A good combination for toning and correcting amenorrhea or dysmenorrhea is a combination of two parts angelica and one part each of false unicorn root (chamaelirium), cramp bark, blue cohosh and wild ginger. For arthritic and rheumatic complaints, combine equal parts angelica root, guiacum, prickly ash, cinnamon and licorice. For colds and flus, combine angelica with other diaphoretic herbs such as ephedra, mint or lemon balm, garlic and a half part licorice to smooth out the action.

Aniseed
Pimpinella anisum
COMMON NAME: Anise
FAMILY: Umbelliferae
PARTS USED: Seeds
ENERGY AND FLAVORS: Spicy, warm
SYSTEMS AFFECTED: Stomach, lungs, liver, kidney
BIOCHEMICAL CONSTITUENTS: Volatile oil, coumarins, lipids, fatty acids, sterols, proteins and carbohydrates
PROPERTIES: Stimulant, carminative, antispasmodic, expectorant, emmenagogue, diaphoretic
DOSE: 3 to 9 grams or one teaspoon of the crushed seeds steeped in a cup of boiling water, covered. Take two or three times daily or as needed.
USED FOR: Gas, nausea, abdominal pains, coughs and colds
NOTES: Aniseed is used to warm the abdomen, prevent and expel gas, aid digestion, and relieve belching, nausea and abdominal pains. A good tea for gas, indigestion, bloating and nausea is that made from combining a pinch each of powders of aniseed, ginger, cardamom,

cinnamon and an even smaller pinch of black pepper, and then steeping the combination in boiled hot water or scalded raw milk. A cup can be taken after meals or throughout the winter to promote digestion and counteract coldness. Aniseed is commonly used as a flavoring agent and substituted for licorice.

Arnica

Arnica montana

COMMON NAME: Leopard's bane

FAMILY: Compositae

PARTS USED: Flower heads

ENERGY AND FLAVORS: Poisonous, warm energy

SYSTEMS AFFECTED: Blood, circulation

BIOCHEMICAL CONSTITUENTS: Sesquiterpene lactone helenalin, which accounts for its most active antiinflammatory action

PROPERTIES: Stimulant, analgesic

DOSE: Externally use freely as an oil or liniment

USED FOR: Bruises, painful injuries

NOTES: Arnica is primarily used as an external rubbing oil or alcoholic liniment for injuries and bruises. As such, it is very effective. To make oil of arnica, simply macerate fresh or dried arnica leaves and flowers in warm sesame or olive oil for three days, then squeeze and strain through a cloth. Bottle for external use on aches, strains, bruises or injuries in which the skin has not been broken. Arnica liniment is made in a similar manner except that rubbing alcohol, vodka or gin replaces oil.

Internally, it should only be taken in minute or homeopathic dosage and is best prescribed by an experienced practitioner.

Artichoke

Cynara scolymus

COMMON NAME: Globe Artichoke

FAMILY: Compositae

PARTS USED: The leaf; the fruit is used as food

ENERGY AND FLAVORS: Cool, bitter

SYSTEMS AFFECTED: Liver, heart

BIOCHEMICAL CONSTITUENTS: An acid substance called cinarin, along with inulin, enzymes, tannin, and sugars

PROPERTIES: Hepatic, biliary fluidifying, cholagogic, diuretic, antirheumatic, digestive, anticholesterol, fat reducing. Artichoke originates from the Mediterranean area, where it is found wild on the island of Crete. It has a long traditional usage as a general detoxifier especially for diseases of the liver.

DOSE: One teaspoon of the leaves steeped for 20 minutes in 1 cup of boiling water—1 cup three times daily. It is intensely bitter and may be dried and powdered and put into gelatin capsules.

USED FOR: Liver and gallbladder problems, lower cholesterol, rheumatic conditions, in small doses before meals for digestive weakness, obesity

Asafoetida
Ferula assafoetida

COMMON NAMES: Devil's dung, Gum asafetida

FAMILY: Umbelliferae

PARTS USED: Gum resin

ENERGY AND FLAVORS: Spicy, acrid, hot

SYSTEMS AFFECTED: Liver, stomach and digestion

BIOCHEMICAL CONSTITUENTS: Essential oil, resin, ferulic acid, glue, sec-butylpropenyl disulfide, farnesiferol

PROPERTIES: Digestant, carminative, aromatic, antispasmodic, expectorant

DOSE: 100 milligrams to 1 gram of the powdered gum steeped in boiling water or added to food

USED FOR: Gas, weak digestion, food sensitivities, hysteria and mood swings, *Candida albicans* overgrowth, hypoglycemia, colds and coughs

NOTES: Asafoetida is routinely used as a carminative and substitute for garlic in many Asian countries. In both India and China it is often favored over garlic, which is looked down upon by Brahmin, Taoist and Buddhist priests probably because of the strong odor it leaves on the breath. Asafoetida has a similarly strong odor and flavor but will not remain on the breath. In Western countries, it is an important ingredient in Worcestershire sauce.

Asafetida, having warming antispasmodic properties, is useful for hysterical symptoms, hypoglycemia, *Candida albicans* overgrowth, coldness, coughs and bronchitis. Called "hing" in Sanskrit, it is the primary ingredient in "hinga-shtak," the most famous digestive formula in India. In this form it is taken as a pill or powder, or it is mixed with food to prevent gas, aid digestion and alleviate the mood drop and loss of energy that follow eating certain foods. Thus asafoetida, or hinga-shtak, are effective as carminatives in regulating chi and helping to overcome food allergies.

Asparagus

Asparagus cochinchinensis

COMMON NAME: Sparrowgrass

FAMILY: Liliaceae

PARTS USED: Sprouts and the root

ENERGY AND FLAVORS: Sweet, bitter, cool

SYSTEMS AFFECTED: Lungs and kidneys

BIOCHEMICAL CONSTITUENTS: Steroidal glycosides and bitter glycosides, asparagine, sucrose, starch and mucilage

PROPERTIES: Nutrient tonic, diuretic, laxative, cardiac tonic, mild sedative, demulcent tonic

DOSE: Of the root, take 6 to 15 grams in decoction

ASPARAGUS SHOOTS USED FOR: Bladder infections

ASPARAGUS ROOT USED FOR: Consumption; AIDS, lung and throat dryness; gynecology; female hormones; to foster patience, love and compassion

NOTES: Asparagus shoots are well-known as a delicious springtime food. The root is considered one of the finest "Yin tonics" in Chinese traditional medicine. Among traditional Chinese pharmacists it is a custom to reserve the sweetest and best-quality asparagus root for themselves, family and close friends. This is because it is believed that the root of this herb, taken in small amounts regularly, will increase feelings of compassion and love (probably because of the steroidal glycosides).

In India, "shatavari," as it is called, is similarly used as a hormonal tonic for the female reproductive system. It is prescribed for women to promote fertility, relieve menstrual pains, increase breast milk and generally nourish and strengthen the female reproductive system.

It is also used as a nutritive tonic for the lungs and consumptive diseases. As such, it is excellent for advanced wasting diseases such as TB and AIDS. Similarly, it should be prescribed for dry throat and lungs, blood-tinged sputum.

For "kidney Yin deficiency," severe adrenal deficiency, or what we may otherwise experience as "burnout" or chronic exhaustive syndrome, asparagus root makes an excellent tonic. Some associated symptoms for this not uncommon condition include fatigue, exhaustion and aching lower back, knees and joints. It is also effective for sports burnout, with attendant exhaustion and fatigue.

The root is contraindicated for individuals with edema, obesity and damp conditions, unless combined with spices such as pepper, cinnamon and ginger.

Balm of Gilead

Populus balsamifera, (var. *balsamifera candicans*), *P. tremula,* and other species

COMMON NAMES: Quaking aspen, White poplar
FAMILY: Salicaceae
PARTS USED: Resinous leaf buds, bark
ENERGY AND FLAVORS: Neutral to warm energy, spicy, acrid flavor
SYSTEMS AFFECTED: Lungs
BIOCHEMICAL CONSTITUENTS: Phenolic glycosides, salicin, cineole, acurcumene, resins, phenolic and gallic acids, tannins and other substances
PROPERTIES: Expectorant, stimulant, antipyretic and analgesic
DOSE: In syrup, for coughs and upper respiratory problems, use in tablespoon doses as needed; as a tincture use 4 to 15 drops
BALM OF GILEAD USED FOR: Coughs
QUAKING ASPEN BARK USED FOR: Reducing headaches, relieving pains and lowering fevers
NOTES: This is the herb mentioned throughout the Bible (Genesis 37:25, 43:11; Jeremiah 8:22, 46:11, 51:5; Ezekiel 27:17). *Populus balsamifera* is a large tree (to 100 feet). The buds are commonly used in cough syrups and mixtures as an expectorant. A good combination for a syrup is equal parts balm of gilead buds, elecampane, wild cherry bark and half part licorice mixed with honey. The buds can also be made into a rubbing ointment for muscular aches and pains.

Poplar bark, containing some salicylic acid, is similar to willow bark in the relief of fevers, and various muscular and arthritic aches and pains. It can be combined with willow and rosemary for these purposes.

Baptisia

Baptisia tinctoria
COMMON NAMES: Wild indigo, Indigoweed

FAMILY: Leguminosae

PARTS USED: Root, leaves

ENERGY AND FLAVORS: Bitter, extremely cold, toxic

SYSTEMS AFFECTED: Liver, blood

BIOCHEMICAL CONSTITUENTS: Baptitoxine (baptisine), two glucosides; baptin, a cathartic; a yellowish resin

PROPERTIES: Alterative, antibiotic, antiseptic, emmenagogue, emetic

DOSE: Boil one-half ounce of the dried root in a pint of water for ten minutes. Of this, take only one tablespoon every three or four hours. If there is nausea or sick feeling, diminish the dose accordingly. For children, give half or less according to size and age; of the tincture, take two to five drops.

USED FOR: Putrid infections, blood poisoning, meningitis, swollen glands (scrofula), malignant sores

NOTES: Baptisia is one of the most powerful antiinflammatories with strong antibiotic and probably antiviral properties. It is generally used for the most severe and inflamed discrasias (infections), blood poisoning, putrid ulcerations, severe disintegration of tissues caused by capillary congestion, malignant ulcers, mouth sores, sore nipples, swollen glands, sore throat, diphtheria, scarlatina, erysipelas, tonsillitis, typhoid dysentery, typhoid pneumonia, cerebrospinal meningitis, fetid leucorrhea, and ulceration of the cervix. Foul discharges with a dark, purplish discoloration definitely call for baptisia. It combines well with other antiinflammatory herbs including echinacea and goldenseal. An ointment can be made with equal parts bloodroot and baptisia to be applied several times daily as a treatment for inflamed tumors, cancers, boils and ulcers. Of course, experienced professional advice should first be obtained.

Barberry

Berberis vulgaris

COMMON NAME: Pipperidge bush

FAMILY: Berberidaceae

NOTE: All indications are the same as for OREGON GRAPE ROOT.

Barley

Hordeum vulgare

COMMON NAMES: Pearl barley, Prelate

PARTS USED: Seed (grain)

ENERGY AND FLAVORS: Neutral to cool energy, sweet flavor

SYSTEMS AFFECTED: Spleen-stomach, lungs, colon

BIOCHEMICAL CONSTITUENTS: Proteins, prolamines, albumin, sugars, starch, fats, B vitamins. The germinated seeds contain alkaloids hordenine and gramine

PROPERTIES: Nutrient, diuretic, demulcent

DOSE: Taken freely as food

USED FOR: Colitis, swelling and tumors, jaundice

NOTES: Barley is used as a mucilaginous porridge during convalescence, diarrhea and bowel inflammation (colitis). In Chinese traditional medicine it is used as an antiinflammatory diuretic, for relieving gallbladder problems, reducing swelling and tumors, clearing jaundice. Dry-roasted barley can be ground and drunk as a healthful beverage substitute for coffee. Boiled in water and drunk as a tea, it is used to help clear the skin of pimples and lesions. For eczema and acne, a combination of barley flour and aloe vera gel can be applied as a facial mask before going to bed. It is then washed off in the morning.

Bayberry
Myrica cerifera, M. pensylvanica

COMMON NAMES: Candleberry, Waxberry, Wax myrtle

FAMILY: Myricaceae

PARTS USED: Bark

ENERGY AND FLAVORS: Spicy, astringent, warm

SYSTEMS AFFECTED: Stomach-spleen, lungs, liver

BIOCHEMICAL CONSTITUENTS: Volatile oil, starch, lignin, albumin, gum, tannic and gallic acids, acrid and astringent resins, an acid resembling saponin

PROPERTIES: Stimulant, astringent, expectorant, diaphoretic

DOSE: Of the powdered bark 1–4 grams; of the tincture 10–20 drops

USED FOR: Colds, flus and fevers; astringent for hemorrhoids; dentifrice

NOTES: The most renowned use of bayberry bark is in "Dr. Thompson's Composition Powder." In the past it was commonly used by many doctors upon the first sign of colds, coughs and flus. There are still many favored versions of composition powder—my own is called Herbal Uprising and integrates licorice root as one of the ingredients (see the chapter entitled "Making an Herbal Formula"). The use of bayberry in this formula acts as a stimulant to rally the body's defenses and resistance to disease. Bayberry is used wherever an astringent is indicated. When unavailable, oak bark can be used in its place although this does not have the stimulating properties of bayberry bark.

Steep one teaspoon in a cup of boiling water, cover and allow to stand until cool enough to drink. Honey may be added to taste. It will effectively induce perspiration, improve circulation and tone all the tissues it contacts. In large doses it serves as an emetic. It may be used as a gargle for sore throats. A fomentation made from this tea can be applied externally at night to relieve, cure and even prevent varicose veins.

Bayberry bark is used to treat prolapsed uterus and excessive menstrual bleeding, and may be used in a douche to treat vaginal discharge. It has also been valued for stopping hemorrhage of the bowels, lungs and uterus. The powder may be taken in gelatin capsules, two at a time as needed. Direct application of the powder to the gums is good for managing pyorrhea.

Bilberry

Vaccinium myrtillus

COMMON NAMES: Whortleberry, Huckleberry, Blueberry, Hurtleberry

FAMILY: Vaciniaceae

PARTS USED: Leaf and berries

ENERGY AND FLAVORS: The leaves are cool and astringent, while the berries are cool, nourishing and sweet

SYSTEMS AFFECTED: Liver

BIOCHEMICAL CONSTITUENTS: The berries contain flavonoid compounds called anthocyanosides, which in the fresh fruit comprise approximately 0.1% to 0.25%

PROPERTIES: Astringent, diuretic, refrigerant

DOSE: The berries can be freely eaten

USED FOR: Strengthening vision, macular degeneration, cataracts, glaucoma, diabetic retinopathy, adult-onset diabetes

NOTES: Bilberries attracted heightened interest when World War II British Royal Air Force pilots reported improved visual acuity on nighttime raids after consuming them. Subsequent studies confirmed their effectiveness in improving nighttime vision, faster restoration of vision after a glare, as well as in the treatment of many other eye disorders, including diabetic retinopathy, macular degeneration, cataracts, and glaucoma, as well as of varicose veins. They are available in Planetary Formula's Bilberry Eye Complex, which combines them with Chinese lycii berries, chrysanthemum flowers, and other herbs as a formula for the eyes.

The dried berries have a long traditional use in the treatment of diarrhea and dysentery. The leaves of this berry, as well as of the closely related huckleberry, are very effective as a tea for regulating blood sugar in the treatment of mild adult-onset diabetes.

Bistort
Polygonum bistorta
COMMON NAMES: Snakeweed, Adderwort, Dragonwort
FAMILY: Polygonaceae
PARTS USED: Root
ENERGY AND FLAVORS: Astringent, bitter, cool
SYSTEMS AFFECTED: Liver, intestines
BIOCHEMICAL CONSTITUENTS: Up to 20% tannins
PROPERTIES: Astringent, hemostatic, antidiarrheal, antimucus
DOSE: 2–3 grams of the powder
USED FOR: Bleeding, vaginal discharge, gum disease
NOTES: Bistort is a strong astringent that helps to stop bleeding and diarrhea and relieves dry mucus conditions. It can be used as a mouthwash with bayberry bark, myrrh and peppermint for pyorrhea. A powder, combined with bayberry, myrrh, echinacea and cinnamon makes an excellent natural tooth powder to counteract gum disease. As a douche, bistort will counteract vaginal discharge.

Blackberry
Rubus fruticosus and other species
FAMILY: Rosaceae
PARTS USED: Berries, leaves and root bark
ENERGY AND FLAVORS: Berries are sweet, the leaves and bark are astringent, cool energy
SYSTEMS AFFECTED: Liver, kidneys
BIOCHEMICAL CONSTITUENTS: Berries contain isocitric and malic acids; sugars, pectin, monoglycoside of cyanidin, vitamin C and A. The root and leaves contain tannins.
PROPERTIES: Berries are a cooling, Yin tonic; the leaves and root bark are antipyretic, astringent and hemostatic

DOSE: Standard infusion of the leaves or decoction of the root bark; the berries can be eaten to one's content

BLACKBERRIES USED FOR: Anemia

LEAVES USED FOR: Fevers, colds, sore throats, vaginal discharge

ROOT BARK USED FOR: Diarrhea, dysentery

NOTES: Blackberries are a Yin, blood-nourishing tonic. The leaves are used for mucus discharges, fevers, colds and sore throats. The root bark is one of the best remedies for diarrhea, dysentery and bleeding.

Black cohosh

Cimicifuga racemosa

COMMON NAMES: Black snakeroot, Bugbane, Rattleroot

FAMILY: Ranunculaceae

PARTS USED: Root

ENERGY AND FLAVORS: Sweet, pungent, slightly bitter, cool

SYSTEMS AFFECTED: Liver, spleen, stomach, large intestine, nervous system

BIOCHEMICAL CONSTITUENTS: Various glycosides including actaeine and cimicifugin; racemosin, estrogenic substances, triterpenes, isoferulic acid, tannin

PROPERTIES: Antispasmodic, expectorant, emmenagogue, diaphoretic, alterative

DOSE: Standard decoction or 3–9 grams in formula; of the tincture, 10–30 drops

USED FOR: Nervousness, spasms, neuralgia, menstrual pains, just before or during labor, asthma and coughs

NOTES: Black cohosh is used for all nervous conditions. It is used to relieve nerve pains, heaviness, numbness and neuralgia generally. It is also commonly used as an emmenagogue to relieve menstrual pains and the pangs of childbirth. Ideally, it should be given in combination with other similar herbs.

For nervousness and insomnia combine equal parts black cohosh root, skullcap, wood betony, passion flower, valerian and half part cayenne pepper. For menstrual pains and the pangs of childbirth, combine it with blue cohosh, raspberry leaf, camomile and ginger. To relieve arthritis it can be combined with equal parts angelica root, prickly ash and guiacum. For asthma and bronchial spasms, it is combined with wild cherry bark, elecampane root and mullein.

Since it has a reputation of facilitating delivery, 10 to 15 drops of the extract can be taken three times daily a week before delivery due date or during the actual time of delivery itself.

Black cohosh was one of the primary ingredients in the once famous proprietary product called Lydia E. Pinkham's Vegetable Compound, commonly used for the treatment of "female complaints." Clinical research from Germany and corroborated by herbalists worldwide has shown its estrogen-like activity. In fact, one study by Lehmann-Willenbrock and Riedel of women who had had a complete hysterectomy with accompanying menopausal symptoms found that extract of black cohosh was as effective as various estrogenic drugs in relieving symptoms. Black cohosh is highly effective at relieving symptoms of menopausal hot flashes in women. It is especially effective when combined with various synergistic herbs, such as vitex and *dang gui* in formulas. Planetary Formula's *Meno-change* is a representative menopause product that contains these herbs.

Black haw

Viburnum prunifolium
COMMON NAMES: American sloe, Stagbush
FAMILY: Caprifoliaceae
PARTS USED: Stem and root bark
ENERGY AND FLAVORS: Bitter, cool
SYSTEMS AFFECTED: Liver, nervous system
BIOCHEMICAL CONSTITUENTS: Coumarins, scopoloteine, amentoflavone, arbutin, oleanolic and ursolic acids, salicin, tannin
PROPERTIES: Antispasmodic, uterine tonic, nervine, antidysentery
DOSE: Standard decoction or 3–9 grams in formula; tincture 10–30 drops
USED FOR: Menstrual pains, menopause, miscarriage, nervousness, diarrhea
NOTES: Equal or more powerful than its relative cramp bark (*V. opulus*), black haw is also used as a uterine tonic to ease menstrual pains and to prevent miscarriage. It can be used as an adjunctive antispasmodic agent to treat asthma, palpitations, heart disease and mood swings. Finally, because of its tannin content, it can be used to stop diarrhea.

Blessed thistle

Cnicus benedictus
COMMON NAME: Holy thistle

FAMILY: Compositae

PARTS USED: Aerial portions

ENERGY AND FLAVORS: Sweet, bitter, cool

SYSTEMS AFFECTED: Liver, spleen-stomach

BIOCHEMICAL CONSTITUENTS: Tannin, cnicine (a bitter principal), a sesquiterpenoid lactone, mucilage and trace of essential oil

PROPERTIES: Alterative, stomachic, astringent, antiseptic, bitter, hemostatic, vulnerary

DOSE: Standard infusion or mild decoction

USED FOR: Liver congestion, stomach problems, loss of appetite, dyspepsia, fevers, bleeding, hepatitis and jaundice

NOTES: Blessed thistle is used primarily for the stomach and liver. It treats liver congestion, loss of appetite, dyspepsia and mucus conditions. It also lowers fevers, resolves blood clots, relieves jaundice and hepatitis and stops bleeding.

Because the liver is so often affected during abnormal periods, blessed thistle is commonly used in combination with other gynecological herbs. One combination that can be used is equal parts blessed thistle, blue cohosh root, false unicorn root, cramp bark, half part ginger.

A near relative, milk thistle (*Silybum marianum*), is used as a protective hepatotonic and will help to heal a damaged liver. Common artichoke leaves, another member of the thistle family, can be made into a tea to help restore the liver to normal function.

Bloodroot

Sanguinaria canadensis

COMMON NAMES: Redroot, Red Indian paint, Tetterwort

FAMILY: Papaveraceae

PARTS USED: Root

ENERGY AND FLAVORS: Bitter, acrid, hot, toxic

SYSTEMS AFFECTED: Lung, heart, liver, blood

BIOCHEMICAL CONSTITUENTS: Isoquinoline alkaloids, including sanguinarine, berberine, coptisine, and others

PROPERTIES: Expectorant, stimulant, alterative, antibiotic, diuretic, febrifuge, sedative, emetic in larger doses

DOSE: 0.5–2 grams of the powdered root; of the tincture, use 1–10 drops.

USED FOR: Coughs, sore throat, skin eruptions, skin cancer, athlete's foot, gum disease

NOTES: Bloodroot is primarily used as an expectorant for acute and chronic coughs, sinus congestion, laryngitis, sore throat, asthma with thick white phlegm, and croup. For pneumonia use doses of one to two drops taken repeatedly throughout the day. It also combines well in cough syrups with eucalyptus, wild cherry bark, elecampane and honey.

Externally it is applied as tincture, powder, or most often as an ointment for the treatment of a wide variety of skin affections, including athlete's foot and other fungoid conditions, skin cancers and burns. Most recently it has been used as part of a dentifrice in a small amount with cinnamon bark, bayberry bark, prickly ash, and other agents to treat gum disease and sensitive teeth. Bloodroot is used in a salve often called black paste for removing tumors, skin cancers, moles, and other topical excrescences. For more information, see "Treatments for Specific Ailments," page 263.

Blue cohosh
Caulophyllum thalictroides
COMMON NAMES: Papooseroot, Squawroot
FAMILY: Berberidaceae
PARTS USED: Rhizome
ENERGY AND FLAVORS: Acrid, bitter, warm, mildly toxic
SYSTEMS AFFECTED: Liver
BIOCHEMICAL CONSTITUENTS: Alkaloids, a fungicidal saponin, glycosides, gum, starch, salts, phosphoric acid and a soluble resin
PROPERTIES: Emmenagogue, antispasmodic, diuretic, diaphoretic, anthelmintic
DOSE: One-half ounce ounce of dried herb simmered in a pint of water; in formula, 3–9 grams; of the tincture, 10–20 drops
USED FOR: Menstrual irregularities, genito-urinary disorders, worms
NOTES: Blue cohosh is primarily used for menstrual irregularities, amenorrhea and dysmenorrhea, and also to ease the pangs of childbirth.

While not related, both black and blue cohosh are often found growing in close proximity and both have similar emmenagogic, antispasmodic properties. Black cohosh is thought to have more estrogenic action while blue cohosh is more of an actual blood mover.

A gynecological formula for delayed or stopped menses is equal parts blue cohosh, black cohosh, angelica, cramp bark, wild ginger and half part ginger. Take as a tea or powder three times daily for at least three months, stopping only during the actual period itself.

While, as the name "papoose root" suggests, it can be used immediately before or during childbirth, usually as a tincture to ease childbirth, it should not be used during the first and second trimesters of pregnancy.

Blue flag

Iris versicolor
COMMON NAMES: Flag lily, fleur-de-lis, liver lily, poison flag, wild iris
FAMILY: Iridaceae
PARTS USED: Rhizome
ENERGY AND FLAVORS: Bitter, acrid, cool
SYSTEMS AFFECTED: Liver
BIOCHEMICAL CONSTITUENTS: Salicylic and isophthalic acids, volatile oil, iridin, a glycoside, gum, resin, sterols
PROPERTIES: Alterative, antiinflammatory, cathartic, diuretic, stimulant
DOSE: Of the powdered root, 1 gram; of the tincture, 10–20 drops
USED FOR: Liver congestion, glandular congestion, hepatitis and jaundice, skin diseases, reduced appetite
NOTES: Blue flag is primarily a remedy for ailments of the liver, urinary and glandular systems. Full doses will produce prompt and rapid bowel evacuation of thin discharges, which can be debilitating on those who are in a weakened state. Thus it is primarily a remedy for excess, hypermetabolic Yang conditions, relieving stagnation generally throughout the system. As a cathartic it should always be combined with other antigriping and warming agents such as ginger. It is excellent to include in small measure for relieving liver stagnation, and consequently treating a variety of chronic skin affections including herpes simplex, acne and psoriasis. It is also used in the treatment of hepatitis, jaundice and chronic rheumatism. Finally, recent studies have demonstrated its effectiveness in the treatment of obesity, as it tends to reduce one's craving for food (probably because the body is kept active in eliminating).

Bogbean

Menyanthes trifoliata
COMMON NAMES: Buckbean, Marsh trefoil
FAMILY: Gentianaceae and Menyanthaceae

PART USED: Leaves

ENERGY AND FLAVORS: Cool, very bitter

SYSTEMS AFFECTED: Liver

BIOCHEMICAL CONSTITUENTS: A glucoside called menyanthin, bitter principle, volatile oil

PROPERTIES: Bitter tonic, antiinflammatory, antirheumatic, cathartic. Bogbean is used similarly to gentian for indigestion and anorexia. As an antiinflammatory, it can be used for arthritis, rheumatic conditions, muscular weakness and fibromyalgia, chronic infections, exhaustion and debility. For arthritic conditions, it can be combined with black cohosh and sarsaparilla.

DOSE: Of the fluid extract, 10–30 drops three times daily. The tea is made by steeping 1 ounce in 1 pint of boiling water, covered. Take ½ cup three times daily before meals. Or 1 teaspoon simmered for 10 minutes in 1 cup of water. Take ½ cup 20 minutes before meals as a tonic.

USED FOR: Rheumatic conditions, swollen glands, dropsy, gout, skin diseases, liver diseases

NOTES: As with many severely bitter herbs, bogbean stimulates the production of hydrochloric acid and can be a gastrointestinal irritant, aggravating ulcers, diarrhea, dysentery or colitis. It is also used for liver conditions, and in a somewhat larger dose as a cathartic laxative. Bogbean has a history of being smoked like tobacco. A large dose causes vomiting.

Boldo

Peumus boldus

FAMILY: Apiaceae or Umbelliferae

PARTS USED: Leaves, bark

ENERGY AND FLAVORS: Cold, bitter

SYSTEMS AFFECTED: Liver, gallbladder

BIOCHEMICAL CONSTITUENTS: Alkaloid, boldine, volatile oil

PROPERTIES: Chologogue, hepatic, bitter aromatic, vermifuge, mild diuretic, urinary antiseptic. Boldo is a native tree or shrub of Chile and Peru. It is used for liver and gallbladder diseases, including gallstones. It is also used for urinary tract infections, for intestinal parasites, and as an antiinflammatory for rheumatic and arthritic problems.

DOSE: 1 teaspoon of the leaves or bark simmered in 1 cup of water for 20 minutes; 1 cup two or three times daily

USED FOR: Liver and gallbladder diseases, gallstones, urinary tract infections, intestinal parasites, arthritic and rheumatic conditions

Boneset
Eupatorium perfoliatum

COMMON NAMES: Feverwort, Thoroughwort

FAMILY: Compositae

PARTS USED: Aboveground portions

ENERGY AND FLAVORS: Cool energy, bitter flavor

SYSTEMS AFFECTED: Liver, lungs

BIOCHEMICAL CONSTITUENTS: Sesquiterpene lactones, eupafolin, euperfolitin, eufoliatin, eufoliatorin, eperfolide and others; immunostimulatory polysaccharides; flavonoids, quercetin, kaempferol, hyperoside, astragalin, rutin, eupatorin; diterpenes including dendroidinic acid, hebenolide; vitamin C, volatile oil and sterols

PROPERTIES: Febrifuge, diaphoretic, expectorant, laxative

DOSE: Standard infusion; of the powder, 0.5–20 grains

USED FOR: Fevers, colds and flu, tightness of the liver and abdomen

NOTES: Boneset is a pure relaxant working on the muscular structures, stomach, gall ducts, bowels and uterus. Besides working internally it exerts a decided action upon the periphery including the skin. Its main use is for fevers and flu.

Taken as a cold infusion it works as a soothing and relaxing agent to the stomach and liver, aiding the secretion of bile and providing a mild laxative effect. By aiding liver detoxification it helps clear the skin, relieve thirst and intermittent and bilious fevers.

As a warm infusion it serves as a reliable diaphoretic, providing a slow and gentle perspiration for the treatment of flu, colds and liver fever sometimes known as "breakbone fever" or dengue. It also relieves the aching pains of rheumatism.

Borage
Borago officinalis

COMMON NAME: Burrage

FAMILY: Boraginaceae

PART USED: Leaves

ENERGY AND FLAVORS: Cool, bitter, sweetish and mildly acrid flavor

SYSTEMS AFFECTED: Lungs, heart

BIOCHEMICAL CONSTITUENTS: Pyrrolizidine alkaloid, including an intermedine, and their acetyl derivatives with amabiline and supinin, choline. This group of alkaloids, and certain plants (some species of spring-harvested comfrey, groundsel and senecio species, coltsfoot) that contain them, are currently suspected as possible causes of liver toxicity and cancer. Though used by traditional people around the world for thousands of years, borage is not the type of nutritive tonic herb that one would want to take regularly over a period of months. Rather, it is more of an occasional acute remedy for fevers and might be considered safe to use as a sole agent for no more than three to seven days maximum. Other ingredients include mucilage, tannin, traces of essential oil.

PROPERTIES: Refrigerant, febrifuge, aperient, galactagogue, pectoral

DOSE: Standard infusion; of the tincture, 10–15 drops

USED FOR: Fevers, lung congestion, heart problems, increasing mothers milk.

NOTES: Borage is used for heart and lung congestion, fevers and to promote mother's milk. Its demulcent properties make it effective against ulcers both internal and external. The seeds, like evening primrose, have been found to be a rich source of gamma linolenic oil.

Buchu

Agathosma betulina

FAMILY: Rutaceae

PART USED: Leaves

ENERGY AND FLAVORS: Pungent, warm

SYSTEMS AFFECTED: Bladder, stomach, lungs

BIOCHEMICAL CONSTITUENTS: Essential oil with barosma camphor

PROPERTIES: Diuretic, stimulant, aromatic, carminative, diaphoretic

DOSE: Standard infusion; in formula, 3–9 grams; of the tincture, 10–30 drops

LEAVES USED FOR: Cystitis and urinary infections

NOTES: Buchu leaves are one of the best diuretics known. The herb originates in South Africa where it is commonly used by the Hottentots. It is mostly used for acute and chronic urinary disorders, including inflammation of the urethra, nephritis, cystitis and catarrh of the bladder.

As with most diuretics, buchu works better if it is taken as a cool water infusion. Since it is commonly combined with uva ursi, for urinary infections, it is worth noting that neither of these herbs should be subjected to boiling as this dissipates their active principles and volatile oils.

When given warm it is a stimulating diaphoretic useful in the treatment of enlarged prostate and irritation of the urethra. Make an infusion using one ounce of buchu leaves to a pint of water. For an after-dinner tea to replace coffee, combine:

Buchu leaves—2 parts
Uva ursi—2 parts
Orange peel—1 part
Peppermint—1 part
Camomile—1 part

Buckthorn
Rhamnus cathartica
COMMON NAME: Common buckthorn
PART USED: Bark
ENERGY AND FLAVORS: Cold, bitter
SYSTEMS AFFECTED: Colon, stomach, spleen, liver
BIOCHEMICAL CONSTITUENTS: Various glycosides, rhamnoemodine and shesterine in the berries; the bark contains rhamnicoside and other anthraquinone derivatives
PROPERTIES: Laxative, depurative, alternative, diuretic
DOSE: One teaspoon of the bark in one-half cup of cool water, let stand for 12 hours before drinking; tincture, 5–20 drops
USED FOR: Constipation
NOTES: Buckthorn is used as a mild laxative, relieving dropsy, liver congestion, constipation, hemorrhoids, colic and obesity. It is milder than its near-relative cascara. It is safe to use for chronic constipation over an extended period. It is frequently added to alternative formulas for its mild laxative effects, helping to carry the blood and liver toxins out of the body with greater efficiency. The berries, made into a syrup with honey or sugar, allspice and ginger, are one of the finest laxatives to give to children.

It is also good to use for ulcerative colitis and acute appendicitis.

Bugleweed
Lycopus virginicus
COMMON NAME: Water horehound
FAMILY: Labiatae
PART USED: Herb
ENERGY AND FLAVORS: Bitter
SYSTEMS AFFECTED: Thyroid, heart, lungs
BIOCHEMICAL CONSTITUENTS: Various phenolic acid compounds: caffeic, rosmarinic, chlorogenic and ellagic acids
PROPERTIES: Sedative, antiinflammatory, astringent, antitussive
DOSE: Of the fluid extract, take 10–30 drops three times daily; of the whole herb, make an infusion of 1 ounce to 1 pint of boiling water. Take 1 cupful three times daily.
USED FOR: Hyperactive thyroid, sedative, bleeding from the lungs, tuberculosis

Burdock
Arctium lappa
COMMON NAMES: Lappa, Bardane, Beggar's buttons
FAMILY: Compositae
PARTS USED: Root, seeds, leaves
ENERGY AND FLAVORS: Bitter, slightly sweet, cool
SYSTEMS AFFECTED: Lungs, stomach, kidney, liver
BIOCHEMICAL CONSTITUENTS: Essential oil, nearly 45% inulin
PROPERTIES: Alterative, diuretic, diaphoretic, nutritive
DOSE: Of the crushed seeds, make a standard infusion; of the root, make a strong decoction
USED FOR: Skin diseases, blood purification, urinary problems, blood tonic
NOTES: Burdock has an abundance of minerals, especially iron, that makes it especially valuable for the blood. It is a good blood purifier and is used for arthritis rheumatism, sciatica and lumbago. The seeds and leaves are a strong surface purifier and are used for treating skin disorders.

Burdock is used to promote kidney functions and helps these organs to filter the blood, eliminating harmful acids.

The diaphoretic property of burdock is due to the presence of a volatile oil. When taken internally, this oil is eliminated from the sweat glands, thus removing toxic wastes. Sweating has a cooling effect on the body; burdock seed is therefore used to clear fevers and heat conditions (Yang diseases) such as boils, styes, carbuncles, canker sores and infections. To induce sweating, drink a cup of burdock seed tea before taking a hot bath.

Chinese burdock is used to eliminate excess nervous energy, and the root is also considered to have aphrodisiac properties. It is commonly eaten as a carrotlike vegetable by the Japanese, who call it "gobo."

Burdock is an excellent remedy for skin diseases, taken alone or with other blood purifiers such as dandelion and sarsaparilla.

Butcher's-broom
Ruscus aculeatus
COMMON NAME: Kneeholly
FAMILY: Liliaceae
PARTS USED: Herb and root
ENERGY AND FLAVORS: Cool, sweetish and slightly acrid
SYSTEMS AFFECTED: Kidneys, bladder
BIOCHEMICAL CONSTITUENTS: Ruscogenin and other saponin glycosides similar to those of wild yams (*Dioscorea villosa*).
PROPERTIES: Diuretic, diaphoretic, aperient
DOSE: A decoction of the twigs or root is taken as a warm infusion. A decoction of the root with honey added to taste is effective for clearing the lungs of phlegm and improving breathing.
CONTRAINDICATION: Because it may have an adrenergic effect of the veins (causing vascular contraction), caution should be used in the presence of hypertension.
USED FOR: Swelling of the legs and feet, urinary obstruction, urinary stones, healing fractures, opening the lungs

Cajuput
Melaleuca leucadendron
COMMON NAMES: Cajeput, White tea tree, Tea tree
FAMILY: Myrtaceae
PART USED: Distilled oil
ENERGY AND FLAVORS: Warm, spicy
SYSTEMS AFFECTED: Lungs, liver
BIOCHEMICAL CONSTITUENTS: Terpenoids, cineole (from 50–65%), nero-

lidol, limonene, benxaldehyde, valeraldehyde, dipentene and various sesquiterpenes.

PROPERTIES: Stimulant, antiseptic, antispasmodic, diaphoretic, expectorant, analgesic

USED EXTERNALLY FOR: Fungus infections, bruises and injuries, arthritic aches and pains, itches and bites on the scalp for dandruff

NOTES: Cajuput is native to Australia and Southeast Asia and has become better known in the market as Tea-tree oil, of which there are actually many varieties. The oil can be used externally as an antifungus treatment for various types of itch, including athlete's foot, or as a liniment for a wide variety of problems. It has numerous applications: Mix ten drops with shampoo and leave on the head for ten minutes to get rid of head lice and nits, relieve an itchy scalp, or restore oily, dry hair; it can be used as a substitute for eucalyptus oil in a steam bath or vaporizer to clear blocked sinuses; it is also applied directly for nasal and mouth sores; three drops mixed in water makes an effective mouthwash for dental plaque and bad breath; it can be rubbed on for muscle aches, boils, abrasions and bruises, dermatitis, pimples and acne, minor burns, sunburn, cradle cap, tropical ulcers, plantar warts, coral cuts, rashes, bites, fingernail infections, cuts and itches, congestion and coughs, arthritis. Internally, one-quarter to one-half teaspoon can be taken in warm water to promote perspiration for the early treatment of colds and flus; this is also an effective treatment for *Candida albicans* overgrowth. The same can be gargled as a treatment for sore throat. Thus this single oil can be carried as a virtual herbal first-aid treatment for most acute diseases.

CAUTION: Use primarily externally; internal use should be confined to a limited period of time and should begin with taking only a single drop and gradually working up to the one-quarter to one-half teaspoon amount. It should definitely be avoided during pregnancy. For those with sensitive skin, dilute pure tea-tree oil with ten parts vegetable oil before applying.

Calamus

Acorus calamus
COMMON NAMES: Sweet flag, Sweet sedge
FAMILY: Araceae
PART USED: Rhizome
ENERGY AND FLAVORS: Acrid, slightly warm, aromatic

SYSTEMS AFFECTED: Heart, liver, spleen-stomach

BIOCHEMICAL CONSTITUENTS: essential oil, amino acid, organic acid, sugars

PROPERTIES: Stimulant, carminative, antispasmodic, expectorant, emetic

DOSE: One teaspoon of the dried root steeped in a cup of water; of the tincture, 10–30 drops; in formula, 3–9 grams

USED FOR: Lack of mental focus, stomach problems, acidity, an aid to quit marijuana and tobacco smoking

NOTES: Calamus is an invaluable remedy for hyperacidity associated with the stomach and intestines. It has a beneficial effect on the liver and can also be used in the treatment of flatulence, colic, dyspepsia and most diseases of the stomach, intestines and liver.

Calamus root has been used by people of Asian cultures since ancient times. In India, it is commonly sold as a condiment-spice like ginger and is used for diseases of the nervous system. Ayurvedic medicine emphasizes the use of calamus root to increase mental focus (probably by focusing the digestive power), and as such it is used as an antidote to smoking marijuana (some even include some dried and ground calamus in their marijuana mixture). Perhaps it is from this tradition that it has been found that chewing calamus root would aid in quitting the tobacco habit as the combination of the two seems to cause a mild nausea and distaste for tobacco. The combination of gotu kola for clearing the mind and relieving mental tension and calamus for helping to focus it is standard treatment for the central nervous system in Ayurveda.

In China, calamus root is considered to have antiarrythmic, hypotensive, vasodilatory, antitussive, antibacterial and expectorant properties. It has been shown to be of low toxicity in animals and adverse reactions are rare. Though recent studies have revealed the presence of B-asarone, a carcinogen, the American variety is considered superior to the European because it seems to lack this ingredient. While calamus is frequently mentioned in the Bible, it likely refers to another plant species, not A. calamus.

The Native Americans would chew the root while running long distances to increase endurance and stamina. Eventually it is added to the bath to quiet the nerves and induce a state of tranquillity. Tincture of calamus is useful as a parasiticide when directly and frequently applied to lice and scabies infestations.

Calamus does have emmenagogic properties and should be avoided during pregnancy.

Calendula

Calendula officinalis

COMMON NAME: Calendula marigold

FAMILY: Compositae

PART USED: Flower heads

ENERGY AND FLAVORS: Spicy, bitter, neutral

SYSTEMS AFFECTED: Liver, heart, lungs

BIOCHEMICAL CONSTITUENTS: Essential oil containing carotenoids, saponin, resin and bitter principle

PROPERTIES: Vulnerary, emmenagogue, diaphoretic, alterative, astringent

DOSE: In formula, 3–9 grams; in tea, 1 teaspoon infused in a cup of boiling water; as a tincture, 10–30 drops

USED AS AN OIL OR SALVE FOR: Bruises and injuries, burns, earaches, shingles, eruptive skin diseases

NOTES: Calendula, used as an oil, in a salve or as a poultice, will effectively treat burns, stop bleeding, soothe pain of injuries and irritation, and promote the healing of wounds, burns and tissues. An infusion is taken internally for fevers, ulcers, menstrual cramps and eruptive skin diseases such as measles. The strong tea, or even better, a poultice or juice of the petals, topically applied, is an effective treatment for shingles. The oil can also be directly placed in the ear, one or two drops with a wad of cotton, to cure earache.

Calendula should not be taken internally during pregnancy.

California poppy

Escholtzia californica

FAMILY: Papaveraceae

PARTS USED: Whole plant

ENERGY AND FLAVORS: Cool, bitter

SYSTEMS AFFECTED: Liver, heart

BIOCHEMICAL CONSTITUENTS: Mild pain-relieving opiate alkaloids, completely free of any toxicity; also contains zinc

PROPERTIES: Sedative, analgesic, hypnotic, antineuralgic. Considering that the most powerful pain-relieving herbs (such as opium poppies, which can be used whole to relieve pain) have been preempted by the medical establishment, it is advantageous for herbalists to recognize and use California poppy as an effective pain analgesic. It can be used for insomnia, anxiety, agitation, emotionalism, melancholia, depression, headache, migraine, neuralgia and psoriasis.

Dose: 1–2 teaspoons of the herb steeped in 1 cup of boiling water or 15–30 drops of the tincture

Used for: Pain, insomnia, neuralgia

Camomile

Chamomilla recutita (Matricaria Chamomilla, M. recutita)

Common Name: Hungarian camomile, Single camomile

Family: Compositae

Part Used: Flower heads

Energy and Flavors: Bitter, spicy, aromatic, neutral

Systems Affected: Liver, stomach, lungs

Biochemical Constituents: Essential oil comprised of blue-colored azulene; also coumarin, flavonic heterosides, tannic acid

Properties: Calmative, nervine, antispasmodic, anodyne, diaphoretic, emmenagogue, carminative

Dose: Standard infusion; of the tincture, 10–30 drops

Used for: Nervousness and irritability, digestive disorders, teething and irritable children, menstrual cramps, back pains

Notes: Camomile is one of the most widely used herb teas, highly regarded for its digestive and calming properties. Camomile, sometimes known as the "Band-Aid for the stomach," should be one of the first herbs considered for all digestive complaints. It is a good remedy for a number of diseases ranging from the common cold and flu to digestive disorders, diarrhea, menstrual cramps, nervousness and insomnia.

An excellent remedy for menstrual cramps is an infusion of camomile flowers with a few slices of raw ginger. This same combination is good for all the above-mentioned diseases. A strong infusion using one ounce to a pint of water is one of the most effective treatments to relieve pains, including the pain of a slipped disc in the back, sciatica, and gout.

Camomile tea, with its high assimilable calcium content, seems to be effective for irritable children and teething, colicky infants.

There are different varieties of camomile, all with similar properties, but the stronger bitter German camomile has the greater antiinflammatory properties. Camomile also makes a good rinse for blond hair.

Camphor

Cinnamomum camphora

COMMON NAMES: Gum camphor, Laurel camphor

FAMILY: Lauraceae

PART USED: Gum resin extracted from the leaves

ENERGY AND FLAVORS: Spicy, bitter, warm, toxic internally

SYSTEMS AFFECTED: Heart, lung, liver

BIOCHEMICAL CONSTITUENTS: Contains a dextrorotatory ketone (d-camphora), a volatile oil and other substances

PROPERTIES: Stimulant, rubefacient, diaphoretic, parasiticide, analgesic, antiseptic

DOSE: Internally not more than one to three drops; externally it should only be used diluted in oil as described, as it can be absorbed through the skin and create some systemic toxicity

USED FOR: A liniment for upper respiratory tract congestion, chilblains, muscular aches and pain

NOTES: Camphor is primarily an oil created by dissolving the crystals in olive oil or some other neutral oil. It is then rubbed over the lung area for acute and chronic lung and bronchial affections, directly applied to the feet or hands to treat chilblains, used on cold sores and as a liniment for the treatment of muscular aches and pains. Since it is toxic and potentially fatal, only small doses should be taken internally. As such it is used for colds, diarrhea and other similar complaints. Toxic symptoms include vomiting, convulsions, palpitations.

Cascara sagrada

Rhamnus purshiana

COMMON NAMES: Sacred bark, Chittem bark

FAMILY: Rhamnaceae

ENERGY AND FLAVORS: cold, bitter

SYSTEMS AFFECTED: Colon, spleen, stomach, liver

BIOCHEMICAL CONSTITUENTS: Anthraquinone glycosides, bitter principle, tannins and resin

PROPERTIES: Laxative, bitter tonic, nervine, emetic

DOSE: Of the powdered bark, take one-quarter to one level teaspoonful in the evening; of the tincture, take 10–30 drops once or three times daily. To prevent "griping" pains, combine with ginger-root.

USED FOR: Constipation, liver congestion

NOTES: The bitter principle of cascara bark stimulates the secretions of the entire digestive system including the liver, gallbladder, stomach and pancreas. It is one of the safest tonic-laxative herbs known and can be used on a daily basis for chronic constipation if needed. It is also useful for colitis, hemorrhoids, liver failure and jaundice. Only bark that has been dried and aged for at least one year should be used.

Castor-oil plant

Ricinus communis

COMMON NAMES: Castor bean, Palma Christi

FAMILY: Euphorbiaceae

PARTS USED: Oil extracted from the bean

ENERGY AND FLAVORS: Bittersweet, neutral energy, toxic

SYSTEMS AFFECTED: Liver, spleen

BIOCHEMICAL CONSTITUENTS: Fixed oil consisting of glycerides of ricinoleic, isoricinoleic acids and to a lesser amount stearic, linoleic and dihydroxystearic. The poisonous aspect of the seeds (ricin) is left behind in the meal after pressing.

PROPERTIES: Demulcent, purgative

DOSE: 1–2 tablespoons before bed

USED FOR: Constipation, externally, for dissolving growths, warts, cysts and various excrescences

NOTES: Taken internally castor oil is one of the most reliable laxatives and is especially useful as a treatment for food poisoning. It is also taken along with anthelmintics to aid in expelling worms. Topically it is useful to dissolve cysts, growths and warts and to soften bunions and corns on the feet. It is also valuable as a castor-oil fomentation over the liver. This is done by generously rubbing castor oil over the entire abdomen and then applying a hot, damp towel wrung out in ginger tea and a heating pad or hot-water bottle over the region of the liver. This is applied for about 30 minutes daily to aid in decongesting the liver and to help detoxify the body.

Castor oil is not recommended for use during pregnancy.

Catha

Catha edulis

COMMON NAMES: Khat, Kat, Flower of paradise

FAMILY: Celastraceae

PARTS USED: Leaves and new shoots

ENERGY AND FLAVORS: Astringent, slightly sweet

SYSTEMS AFFECTED: Kidney–adrenals, especially the sympathetic nervous system

BIOCHEMICAL CONSTITUENTS: Contains khatamines, cathinone, norpseudoephedrine, and related phenyalkylamines. There is also another group of alkaloids found in the fresh leaves called cathedulins. Besides these, the plant also contains volatile oils, flavonoids, sterols, and triterpenes, as well as proteins, vitamins, and minerals. It is the phenylalkylamines (called cathines), that are responsible for the central nervous system stimulant activity.

PROPERTIES: Stimulant and tonic, similar to the use of coca leaves in South America.

The chewing of khat as a stimulant is common in many countries of east Africa through the Arabian peninsula, where it is used by craftsmen, laborers, and farmers to reduce physical fatigue; the masticated material appears as a bulge in the cheek of the consumers. The juice is swallowed, while the plant residue is ejected. Khat is so endemic in these countries that chewing it is employed during weddings and burials and drinking it as a beverage, during family events. In fact, in many of these countries, many houses have a special room called a *muffraj* that is specially set aside for khat chewing. According to Rudolf Fritz Weiss, M.D., (*Herbal Medicine*, 1988, Arcanum Press), it is a small shrub whose leaves are commonly chewed fresh by the elderly for a variety of diseases associated with old age. He further states that it is chemically close to such central stimulants as ephedrine and amphetamines. It loses most of its potency upon drying, however. It can be cultivated in the garden. In Europe, some companies use it for appetite suppression in weight-loss products.

Caution against overindulgence is appropriate, since in those countries catha dependence is a well-known fact. Khat is high in polyphenolic tannins and can cause gastrointestinal disturbances, including constipation. It can also cause periodontal diseases, mucosal lesions, and an increased risk of esophageal cancer. Habitual use, like that of *ma huang,* can lead to chronic elevation of the blood pressure. In one country where it is used by 90% of men and 10% of women, purchase of the drug consumes up to one third of earned wages. Interfamily problems occur as a result of higher irritability by the user, who becomes silent and withdrawn when its effects wear off.

USED FOR: Stimulation to reduce the feeling of fatigue, weight loss

Catnip

Nepeta cataria
COMMON NAME: Catmint
FAMILY: Labiatae
PART USED: Leaves
ENERGY AND FLAVORS: Spicy, bitter, cool
SYSTEMS AFFECTED: Lungs, liver, nerves
BIOCHEMICAL CONSTITUENTS: Essential oil comprised of cavracol, citro-nellol, nerol, geraniol, pulegone, thymol and nepetalic acid along with tannins
PROPERTIES: Diaphoretic, sedative, nervine, carminative
USED FOR: Insomnia, fevers and colds, diarrhea
NOTES: Catnip is famous for its sedative effects on the nervous system. It gently relieves the "congestion" affecting the nerves as a result of built-up emotional tensions.

Catnip is a good cure for diarrhea and is frequently used in enemas to relax and gently restore the tone of the bowels. Because of its mild, gentle nature, catnip, like lemon balm, is excellent to give for nervousness and hyperactivity of children as well as a diaphoretic tea to relieve fevers and colds. For such conditions, it combines well in a tea along with equal parts camomile, spearmint and lemon balm.

It is best taken as a tea; steep one ounce of the dried leaves, covered, in a pint of boiling water until cool enough to drink. Take before retiring in the evening, alone or with passion flower and/or lemon balm, for insomnia.

Cat's-claw

Uncaria tomentosa
COMMON NAME: Una de gato
FAMILY: Rubiaceae
PARTS USED: Edible inner bark of the vine
ENERGY AND FLAVORS: Cool, bitter

SYSTEMS AFFECTED: Liver

BIOCHEMICAL CONSTITUENTS: Oxindole-alkaloids, *N*-oxide, rhyncophylline, *N*-oxide, carboline alkaloid, hirustine *N*-oxide triterpenes, polyphenols, phytosterols (stigmasterol and campsterol). Some studies have isolated the alkaloid isoteropodine as the primary constituent, but much more needs to be learned about this important botanical.

PROPERTIES: Antiinflammatory, antirheumatic, antioxidant, antiviral, antitumor, antimicrobial, contraceptive, cytostatic, immune tonic.

This is considered one of the most powerful botanicals of the Amazon Peruvian rain forest. The natives have a wide use of applications for it, ranging from such acute conditions as headaches, colds, influenza, and fevers to the treatment of gastrointestinal problems (especially colitis, irritable bowel syndrome, Crohn's disease, and ulcers), tumors, arthritis, fibromylagia, asthma, and cardiovascular diseases, and as an immune tonic. This latter property has made it particularly useful for the treatment of AIDS. Cat's-claw is also a rich source of proanthocyanidin (pycnogenol), which is a powerful antioxidant and free radical scavenger. By detoxifying the gastrointestinal tract, cat's-claw is also helpful in fostering the replenishment of friendly bacteria. Cat's-claw is available in Planetary Formula's Cat's Claw Combination.

DOSE: Cat's-claw is available in dried and powdered form made into gelatin or compressed capsules. It can also be made into a tea using 1 tablespoon of the bark simmered in 1 cup of water. Take 1 cup three times daily or the equivalent dose in other forms.

USED FOR: Colitis; Crohn's disease; influenza, colds, fevers (as an antiviral); AIDS; cancer; arthritis; cardiovascular conditions

Ceanothus

Ceanothus americana

COMMON NAMES: Red root, New Jersey tea

FAMILY: Rhamnaceae

PARTS USED: Roots

ENERGY AND FLAVORS: Bitter, astringent, cool

SYSTEMS AFFECTED: Lymphatic system, liver, spleen

BIOCHEMICAL CONSTITUENTS: Various alkaloids

PROPERTIES: Lymphatic stimulant, expectorant, antispasmodic, astringent. Ceanothus can be used for lymphatic cleansing, enlarged spleen and liver, colds, bronchitis, whooping cough, tonsillitis, diphtheria, sinus conditions, nosebleeds, uterine bleeding, and hemorrhoids. Red root increases platelet counts that may have been lowered as a result of chemotherapy. It also improves digestion and assimilation and firms up stools.

DOSE: A decoction of 1 ounce to 1 pint of boiling water simmered for 20 minutes. Take ½ cup three times daily; or 10–30 drops of the fluid extract.

USED FOR: Lymphatic congestion, enlarged spleen or liver, bronchitis, uterine bleeding, hemorrhoids, increasing the platelet count as a result of chemotherapy, cancer

Celandine

Chelidonium majus

COMMON NAMES: Greater celandine

FAMILY: Papaveraceae

PART USED: Aerial portions

ENERGY AND FLAVORS: Bitter, cool

SYSTEMS AFFECTED: Liver, colon

BIOCHEMICAL CONSTITUENTS: Various alkaloids including allocryptopine, berberine, chelamine, chelidonine, coptisine, sanguinarine, sparteine and others. The root contains choline, histamine, tyramine, saponins, chelidoniol, chelidonic acid, carotene and vitamin C.

PROPERTIES: Alterative, diuretic, purgative, antispasmodic, diaphoretic, anodyne, narcotic

DOSE: The dried herb is used in infusion of one-half ounce to a pint of boiling water. The tincture and fluid extract is best made from the fresh plant and 5–10 drops are taken as a single dose three times daily. Some mild side effects include dry mouth and occasional dizziness.

USED FOR: Liver congestion, hepatitis, gallstones, asthma and spasmodic coughs, skin problems

EXTERNALLY FOR: Cataracts (with milk), warts (the fresh juice of the herb)

NOTES: Celandine is primarily used as a liver detoxifying herb for the treatment of hepatitis, jaundice, cancer, psoriasis, eczema and skin problems. In addition to its blood-purifying properties, celandine also relieves muscle spasms and bronchospasms. It also seems to counteract mucus in the lungs and bronchioles, making it a possible treatment for asthma. It mildly lowers arterial blood pressure, produces diuresis, and delays the development of anaphylactic shock. The Chinese have done extensive studies demonstrating its effectiveness for the treatment of bronchitis and whooping cough.

The fresh juice mixed with milk is directly applied to remove cataracts and white spots that form on the cornea of the eye. The fresh acrid juice can also be directly applied to remove warts.

Chaparral

Larrea tridentata
FAMILY: Zygophyllaceae
PART USED: Leaves
ENERGY AND FLAVORS: Bitter, acrid, slightly salty, cool
SYSTEMS AFFECTED: Kidneys, lung, liver
BIOCHEMICAL CONSTITUENTS: Contains a powerful antioxidant, NDGA (nordihydroquaiaretic acid), which is partially responsible for its antitumor properties. It also has vasodepressant effects and will increase ascorbic acid in the adrenals.
PROPERTIES: Alternative, blood purifier, antibiotic, antiseptic, parasiticide, expectorant, antitumor, diuretic
DOSE: One half-ounce infused in a pint of boiling water or 3–6 grams of the dried leaves infused in boiling water; of the tincture, 10–30 drops. It should be taken at least three times daily.
USED FOR: Blood purifier, cancer and tumors, antioxidant, arthritis and rheumatic pains, colds and flus, diarrhea, urinary tract infections
NOTES: Chaparral is one of the best herbal antibiotics, being useful against bacteria, viruses and parasites, both internally and externally. It may be taken internally for colds, flus, inflammation of the respiratory and intestinal tracts, diarrhea and urinary tract infections.

It can be taken internally either as a tincture, powder or tea. Its antibiotic, alterative properties are heightened when combined with other alterative herbs such as echinacea, goldenseal, garlic or usnea.

It is considered an effective anticancer herb taken either alone or in combination with other alteratives such as red clover blossoms, dandelion, echinacea, poke root, sarsaparilla, barberry root, stillingia, burdock root and buckthorn bark.

Externally it is an antiseptic healing herb when applied as a poultice or fomentation directly on wounds and injuries. A liniment made by steeping the leaves in rubbing alcohol can be directly applied on bruises and injuries as well as warts.

Chelone
Chelone glabra
COMMON NAMES: Turtlehead, Balmony
PARTS USED: Whole plant
ENERGY AND FLAVORS: Bitter, cool energy
SYSTEMS AFFECTED: Liver
BIOCHEMICAL CONSTITUENTS: Not known
PROPERTIES: Hepatic, chologogue, laxative, digestive tonic
DOSE: 1 teaspoon simmered for 10 minutes in 1 cup of water; ½ cup
    20 minutes before meals
USED FOR: Liver diseases (such as hepatitis), gallstones, jaundice, poor
    digestion, loss of appetite

Cherry stems
Prunus cerasus
COMMON NAME: Cherry stipules
PARTS USED: Stems of the fruit
ENERGY AND FLAVORS: Astringent, cool, bitter
SYSTEMS AFFECTED: Bladder
BIOCHEMICAL CONSTITUENTS: Potassium salts, organic acids, polyphenols
PROPERTIES: Diuretic, antiinflammatory and mild astringent. Cherry
    stems have been used for centuries throughout Europe as a tradi-
    tional treatment to increase diuresis and overcome urinary tract in-
    fections.
DOSE: Simmer 1 tablespoon of the fruit stalks in 1 cup of water; take
    three times daily
USED FOR: Cystitis

Chickweed
Stellaria media
COMMON NAME: Starweed
FAMILY: Caryophyllaceae
PART USED: Aerial portion
ENERGY AND FLAVORS: Sweet, mildly bitter, cool energy
SYSTEMS AFFECTED: Lungs, stomach
BIOCHEMICAL CONSTITUENTS: Saponins, which exert an antiinflammatory
    action similar to cortisone but much milder and without the harmful
    side effects. This action has made a direct application of chickweed
    oil on skin rashes widely used and appreciated by herbalists.

PROPERTIES: Demulcent, emollient, expectorant, antitussive, antipyretic, alterative, vulnerary

DOSE: Standard infusion using one ounce of the dried or two ounces of the fresh herb; one cup is taken three times daily or as needed

USED EXTERNALLY FOR: Skin irritations, itch and rashes

INTERNALLY FOR: Weight loss, as a potherb, demulcent for sore throat and lungs

NOTES: Chickweed is a common wayside weed with great value in treating blood toxicity, fevers, inflammation and other hot diseases. It is mild enough to be eaten safely as a potherb.

Its most common use is as an oil or salve applied directly to skin rashes, eczema and psoriasis. For this the whole fresh or dried herb is macerated in olive oil for four days. It is then squeezed out through a cloth and is ready to use.

Another traditional use for chickweed is for weight reduction. Whether this is due to any direct elimination of fat, its filling demulcent properties, its mild diuretic and laxative properties or a combination of all three would be difficult to prove.

Externally, a poultice of the steamed herb is applied to resolve boils and abscesses.

Cleavers

Galium aparine

COMMON NAMES: Clivers, Goose grass, Bedstraw

FAMILY: Rubiaceae

PARTS USED: Aerial portions

ENERGY AND FLAVORS: Bitter, cool

SYSTEMS AFFECTED: Bladder, gallbladder

BIOCHEMICAL CONSTITUENTS: A glycoside, asperuloside and other iridoids, also anthraquinone derivatives

PROPERTIES: Diuretic, alterative, aperient, mild astringent

USED FOR: Urinary tract infections, venereal diseases, skin diseases, hepatitis, externally for burns and rashes.

NOTES: Cleavers is one of the most effective diuretic blood purifiers known. It is very effective for the treatment of all urinary and reproductive-organ inflammations as well as hepatitis and venereal disease. It is used to treat enlarged lymph glands, cystitis, psoriasis and skin diseases and eruptions. Externally, it makes an effective poultice for scalds and burns. Its cooling properties also make it appropriate for the treatment of fevers.

A tea is made by infusing one ounce of cleavers in a pint of water. Either the tea or a teaspoon of the tincture taken three times daily makes an effective course of treatment.

Collinsonia

Collinsonia canadensis
COMMON NAME: Stoneroot
FAMILY: Labiatae
PART USED: Root
ENERGY AND FLAVORS: Spicy, sour, warm
SYSTEMS AFFECTED: Liver, pericardium, lung, colon, veins
BIOCHEMICAL CONSTITUENTS: Saponin, alkaloid, tannin, resin
PROPERTIES: Astringent, diuretic, emmenagogue, alterative
DOSE: Standard decoction of the root of which a cup of tea is taken three times daily; of the tincture, 10–30 drops
USED FOR: Hemorrhoids, varicose veins, diarrhea
NOTES: The main use for collinsonia is the treatment of hemorrhoids. This is because it has the ability to strengthen the veins of the body and thus works directly on strengthening the portal vein of the rectum and varicose veins generally.

It is also useful for treating diarrhea.

Coltsfoot

Tussilago farfara
COMMON NAMES: Horsehoof, Coughwort
FAMILY: Compositae
PARTS USED: Leaves and flowers
ENERGY AND FLAVORS: Bitter, sweet, neutral
SYSTEMS AFFECTED: Lungs
BIOCHEMICAL CONSTITUENTS: About 8% mucilage, including various polysaccharoids based on glucose, galactose, fructose, arabinose and xylose; inulin; flavonoids, rutin, hyperoside and isoquercetin; tannin
PROPERTIES: Antitussive, expectorant, demulcent, antiinflammatory, astringent
DOSE: Standard infusion of one ounce of the dried herb to a pint of boiling water
USED FOR: Lung complaints, coughs
NOTES: Coltsfoot is a traditional herb used for coughs and irritating upper-respiratory problems by people throughout the world includ-

ing Europe and China. It is specific for all chronic cases of emphysema and silicosis, both exhibiting signs of persistent cough. Since these problems are often heightened upon first awakening in the morning, it is a good idea to have coltsfoot tea prepared and stored in a thermos the night before.

Coltsfoot does contain extremely small traces of pyrrolizidine alkaloids, which have been found to cause liver toxicity and cancer. However, the amount is extremely small and it is likely that other beneficial properties of the herb counter any potential liver cancer effects. The amount found in the dried plant is minuscule enough (0.00–0.015%) to be disregarded as any potential threat to health. Nevertheless, its use has been banned in West Germany. In any case, it would be wise not to use this herb during pregnancy as these alkaloids seem to have a particularly harmful effect on the liver of fetuses and newborn infants.

Comfrey
Symphytum officinale
COMMON NAME: Knitbone
FAMILY: Boraginaceae
PARTS USED: Leaf and root
ENERGY AND FLAVORS: Bitter, sweet, cool energy
SYSTEMS AFFECTED: Lungs, stomach, kidneys, bone and muscles
BIOCHEMICAL CONSTITUENTS: Allantoin, mucilage, tannins, starch, inulin, traces of oil and liver-toxic pyrrolizidine alkaloids. The root contains steroidal saponins, which at least partially accounts for its antiinflammatory and pain-relieving properties.
PROPERTIES: Tonic, demulcent, expectorant, vulnerary, astringent
DOSE: Standard decoction, or one teaspoon of the tincture three times daily
USED FOR: Promoting healing, broken bones, lungs, diarrhea, hemorrhage and bleeding, lack of pepsin for protein digestion
NOTES: Comfrey is indicated for any rapid wound or bone healing. As such it can be used both internally and externally with outstanding results in the healing of fractures, wounds, sores and ulcers. The allantoin in comfrey increases cell proliferation, which accounts for its rapid-healing powers.

The astringent property makes it useful for stopping hemorrhage, whether it be from the stomach, lungs, bowels, kidneys or hemorrhoids. To treat bleeding, use a strong decoction of the root, using one-half to one ounce of the root every two hours until bleeding has stopped.

Comfrey will help the pancreas in regulating blood sugar levels. It helps relieve irritations associated with the gallbladder, kidneys, bladder, small intestines and stomach. It helps promote the secretion of pepsin and is a general aid to digestion.

Its demulcent properties, especially of the root, have been used to sooth lung troubles and coughs. Comfrey root has the highest content of mucilage of any of the herbs.

Comfrey is extremely prolific in terms of its effects in promoting the rapid healing of tissues as well as its growth habits in the garden. A small piece of the root will reproduce itself in a short period.

A common addition to herb formulas, especially for the treatment of lung ailments, is comfrey mucilage. Soak two ounces of dried comfrey root overnight in one quart of water. Simmer in a covered container for thirty minutes, strain, filter and squeeze through a muslin or linen cloth. Return the extract to the cleaned vessel and add six ounces of honey and two ounces of vegetable glycerine, and simmer for another five minutes. Cool and store in a wide-mouthed jar. Take two tablespoons every hour for acute diseases (including internal hemorrhage), or two to four times daily for chronic ailments.

There has been some controversial research in which the regular long-term ingestion of Russian comfrey root is claimed as containing certain pyrilizidine alkaloids which have been known to cause liver veno-occlusive disease in humans. In this condition the small and medium veins of the liver become obstructed which results in liver disfunction, cirrhosis and possibly death. Since pregnant women, developing fetuses and infants seem to be particularly vulnerable to these alkaloids, it may not be advisable for these to take comfrey root at all and certainly not for any prolonged period.

This information is still a point of controversy among herbalists for many reasons. While it has been demonstrated that feeding 6-week-old rats 30% to 50% of their total diet of comfrey root did cause tumors to develop, humans have never manifested tumors from regular, long-term ingestion of comfrey plants with pyrilizidine (PA's) alkaloids. Instead, humans tend to develop liver veno-occlusive disease. It is known that animals have quite different metabolisms than humans. What is often poisonous and toxic to one is quite safe and harmless to the others. Further, it is unlikely that 6-week-old rats would naturally consider comfrey root as a food worthy to constitute nearly 50% of their total dietary input. This is in view of the literally millions of people worldwide who have popularly and widely used comfrey for a variety of common ailments.

Independent laboratory analysis of three specimens of comfrey root conducted by a grower in Washington State revealed one without any PA's whatsoever, while the other two only showed extremely minute trace amounts, hardly enough for serious concern. When evaluating such data, it is important to keep in mind that high concentrations of many foodlike substances taken over a prolonged period will eventually reveal some minor toxic component which would not be evident with normal consumption.

The problem with applying this type of scientific methodology with comfrey is similar to so many benign healing herbs such as a sassafras. In the case of sassafras, it is known to contain safrole, which despite its presence in varying amounts in such common foods and spices as basil, black pepper and nutmeg, is nevertheless considered to be carcinogenic to humans in its pure form. Sassafras is condemned much as comfrey is, based upon the presence, even in a minute amount, of safrole, a substance that is known to induce cancer in laboratory animals and humans when used in its pure form.

Plants have a dynamically complex biochemistry. In many instances this allows for small amounts of substances, which when isolated and concentrated might otherwise be poisonous in their whole lifeform, to be quite safe and harmless. This must certainly be one possible explanation for the fact that, despite the carcinogenicity of safrole, in the Southeastern U.S. where sassafras is taken as a regular and common beverage there is one of the lowest incidents of cancer anywhere on the North American continent. It is also a possible reason for the lack of any conclusive cases or historical records of liver veno-occlusive disease among humans who have been known to take fairly large long-term doses of comfrey root or leaf to treat a variety of diseases.

It might be pointed out that the possible toxicity of comfrey only applies to internal ingestion, not to its most valuable external use as a poultice for broken bones, wounds and ulcers. Further, I have had wide experience using it myself, observing only the most positive effects in its use either externally or internally. Recent studies have shown that not all comfrey leaf possesses pyrrolizidine alkaloids, and that which is harvested in late summer or fall seems to have only minute traces. The root has higher amounts than the leaf.

Corn silk
Zea mays
COMMON NAMES: Yumixu—Chinese, Stigmata maydis
FAMILY: Gramineae
PART USED: Tassels of the corn flower
ENERGY AND FLAVORS: Sweet, bland, neutral
SYSTEMS AFFECTED: Bladder, small intestines, liver
BIOCHEMICAL CONSTITUENTS: Saponins, allantoin, various sterols including B-sitosterol and stigmasterol. Vitamins including C and K.
PROPERTIES: Diuretic, lithotriptic (dissolves stones), demulcent, cholagogue
DOSE: Standard infusion using one ounce of the fresh or dried silk steeped in a pint of boiling water; one cup taken three times daily. Of the tincture, take 10–30 drops three times daily.
USED FOR: Urinary infections
NOTES: A traditional natural treatment for all urinary tract complaints including cystitis, urethritis and prostatitis. It is also used to clear edema of the body generally.

Cramp bark
Viburnum opulus
COMMON NAMES: Guelder rose, Snowball tree
FAMILY: Caprifoliaceae
PART USED: Bark
ENERGY AND FLAVORS: Bitter, neutral
SYSTEMS AFFECTED: Liver, lungs, heart, small intestine
BIOCHEMICAL CONSTITUENTS: hydroquinones, arbutin, coumarins, tannins; catechins
PROPERTIES: Antispasmodic, sedative, nervine, astringent
DOSE: A decoction is made by simmering one-half ounce of the bark in a pint of boiling water for twenty minutes. One cup of this tea or a teaspoon of the tincture can be taken three times daily.
USED FOR: Menstrual cramps, PMS, threatened miscarriage, asthma, sedative, nervine
NOTES: Cramp bark is useful for the cramps and discomfort of menstru-

ation as well as other uterine problems. Its near relative black haw (*Viburnum prunifolium*) is even more prized. Either or both are combined with false unicorn root (*Chamaelirium luteum*) for the general treatment of all female reproductive disorders. Besides its general tonic effect upon the uterus and the regulation of the menstrual cycle, it is also effective for threatened miscarriage.

Another good acute formula for the treatment of menstrual cramps, PMS and convulsions is equal parts cramp bark or black haw with ginger and angelica root and three parts camomile flowers.

Because of its general nervine and sedative properties, it is a good acute treatment for heart palpitations and rheumatism. Cramp bark can also be used as an antispasmodic in the treatment of asthma.

Cranesbill root

Geranium maculatum

COMMON NAMES: Wild geranium, storksbill, alumroot
FAMILY: Geraniaceae
PART USED: Root
ENERGY AND FLAVORS: Astringent, bitter, neutral
SYSTEMS AFFECTED: Stomach, intestines, liver, heart
BIOCHEMICAL CONSTITUENTS: Tannic and gallic acids, starch, pectin, gum
PROPERTIES: Astringent, hemostatic, styptic, vulnerary
DOSE: Standard decoction or 5–30 drops of the tincture
USED FOR: Diarrhea and dysentery, colitis, bleeding, vaginal discharge
NOTES: Cranesbill is primarily a remedy for diarrhea, colitis, dysentery, especially with associated bleeding. It is also used to stop either internal or external bleeding and to promote healing of burns and torn flesh. It can be topically applied and used as a douche for vaginal discharge and hemorrhoids.

Culver's root

Leptandra virginica (Veronicastrum virginicum)

COMMON NAMES: Black root, Physic root
FAMILY: Scrophulariaceae
PART USED: Root
ENERGY AND FLAVORS: Cold energy, bitter taste
SYSTEMS AFFECTED: Liver
BIOCHEMICAL CONSTITUENTS: Volatile oil, saponins, mannitol, dextrose, tannins and other constituents

PROPERTIES: Cholagogue, laxative, diaphoretic
DOSE: 1–4 grams of the powdered root bark
USED FOR: Liver disorders, constipation
NOTES: Culver's root is an old-time American doctors' remedy for liver
    congestion with accompanying constipation. Thus it is to be consid-
    ered when compounding a formula for the liver, gallbladder, to treat
    constipation, colitis, gallstones and hepatitis.

Cyperus

Cyperus rotundus
COMMON NAME: Sedge root
FAMILY: Cyperaceae
PART USED: Root
ENERGY AND FLAVORS: Spicy, bitter, sweet, slightly warm
SYSTEMS AFFECTED: Liver
BIOCHEMICAL CONSTITUENTS: 0.5% essential oil comprised of cyperol,
    cyperene, cyperone, pinene and sesquiterpenes
PROPERTIES: Carminative, antispasmodic, emmenagogue
DOSE: 3–9 grams
USED FOR: Abdominal pains and cramps, colds and flu, menstrual irreg-
    ularities, depression
NOTES: This common wayside weed, closely related to the famous
    Egyptian papyrus, is widely used in folk practice. Perhaps the only
    reason it has fallen out of vogue among Western herbalists is the
    difficulty of obtaining clean, good-quality dried root. It was eaten for
    food by many of the Native Americans, which attests to its safety as
    a therapeutic agent. It is widely used in Chinese folk practice for
    common acute complaints including simple colds, flus, mucus con-
    gestion, digestive and menstrual disorders. It is an effective remedy
    for alleviating food allergy symptoms associated with candida over-
    growth and other metabolic disorders.

    It is ideal to use with other herbs such as tang quai (*Angelica sinen-
    sis*), vitex berries, or false unicorn root and cramp bark for menstrual
    disorders. Like the Chinese herb bupleurum, cyperus is used in this
    way to "regulate chi," which means that it will aid digestion and
    assimilation and regulate moods. It is also acknowledged as one of
    the best female regulators in Ayurvedic medicine and being especially
    good for relieving menstrual cramps. Various members of this genus
    are found in marshy, river-bottom areas throughout North America
    and other areas of the world.

Damiana

Turnera diffusa
FAMILY: Turneraceae
PART USED: Leaves
ENERGY AND FLAVORS: Spicy, warm
SYSTEMS AFFECTED: Kidney
BIOCHEMICAL CONSTITUENTS: Volatile oil, hydrocyanic glycoside, bitter principle, tannin, resin
PROPERTIES: Yang tonic, aphrodisiac, diuretic, nervine, aperient
DOSE: Standard infusion of one ounce steeped in a pint of boiling water, one cup three times daily; of the tincture, 10–30 drops
USED FOR: Lowered libido, depression, mucus congestion
NOTES: Damiana is primarily used as a mild aphrodisiac either for men or women. It is also useful as an antidepressant and digestive, and as a treatment for mucus congestion and consequent coughs.

Dandelion

Taraxacum officinale
FAMILY: Compositae
PARTS USED: Whole plant
ENERGY AND FLAVORS: Leaves are cool and bitter, the root is bitter, sweet and cool
SYSTEMS AFFECTED: Liver, spleen, stomach, kidney, bladder
BIOCHEMICAL CONSTITUENTS: Lactupicrine, a bitter principle, tannin, inulin and a latexlike substance, polysaccharides, carotene
PROPERTIES: Alterative, cholagogue, diuretic, stomachic, aperient, tonic
DOSE: Standard decoction or 10–30 drops of the tincture
USED FOR: Liver problems, urinary tract infections, skin eruptions, stomach pains, breast cancer, beverage
NOTES: The main benefits of this great herb are exerted upon the function of the liver. Dandelion has the capacity to clear obstructions and stimulate and aid the liver to eliminate toxins from the blood. In this way dandelion root is particularly used as a blood purifying herb, and also partially due to its high mineral content.

The root is also useful for clearing obstructions of the spleen, pancreas, gallbladder, bladder and kidneys. It is of tremendous benefit to the stomach and intestines. To treat stomachaches, drink one-half cup of the infusion every half hour until relief is attained.

In Chinese medicine this condition would be considered as "liver attacking spleen-pancreas," which refers to an imbalance of liver and pancreatic enzymes necessary for digestion. Thus it would seem that dandelion root helps to balance these enzymes that simultaneously benefit digestion, assimilation and elimination.

Even the most serious cases of hepatitis have rapidly been cured, sometimes within a week, with dandelion root tea taken in cupful doses four to six times daily and a light, easily digested diet of vegetable broths and rice and mung bean porridge.

I consider dandelion root a specific for hypoglycemia, but it may need to be combined with other tonic herbs such as ginseng and a little ginger for maximum benefit. A cup of dandelion root tea is taken three times daily along with the recommended balanced diet. Similarly, it can be used to remedy recent onset of diabetes, especially when combined wiht huckleberry leaf in tea.

Dandelion root helps decrease high blood pressure, thus aiding the action of the heart. It can also be helpful in treating anemia by supplying necessary nutritive minerals.

The young dandelion leaves can be eaten fresh as a steamed potherb. With chicory and endive greens it provides a pleasant source of mild vegetable bitter necessary for balanced nutrition. This is especially good in the early spring, which is a time for physical housecleaning, which these plants help to accomplish.

Roasted dandelion root makes a pleasant beverage that can be consumed daily. It combines well with roasted bancha, or "kukicha" tea, or chicory root.

Dandelion leaf tea is one of the finest diuretics known, at least equal to any known drug medicine. Thus dandelion leaf tea can be taken for fluid retention, cystitis, nephritis, weight loss and hepatitis.

Chicory (*Cichorium intybus*) has properties similar to dandelion and can be used for similar purposes, although it has slightly more calming and blood-building properties.

Devil's claw
Harpogophytum procumbens
COMMON NAME: Grapple plant
FAMILY: Pedaliaceae
PART USED: Tuber
ENERGY AND FLAVORS: Cool, bitter (reported to be 6,000 times more bitter than gentian)

SYSTEMS AFFECTED: Liver

BIOCHEMICAL CONSTITUENTS: Kaempferol; luteolin; chlorogenic and cinnamic acids; iridoid glycosides, including procumbide, harpagide, and harpagoside; quinone; harpogoquinone; and various other substances, including ursolic and oleanolic acid derivatives, exters, stachyose, and other sugars

PROPERTIES: Antiinflammatory, antirheumatic, and antiphlogistic

Devil's claw is specifically used for arthritic and rheumatic conditions, sciatica, neuralgia, and headaches. It has been found to be effective for the elderly for rheumatic pains, hyperlipedemia, hypercholesterolemia, and obesity.

DOSE: Because of its extreme bitterness, it is usually taken in tablet form.

CONTRAINDICATIONS: Not to be used during pregnancy

USED FOR: Arthritic and rheumatic conditions, sciatica, neuralgia, headaches, high cholesterol, obesity

Devil's club

Oplopanax horridum

FAMILY: Araliaceae

PART USED: Root bark

ENERGY AND FLAVORS: Cool, bitter

SYSTEMS AFFECTED: Pancreas, spleen

BIOCHEMICAL CONSTITUENTS: According to herbalist, Michael Moore, "it contains neurolidol toregal, dodinene, bulnesol, dodecenol, cadanene, and cedrol (among others), as well as araliasides and panaxosides of varied and unspecified nature." (From *Medicinal Plants of the Mountains West* by Michael Moore, publ. 1993 by Red Crane Books, Santa Fe, New Mexico.)

PROPERTIES: Tonics, antiinflammatory, antidiabetic, antirheumatic.

Devil's claw with its tannins removed has demonstrated the ability to lower blood sugar. It is interesting that many studies have not shown its ability to lower blood sugar in alkaline or crude extracts including water. In fact, water extracts contain elements that actually can raise blood sugar. The hypoglycemic principle is separated when it is precipitated in acetone, hardly a home herbalist's process. The inconsistency of this herb may be because of its similarity to ginseng, of which it is a relative and which also has many similar therapeutic properties but is dependent upon constitutional predisposition.

DOSE: 1 ounce simmered for 30 minutes in 1 pint of water; 1 cup three times daily

USED FOR: Arthritic and rheumatic conditions, *qi* tonic, diabetes

Dill

Anethum graveolens

COMMON NAME: Dillweed

FAMILY: Umbelliferae

PART USED: Aerial portions

ENERGY AND FLAVORS: Spicy, warm

SYSTEMS AFFECTED: Stomach, spleen, liver

BIOCHEMICAL CONSTITUENTS: Essential oil, fatty oil, some acids

PROPERTIES: Carminative, antispasmodic, stomachic, emmenagogue, diuretic, galactagogue, calmative

DOSE: A teaspoon of dill tea for infants or small children as often as needed; for adults, make a standard infusion of the leaves or root and take a cupful three times daily

USED FOR: Abdominal pains and cramps, children's colicky pains, colds, flus and coughs

NOTES: Dillweed is primarily used to treat the frequent symptoms of children's colicky stomach aches and pain. It is also good for adult stomach aches as well as insomnia caused by indigestion. Dill, taken internally as a tea by the mother, will increase breast milk. The root can be boiled and used as a tea for colds, flus and coughs.

Dusty miller

Senecio cineraria (Cineraria maritima)

FAMILY: Compositae

PART USED: Sterilized juice

ENERGY AND FLAVORS: Warm energy

SYSTEMS AFFECTED: Eyes

BIOCHEMICAL CONSTITUENTS: Contains pyrrolizidine alkaloids and should not be used internally

PROPERTIES: The sterilized juice is sold as eye drops by homeopathic pharmacies for clearing the eyes, brightening vision and treating capsular and lenticular cataract of the eye. It is easily made by juicing the fresh plant, squeezing and straining the juice through a fine cloth, adding an equal amount of vegetable glycerine and 20% boric acid as a preservative. This can then be used for eye drops.

USED EXTERNALLY AND APPLIED DIRECTLY TO THE EYES FOR: Strengthening and
  clearing vision and other eye problems, cataracts

Echinacea

Echinacea angustifolia and other species (*E. purpurea, E. pallida,* et al.)
COMMON NAMES: Snakeroot, Coneflower, Prairie
FAMILY: Compositae
PARTS USED: Root, leaves
ENERGY AND FLAVORS: Bitter, pungent, cool
SYSTEMS AFFECTED: Lungs, stomach, liver
BIOCHEMICAL CONSTITUENTS: Essential oil, polysaccharides, echinaco-
  side, a triglycoside of caffeic acid derivative, in *E. angustifolia* and *E.
  pallida* but not in *E. purpurea,* echinacin and other constituents

Echinacea and the Eclectics

Echinacea was intimately associated with the "Eclectics," the great
herbal-medicine movement of nineteenth-century North America.
Eclectic medicine, founded around the 1850s by Dr. Wooster Beach,
specialized in the integration of Native American herbs, homeopathic
medicine and what was then the Western scientific knowledge of the
day. They numbered in the thousands, highly qualified and dedicated
doctors, including women (theirs was the first to admit women into
the medical profession), who published numerous books and respected
scientific journals. Their main college was located in Cincinnati, Ohio,
where, during the Western expansion of the mid-1800s, North American herbalism (perhaps all of Western herbalism) reached its highest
achievement. There was the distinguished work of such esteemed doctors as King, Ellingwood, Cook, Scudder, Felter, and the greatest herbal
pharmacist, John Uri Lloyd, who specially crafted the many herbal
Eclectic medicines that were sold to physicians and used throughout
the country.

  The Eclectics, especially as described in the writings of Dr. John M.
Scudder, were unwittingly pointed in the direction of independently
evolving a system of differential medical diagnosis that was astonish-
ingly close to that of the thousands-of-years-old medical systems that
evolved in China and India. This included the evaluation of the tongue
and pulse and other diagnostic indications.

  By the late 1930s, with the closing of the college in Cincinnati in
1939, they had not yet evolved the principles of complex formulations

used in China and India where it was found necessary to treat complicated disease patterns by combining herbs to work on several organic systems simultaneously. Around the turn of the century, Eclectics discovered and popularized the use of echinacea root as the sovereign anti-inflammatory remedy. Thus this most sacred healing herb of the Plains Indians became widely prescribed by Eclectics until their passing. Probably if it were not for the discovery of the wonder drugs, such as penicillin, echinacea would be one of the herbs of choice for the treatment of all infections and inflammatory conditions.

With the increased use of, and support for, the industrial-based medicines, the Eclectics' influence faded. What survives is the Lloyd Library, probably the greatest herbal medical library in the world. Located in Cincinnati, its numerous stores contain not only all the accumulated herbal knowledge of the Eclectics, but a current catalogue of books and journals on herbal medicine published worldwide. It is in this place, upon the ashes of the Eclectic forebears, that the American Herbalist Guild scheduled its first annual meeting in May of 1990!

Echinacea

Echinacea is the wonder herb for all acute inflammatory conditions. Generally it is mild enough so there are no side effects even after taking large doses. There are paradoxical reactions experienced by a few individuals, but this is usually alleviated by combining echinacea with a very small amount of licorice and ginger. Because of its mild nature, however, it should be taken in small, frequent doses every two hours and accompanied by a simple warm-liquid diet of vegetable broth and thin rice porridge.

I have personally seen echinacea work for even the most severe inflammatory conditions including boils, skin eruptions, pussy sores, venomous bites, gangrene, septicemia, poison oak and poison ivy, syphilis and gonorrhea, as well as any acute bacterial and viral infections. Whenever there is pus or red inflammation in a particular area, echinacea is sure to be effective, usually within three days. Thereafter the frequent dosage described above can be tapered down to only three or four times daily for a week or two after all symptoms have disappeared.

Recent studies in Germany, where echinacea has been in constant use since the early 1930s, have established its usefulness not only for chronic conditions but more acute arthritic diseases, certain cancers, and various viral diseases and possibly even helping in the treatment against AIDS.

DOSE: Of the tea, one-half cup; of the liquid extract, 10–30 drops; of the dried powder, two grams at a time. For acute conditions, every two hours; for chronic conditions, three times daily

USED FOR: All inflammatory conditions

Elder

Sambucus nigra and *S. canadensis*

FAMILY: Caprifoliaceae

PART USED: Primarily the flowers

ENERGY AND FLAVORS: Acrid, bitter, cool

SYSTEMS AFFECTED: Lungs, liver

BIOCHEMICAL CONSTITUENTS: Essential oil, terpenes, glycosides, rutin, quercitrin, mucilage and tannin. The fruits are high in vitamin C.

PROPERTIES: Diaphoretic, alterative, laxative (aged bark), stimulant, anti-rheumatic (berries)

DOSE: Of the flowers, one-half to one ounce steeped in boiling water

GOOD FOR: Colds, flus and fevers

EXTERNALLY FOR: Clearing the skin

NOTES: Elder flowers are commonly used in the first stages of colds and flus. Combine equal parts elder flowers, peppermint and yarrow with a quarter part licorice. Covered, steep approximately one ounce or more of this mixture, with three or four slices of fresh ginger if available, in a pint of boiling water. Drink one or two cups as hot as possible before taking a hot bath and retiring to bed with plenty of warm covers to induce perspiration.

Elder flowers are also used in salves for the treatment of burns, rashes, minor skin ailments and to diminish wrinkles. The leaves are a good detoxifying agent in salves. The bark can be quite strong and toxic as a laxative unless properly aged for a year or more. Finally, the berries are a good general blood purifier and have been used as an effective treatment for arthritic and rheumatic complaints.

Only the black elder is safe to use internally. Red elder (*S. race-mosa*) is toxic.

Elecampane

Inula helenium

COMMON NAMES: Scabwort, Elf dock, Horseheal

FAMILY: Compositae

PART USED: Root

ENERGY AND FLAVORS: Sweet, acrid, bitter, warm

SYSTEMS AFFECTED: Lungs, spleen, stomach

BIOCHEMICAL CONSTITUENTS: Essential oil, bitter principles, resin, inulin

PROPERTIES: Tonic, carminative, expectorant, diuretic, antiseptic, astringent, stimulant, vermifuge

DOSE: Of the dried root, one ounce steeped in a pint of boiling water twenty minutes, one cup three times daily; of the tincture, 10–30 drops, three times daily

USED FOR: Respiratory complaints, chronic coughs, digestive weakness

NOTES: Elecampane root is specific for chronic mucus, coughs and digestion. Therefore it is given for asthma and bronchitis and is beneficial when given on a long-term basis. Its carminative properties aid the digestion and assimilation of food, and for this reason, there is less tendency to form mucus.

Epazote

Chenopodium ambrosioicles

COMMON NAMES: Mexican wormseed, American wormseed

FAMILY: Chenopodiaceae

PART USED: Aerial portions

ENERGY AND FLAVORS: Bitter, cool

SYSTEMS AFFECTED: Liver, GI tract

BIOCHEMICAL CONSTITUENTS: Ascaridole, geraniol, cymene, terpinene, methyl salicylate, butyric acid, triterpenes

PROPERTIES: Anthelmintic, carminative

DOSE: For worms take 1–4 grams of the powdered seeds as a single dose, once or twice a day for three days with a purgative such as cascara, senna or rhubarb root

USED FOR: Gas, worms

NOTES: The seeds have traditionally been used for the treatment of worms including pinworms, roundworms, hookworms and smaller tapeworms. Recently, the Southwestern custom of adding a pinch of the leaves when cooking pinto beans to reduce flatulence significantly has received considerable attention. It seems to be effective. Further, most Central Americans and Indians traditionally grow this plant near their kitchen so it will always be readily available. While a small amount will enhance flavor, too much may cause bitterness. In China, a similar species is used as a tea for the treatment of fevers including those of the malarial kind.

Ephedra

Ephedra gerardiana, E. sinica, E. equisatina, E. distachya, E. helvetica,
    et al.
COMMON NAMES: Chinese species is called ma huang
FAMILY: Ephedraceae
PART USED: Stems
ENERGY AND FLAVORS: Pungent, bitter, warm
SYSTEMS AFFECTED: Lungs, bladder
BIOCHEMICAL CONSTITUENTS: Ephedrine alkaloids
PROPERTIES: Diaphoretic, stimulant, diuretic, decongestant, antirheu-
    matic, astringent
DOSE: 2–6 grams in decoction
USED FOR: Asthma, emphysema, bronchitis, hay fever, allergic rashes
NOTES: As one of the most primeval herbs on the planet, ephedra was
    mentioned as a medicinal plant in the Vedas, the ancient scriptures
    of India. Further, the Chinese have been using them over five thou-
    sand years as a treatment for asthma. The alkaloid ephedrine, first
    isolated by a Chinese scientist in 1924, has antiasthmatic and stimu-
    lant properties. However, studies have thus far established that only
    the Chinese species contains sufficient amounts of the ephedrine al-
    kaloid to generate the specific antiasthma and stimulant effects.

Nevertheless, both the Native American varieties as well as the
    Chinese ma huang have been used for the treatment of arthritic and
    rheumatic problems. Ephedra stimulates the sympathetic nervous
    system, which makes it particularly useful for the treatment of
    asthma, emphysema, bronchitis, whooping cough, hay fever and ur-
    ticaria.

Epimedium

E. pimedium grandiflorum, E. sagittatum
COMMON NAME: Lusty goatherb
FAMILY: Berberidaceae
PART USED: Aerial part of the herb
ENERGY AND FLAVORS: Pungent and warm
SYSTEMS AFFECTED: Liver, kidney, male reproductive organs
BIOCHEMICAL CONSTITUENTS: Icariin, benzene, sterols, tannin, palmitic
    acid, linolenic acid, oleic acid, vitamin E
PROPERTIES: Yang tonic, aphrodisiac, antirheumatic, vulnerary, antitus-
    sive, antiasthmatic

DOSE: 3–15 grams once or twice daily in decoction

USED FOR: Strengthening kidney function, impotence, hypertension, arthritis and lower-back pains, chronic bronchitis and asthma

NOTES: This is an herb commonly associated with Chinese herbal medicine but is grown in many parts of North America as an ornamental. It specifically stimulates the production of androgen hormones, with no effect on estrogen. Therefore, it is ideal for treating male impotence and promoting sperm production. It is also beneficial in the treatment of prostate, testes and levator ani.

Low doses of 3–6 grams will increase urinary output while higher doses of 8–15 grams will treat frequent urination. Because of its effect upon the kidneys, it is good for treating lower-back pains, arthritis, rheumatism and lowering blood pressure.

Finally, it also seems to have antitussive and expectorant properties. Therefore, it is effective for chronic bronchitis and asthma.

Eucalyptus

Eucalyptus globulus

COMMON NAME: Blue gum tree

FAMILY: Myrtaceae

PART USED: Leaves

ENERGY AND FLAVORS: Spicy, warm

SYSTEMS AFFECTED: Lungs, kidneys

BIOCHEMICAL CONSTITUENTS: Essential oil with cineole, ellagic and gallic acid, bitter principle, resin, antibiotic properties, tannin

PROPERTIES: Expectorant, stimulant, antibiotic, antiseptic, rubefacient

DOSE: Of the leaves in infusion, one-half ounce to a pint; of the oil, 1–5 drops

USED FOR: Respiratory complaints, coughs, arthritic aches and pains, as an antiseptic

NOTES: Native to Australia, there are a great number of species of eucalyptus trees. The foliage of some contains many essential oils useful in herbal medicine. Their special value is their ability to control and regulate areas with a high water table, such as bogs and swamps.

The eucalyptus tree was introduced worldwide by a German botanist and explorer, Baron Ferdinand von Muller, director of the Botanical Gardens in Melbourne from 1857 to 1873. These fast growers have been naturalized throughout many areas of the world, including California, Southern Europe, non-tropical areas of South America,

South Africa and India. One negative consequence, however, is that in many areas they threaten to replace indigenous trees.

It was von Muller who first suggested that the oil of the leaves resembled that of cajuput (tea tree oil) and suggested its use as a disinfectant in connection with infectious disease.

Eucalyptus is one of the most powerful natural antiseptics. The aged oil forms ozone, which specifically destroys bacteria, fungi and viruses. An emulsion can be made by mixing equal parts gum Arabic and eucalyptus oil and taking three to five drops every two hours during the acute stages of colds, coughs and flus. An infusion can be made of leaves and taken internally for the same purpose, and most especially for chronic coughs and TB.

Most commonly, the oil is rubbed directly on the chest or back for all respiratory problems. Similarly, it is rubbed as a liniment for the relief of arthritic and rheumatic pains.

Evening primrose
Oenothera biennis
COMMON NAME: Sundrops
FAMILY: Onagraceae
PARTS USED: Leaves, oil from the seed
ENERGY AND FLAVORS: Sweet, cool and nourishing
SYSTEMS AFFECTED: Liver, kidney
BIOCHEMICAL CONSTITUENTS: According to Tyler, the oil contains about 14% of a fixed oil, of which 70% is *cis*-linolenic acid and 9% is gamma-linolenic acid (GLA). GLA is also found in black currant seeds and borage seeds. Oils from all three sources are sold and used interchangeably especially for PMS symptoms.
PROPERTIES: The oil is primarily used as a "Yin tonic" treating inflammatory conditions that arise from a fundamental exhaustion of an organic process. It is especially useful for treating premenstrual syndrome and relieving hypertension and anxiety and associated inflammatory symptoms. Thus it has been used for infantile eczema, painful breasts, hypertension, arthritis, neurotic disorders.
DOSE: Of the oil varies and can range from 250 milligrams or more daily.

Eyebright
Euphrasia officinalis
FAMILY: Scrophulariaceae

PART USED: Aerial portions

ENERGY AND FLAVORS: Bitter, mildly astringent, cool

SYSTEMS AFFECTED: Liver, lung

BIOCHEMICAL CONSTITUENTS: Tannins, iridoid glycosides, including aucubin, phenolic acids, volatile oil

PROPERTIES: Astringent, antiinflammatory, expectorant

DOSE: As indicated.

USED FOR: Conjunctivitis, sinus congestion

NOTES: Eyebright has dry, cooling, antiinflammatory properties. For centuries, it has been used by herbalists for various diseases of the eyes and sinuses. It can be taken either internally or externally in the form of an eyewash. Steep one ounce of the herb in a pint of boiling water, allow to cool and strain. Use an eyecup to rinse the eyes. Dr. Christopher's famous and highly effective eyewash consists of equal parts eyebright, goldenseal, bayberry, raspberry leaves and half part cayenne pepper.

False unicorn

Chamaelirium luteum

COMMON NAME: Helonias

FAMILY: Liliaceae

PART USED: Root

ENERGY AND FLAVORS: Bitter, warm

SYSTEMS AFFECTED: Kidney, spleen, uterus

BIOCHEMICAL CONSTITUENTS: Saponins, glycosides, chamaelirin and helonin, diosgenin

PROPERTIES: Uterine tonic, diuretic, vermifuge, anthelmintic

DOSE: Standard decoction or 10–30 drops of the tincture

NOTES: False unicorn should not be confused with *Helonias bullata*, a Federally listed endangered species.

False unicorn is used for painful and irregular menstruation (dysmenorrhea and amenorrhea), threatened miscarriage and nausea during pregnancy. It is also a good general tonic for the entire genito-urinary tract, good for dyspepsia, anorexia, atony of the sexual organs and aching pain in the lumbosacral region. It is also effective against intestinal worms and parasites.

Garcinia

Garcinia cambogia and *G. indica*

COMMON NAME: Malabar tamarind

FAMILY: Clusiaceae or Guttiferae

PARTS USED: Fruit

ENERGY AND FLAVORS: Cool, sour

SYSTEMS AFFECTED: Spleen, liver

BIOCHEMICAL CONSTITUENTS: Hydroxycitric acid

PROPERTIES: Digestive, alterative, antiinflammatory, vermicide and vermifuge, antidiarrheic, antitumor

DOSE: Garcinia is found in various extracts and commercial products including Planetary Formula's Triphala Herbal Diet. The product marketed as Citrin is a high-quality extract of this herb. It is very safe even for long-term use, but as for all products, follow the recommended protocol.

USED FOR: Weight loss

NOTES: Studies in both India and America have found that the hydroxicitrate of garcinia acts as a botanical analogue to citric acid, which is fundamental to driving the body's metabolic processes through the breakdown and use of carbohydrates and the ultimate synthesis and use of fat. Garcinia is effective because it accelerates fat burning and consequently the buildup of body fat. This is one of the safest herbs to use to inhibit weight gain and to encourage the process of fat burning.

Ginkgo

Ginkgo biloba

COMMON NAMES: Ginkgo nut, Maidenhair tree

FAMILY: Ginkgoaceae

PARTS USED: Leaves and nut

ENERGY AND FLAVOR: Bitter, astringent, neutral energy; nuts are mildly toxic

SYSTEMS AFFECTED: Lungs, kidneys; the leaves have only recently been found to be effective for the brain

BIOCHEMICAL CONSTITUENTS: Flavonoids, including kaempferol, quercitine, isorhamnetine and other glycosides, proanthocyanidines and nonflavonoid terpenes, bilobalide and gingkolides A, B, and C, lignans; essential oil and tannins

PROPERTIES: The nuts are expectorant, antitussive, antiasthmatic, sedative,mildly astringent; the leaf extract seems to have vasoactive properties, especially improving circulation to the brain

DOSE: At least 40 milligrams of the 24% concentrated extract, three times daily for a minimum of three months

USED FOR: Improving blood circulation to the brain, improving peripheral blood circulation, coldness, tinnitus, Alzheimer's and senility, to
improve one's mood and sociability, Raynaud's disease, arthritic and
rheumatic problems, arteriosclerosis, eye weakness caused by poor
circulation, vertigo, anxiety and tension, lung and bronchial congestion

NOTES: While the nut has primarily been used in Chinese medicine for
asthmatic, bronchial and pulmonary conditions, a flavonoid extract
of ginkgo leaf has been discovered to be effective for peripheral blood
circulation and circulation to the brain.

In Europe, several studies were made on geriatric patients. According to herbalist Amanda McQuade, "one study of patients between
the ages of 60 and 80 with senile dementia showed measurable improvement in as little as eight weeks. Treatment with gingko under
four to eight weeks is considered too short to be effective. No side
effects or habituation have been demonstrated using the average dose
of 40mg, three times daily, for three months. Even a single dose of
600mg given experimentally to young women produced no side effects except improved memory."[*]

In her article, Amanda further states how "Gingko is used to treat
or improve memory, mental efficiency, ability to concentrate, sociability and mood especially in the senile and aged." It has been shown
to reduce anxiety, tension, headaches, vertigo, symptoms of senility,
senile dementia, tinnitus, visual problems, Alzheimer's, peripheral
blood disorders such as Raynaud's, postphlebitis and diabetic peripheral vascular disease.

Other uses include those conditions of auditory nerve damage that
can benefit from improved blood flow. In fact, just about any condition that could be ameliorated with increased blood flow is likely to
benefit from the regular use of ginkgo leaf.

The potency of the European extract that has demonstrated effectiveness is a 50-to-1 extract (50 parts of the leaves to make one part
extract). This is then standardized to 24% of the flavone glycosides.
To date, there are literally hundreds of scientific studies attesting to
the benefits of using this 24% concentrated extract.

---

[*]Amanda McQuade, "Strange and Beautiful Gingko," *Let's Live*, vol. 56, #5 (June 1988),
pp. 80–83.

Possible side effects from the use of ginkgo include dermatitis, irritability, restlessness, diarrhea and vomiting, though these are rare.

Goldenseal

Hydrastis canadensis
COMMON NAMES: Puccoon root, Yellowroot
FAMILY: Ranunculaceae
PARTS USED: Rhizome and root
ENERGY AND FLAVORS: Bitter, cold
SYSTEMS AFFECTED: Heart, liver, stomach, colon
BIOCHEMICAL CONSTITUENTS: Hydrastine, berberine, resin, traces of essential oil, chologenic acid, fatty oil, albumin and sugar
PROPERTIES: Alterative, antiinflammatory, bitter tonic, aperient, hemostatic, astringent
USED FOR: Dyspepsia and acid indigestion, gastritis, colitis, duodenal ulcers, menorrhagia and as a general tonic for the female reproductive tract, leucorrhea and penile discharge, eczema and skin disorders
DOSE: One teaspoon of the root simmered in a cup of boiling water ten to twenty minutes or 5–30 drops of the tincture
NOTES: It dries and cleanses the mucus membranes, treats liver diseases such as cirrhosis and hepatitis and is generally used for all inflammations, often combined with other alteratives such as echinacea, garlic, myrrh and chapparal.

Contraindicated during pregnancy and for some cases of hypertension as well as for individuals with internal cold, deficient conditions.

Gravel root

Eupatorium purpureum
COMMON NAMES: Joe-pye weed, Queen of the meadow
FAMILY: Compositae
PART USED: Root
ENERGY AND FLAVORS: Bitter, pungent, neutral
SYSTEMS AFFECTED: Kidney, bladder, stomach and liver
BIOCHEMICAL CONSTITUENTS: Volatile oil, flavonoids, and euparin
PROPERTIES: Diuretic, lithotriptic (dissolves stones), nervine, tonic, antirheumatic, carminative
DOSE: Standard decoction or 3–9 grams; of the tincture, 10–30 drops
USED FOR: Most urinary tract problems, especially those of a more

chronic nature including gravel, stones, hematuria, frequent and nighttime urination. It strengths the nerves of the urinary organs.

Green tea

Thea cinensis, Camellia sinensis

FAMILY: Theaceae

PARTS USED: Young leaves and leaf buds

ENERGY AND FLAVORS: Cool, mildly bitter, pleasant

SYSTEMS AFFECTED: Liver

BIOCHEMICAL CONSTITUENTS: Caffeine, but less than in coffee, and tannins, the main one being epigallocatechin, which, when oxidized in black tea, tend to increase the caffeine bioavailability; flavonoids, including quercitin and kaempferol

PROPERTIES: Stimulant, diuretic, astringent

Because of the tannins in green tea, it is useful for diarrhea. The caffeine content accounts for its stimulant properties. One of the distinguishing uses of tea in contrast to coffee is the traditional one as a stimulant of thought and conversation. Coffee, on the other hand is a more powerful stimulant providing more general alertness and excitement. Perhaps this is only tradition, or perhaps someday we will find a biochemical explanation for this phenomenon. Catechins, other tannins found in green tea, have been shown to have antitumor effects. This is perhaps one of the most interesting recent discoveries about green tea that will certainly encourage more widespread use and appreciation of this beverage.

DOSE: 1 or 2 cups daily

USED FOR: Stimulent, diarrhea, preventing cancer

Guarana

Paullinia cupana

COMMON NAME: Brazilian cocoa

FAMILY: Sapindaceae

PARTS USED: Crushed seeds

ENERGY AND FLAVORS: Bitter, warm energy

SYSTEMS AFFECTED: Kidneys and adrenals

BIOCHEMICAL CONSTITUENTS: Guarana is considered the highest known worldwide source of caffeine. Having 2.5 times the caffeine content of coffee, it therefore also has the entire negative effects and symptoms of heavy coffee drinking. Guarana, like coffee and another caffeine-rich plant, yerba mate, also originates in South America. It is uniquely a rich source of guaranine, another alkaloid like caffeine that can stimulate long, slow endurance.

PROPERTIES: Stimulant, nervine, aphrodisiac, febrifuge, narcotic (slight).
It is used as a mild stimulant but is stronger than coffee.

DOSE: 1–2 teaspoons infused in 1 cup

USED FOR: Stimulant

Gymnema sylvestre
Asclepias geminata

COMMON NAME: Gurmar, Hindi name meaning "sugar taste destroyer"

FAMILY: Asclepiadaceae

PARTS USED: Leaves

ENERGY AND FLAVORS: Cool, sweetish and slightly sour

SYSTEMS AFFECTED: Spleen, pancreas

BIOCHEMICAL CONSTITUENTS: Gymnemic acid, which may be a glucoside that has antisaccharine properties; bitter neutral principle; albuminous and coloring matters; calcium oxalate; parabin; glucose; carbohydrates; some tartaric acid

PROPERTIES: Digestive, tonic, astringent, refrigerant, diuretic

Gymnema has the unique property of inhibiting the taste of sugar. Because it has molecular structure similar to that of sugar, it blocks up to 50% of the absorption of sugar. In doing so, it will not effect the taste of food but will suppress the desire for sweets. This makes it an ideal herb to use for the treatment of diabetes along with the Ayurvedic mineral compound called *shilajit* and/or in combination with GTF chromium to help stabilize blood sugar. To experience its effects, first taste something sweet, then swish gymnema tea in the mouth for 20–30 seconds and taste something sweet again. You will find that the gymnema has blocked the perception of sweetness in the mouth and may therefore block the absorption of sweet in the digestive system, although this is not fully known. As an antidiabetic herb, gymnema apparently works by enhancing the endogenous production of insulin. It is therefore a good herb to take after indulging in sweets to block sugar absorption in those with either type I and type II diabetes. As a result, gymnema can treat of a wide variety of digestive diseases and diseases resulting from the use of sugar, such as hyperactivity, allergies, anemia, cholesterol, diabetes, obesity, urinary tract infections, and hypoglycemia. Gymnema is a regulator and will exert its blood sugar–lowering effects only in cases of diabetes.

DOSE: At least 400 milligrams of gymnema extract per day for those with either type I or type II diabetes

USED FOR: Blocking sugar cravings, diabetes, obesity

Horse chestnut
Aesculus hippocastanum
FAMILY: Hippocasatanaceae
PARTS USED: Bark and fruit
ENERGY AND FLAVOR: Neutral, bitter
SYSTEMS AFFECTED: Intestines
BIOCHEMICAL CONSTITUENTS: Bark—aesculin, ash, and tannin; seeds— phytosterol, starch sugar, and linoleic, palmitic, and stearic acids
PROPERTIES: The bark is tonic, narcotic, and a febrifuge.

The bark is used for intermittent fevers and externally for ulcers and sores. The fruit is used for rectal problems, such as hemorrhoids, as well as for other problems of a rheumatic and neuralgic nature.

DOSE: Of the bark: simmer 1 ounce in 1 pint of water for 20 minutes. Take only 1 tablespoon three or four times daily. Of the fruit: make a tincture with the ground-up fruits and take 5–20 drops three times daily.

USED FOR: Hemorrhoids, rectal diseases

Iceland moss
Cetraria islandica
COMMON NAME: Iceland lichen
FAMILY: Parmeliaceae
PARTS USED: Lichen
ENERGY AND FLAVORS: Sweet, bland, cool
SYSTEMS AFFECTED: Lungs, stomach
BIOCHEMICAL CONSTITUENTS: Mucins, bitter fumaric acids, usnic acids, some iodine, polysaccharides
PROPERTIES: Demulcent, pectoral, antiemetic, nutritive tonic
DOSE: Take freely as needed
NOTES: Iceland moss can be used as a survival food. Medicinally, it is commonly used for lung weakness and other upper-respiratory problems associated with degenerative wasting. It is either decocted or rendered into a syrup together with Irish moss and comfrey root for all these conditions. It should be made into a decoction.

Ipecacuanha

Cephaelis ipecacuanha

COMMON NAME: Ipecac

FAMILY: Rubiaceae

PART USED: Root

ENERGY AND FLAVORS: Bitter, nauseating, cold

SYSTEMS AFFECTED: Lungs, liver

BIOCHEMICAL CONSTITUENTS: Isoquinoline alkaloids, tannins, glycosides, saponins, starch, choline and resins

PROPERTIES: Emetic, expectorant, amoebicide, diaphoretic, stimulant

DOSE: One-half to one teaspoon or as indicated

USED FOR: Vomiting up food poisons, amoebas, phlegm in the lungs

NOTES: Ipecac is easily obtained as syrup of ipecac from most pharmacies. Its primary use is as an emetic against organic noncaustic poisons such as food poisoning. It should never be used for caustic poisons, however, as any attempt to vomit back the poison may result in serious danger to the esophagus. Emesis can also be employed as a way of relieving severe lung and bronchial congestion and for the relief of asthma. Usually a teaspoon is sufficient to produce easy emetic action within 10 to 20 minutes after ingesting. Smaller doses can be used as an expectorant as well as a treatment against intestinal amoebas.

Irish moss

Chondrus crispus

COMMON NAMES: Carrageenin

FAMILY: Gigartinaceae

PARTS USED: Seaweed

ENERGY AND FLAVORS: Sweet, salty, cool

SYSTEMS AFFECTED: Lungs, stomach

BIOCHEMICAL CONSTITUENTS: Polysaccharides, proteins, mucins, amino acids, iodine, bromine and manganese salts

PROPERTIES: Demulcent, nutrient, emollient

Irish moss is used for lung diseases associated with dryness and/or wasting. It is also used topically or internally for ulcers and sores. It is commonly prepared as a syrup with Iceland moss and blackstrap molasses.

DOSE: 3 to 9 grams

USED FOR: Lung diseases associated with dryness, tuberculosis, sores and ulcers

Japanese turf lily

Ophiopogon japonicus
COMMON NAMES: Creeping lily root, dwarf lilyturf
FAMILY: Liliaceae
PART USED: Bulbs
ENERGY AND FLAVORS: Sweet, slightly bitter, slightly cool
SYSTEMS AFFECTED: Heart, lung, stomach
BIOCHEMICAL CONSTITUENTS: Ruscogenin (steroid sapogenin), sitosterol, stigmasterol, sitosterol-D-glucoside, ophioside, sugars, mucilage
PROPERTIES: Demulcent, nutrient tonic, Yin tonic
DOSE: 6–12 grams in decoction
NOTES: This is another grasslike ornamental grown in many gardens throughout the world. Its tonic therapeutic value makes it worth pointing out. Since the flavor of these little bulblets is not at all unpleasant, it is a good idea to consider including a few of them in soups for their therapeutic value.

Japanese turf lily is used for any symptoms associated with dryness, lack of vital fluids, including general depletion of bodily fluids, dryness of the heart, skin and dry stool. It is especially useful for dry cough, asthma or with spitting of blood.

Because of its deep nourishing properties, it gives one a sense of inner well-being, strength, and thus will lessen palpitations, insomnia and general paranoia and fearfulness.

It is contraindicated when one has a particular tendency toward cold sensitivity, diarrhea or loose stools. However, the contraindication is only with regard to long-term use.

Juniper

Juniperus communis
FAMILY: Cupressaceae
PART USED: Berries
ENERGY AND FLAVORS: Spicy, sweet, warm
SYSTEMS AFFECTED: Kidneys and stomach
BIOCHEMICAL CONSTITUENTS: Volatile oil, various sugars, resin, vitamin C
PROPERTIES: Diuretic, carminative, antiseptic, stimulant
DOSE: Steep one teaspoon in a cup of boiling water for twenty minutes, covered, take one cup three times daily; of the tincture, take 10–30 drops three times daily
USED FOR: Urinary problems, gout, rheumatic complaints, flatulence
Avoid internal use during pregnancy.

Notes: Juniper berries are primarily used for the treatment of urinary problems, including urine retention, stones and gravel, lumbar pains, uric acid buildup and gout and rheumatic problems. Four to six drops of the oil taken with honey three or four times a day has been a successful home remedy for these ailments. It is antiinflammatory for arthritic and rheumatic ailments as well as being a useful carminative for indigestion and flatulence. It was traditionally the primary flavoring in gin.

Kava kava

Piper methysticum

Common Name: Kawa

Family: Piperaceae

Part Used: Root

Energy and Flavors: Pungent, bitter, warm

Systems Affected: Liver, kidneys

Biochemical Constituents: Resin including lactones, kawahin, yangonin, methysticin, glycosides, starch

Properties: Antispasmodic, stimulant, diuretic, antifungal, analgesic, muscle relaxant, anesthetic, anticonvulsant

Dose: 2–4 grams or 10–50 drops. To induce a tranquil, euphoric state, up to 150 drops of the fluid extract can be occasionally (not regularly) taken. The Polynesians have found that large, frequent doses of kava kava can cause dry skin and bloodshot eyes. These symptoms disappear after use is discontinued.

Notes: Kava kava is a traditional popular Polynesian herb made from the dried lateral root of the kava tree (called *waka* by the natives). It is used medicinally, ritually, and recreationally by the Polynesian people. Its use, according to herbalist Ed Smith, is as a "mild tranquilizer to relax the mind and clarify the thought processes, soothe the temperament, and induce a mild euphoria with feelings of peace and harmony." This makes it the ideal herb to take before and during intense conferences and negotiations. He further states, "It is usually taken with a group of people together to enhance sociability and evoke feelings of empathy and camaraderie, and is often used to facilitate reconciliation. In Europe, kava is an approved phytomedicine which is used to treat anxiety and despondency." (Ed Smith is a founding member of the American Herbalists Guild and of Herb Pharm Products.)

Planetary Formulas combines kava kava with St.-John's-wort and a traditional Chinese formula for depression and anxiety in a product called Kava–St.-John's-wort Complex.

Khella

Ammi visnaga
FAMILY: Apiaceae or Umbelliferae
PARTS USED: Seeds
ENERGY AND FLAVORS: Warm, spicy, acrid
SYSTEMS AFFECTED: Heart, lungs, bladder, liver, gallbladder
BIOCHEMICAL CONSTITUENTS: Seeds contain a fatty oil including khellin
PROPERTIES: Relaxant and antispasmodic
DOSE: 6–9 grams of the seeds in decoction or ½–1 teaspoon of the alcoholic extract
USED FOR: Asthma, angina, vitiligo, contraception (after intercourse)
NOTES: For heart problems, khella may need to be taken several weeks before its positive effects are seen

First mentioned in the Ebers papyrus circa 1550 B.C., khella is a smooth-muscle relaxant that can relieve spasms of the gallbladder, bile duct, and urinary bladder. As such, it relieves urinary pains from stones, aiding in their elimination, as well as the pain associated with gallstones. It is a well-known preventive for asthma attacks when taken in the evening before retiring. Research on the effectiveness of khella for asthma led to the formulation of many commercial drug products in the 1950s. It may not be so effective, however, during an acute asthma attack. Because of its antispasmodic properties, it is generally useful for all spastic coughs. For upper-respiratory problems, khella works best when combined with other respiratory herbs, such as lobelia, thyme, and wild cherry bark. Also because of its antispasmodic properties, khella is effective for relieving menstrual cramps.

One of its most important uses is for the heart. Since the 1940s, the clinical effectiveness of khella at relieving the symptoms of angina have been well documented. Khellin, derived from the plant, is a safe and effective drug in relieving angina symptoms, improving the heart's ability to tolerate exercise and in normalizing electrocardiogram results.

A closely related species, *A. majus,* is cultivated in India for the treatment of vitiligo (blotchy skin) because of its high concentration of psoralen. (This is also found in a Chinese herb used for the same purpose—*Psoralea corylifolia*, called *bu gu zhi*). Psoralen is also effective for psoriasis; the production of pigment is stimulated when the skin is exposed to ultraviolet light.

Khella also has a long history as a contraceptive. The ground seeds, taken after intercourse, are used to prevent the implantation of the fertilized ovum in the uterus.

Kola nut

Cola acuminata and *C. nitida*

COMMON NAMES: Cola, Guru nut

FAMILY: Sterculiaceae

PART USED: Seed

ENERGY AND FLAVORS: Bitter, warm

SYSTEMS AFFECTED: Kidney-adrenals, heart, liver

BIOCHEMICAL CONSTITUENTS: Caffeine (up to 2.5%), theobronine, tannins, phenolics, coloring matter, betaine, protein, starch

PROPERTIES: Stimulant, diuretic, cardiac tonic, antidepressive, astringent

DOSE: 1–3 grams; of the tincture 5–15 drops

USED FOR: Tiredness and fatigue

NOTES: The active ingredient in kola nut is caffeine. It is used both for its stimulating action as well as its flavor and color in various soft drinks. Its use for depression and fatigue, therefore, is purely symptomatic. A continual reliance on such symptomatic treatments as this and others such as coffee or tea (*Camellia sinensis*) for tiredness and fatigue is bound to deplete further the body's reserves, setting one up for more chronic degenerative conditions. Fatigue and tiredness usually have a cause that should be discovered and treated at a deeper level with diet, herbs and appropriate physiotherapy and lifestyle adjustments.

Lady's mantle

Alchemilla xanthochlora (*A. vulgaris*)

FAMILY: Rosaceae

PART USED: Aerial portions

ENERGY AND FLAVORS: Bitter, astringent flavors with cool energy

SYSTEMS AFFECTED: Uterus, spleen, kidneys

BIOCHEMICAL CONSTITUENTS: Tannin, glycoside, salicylic acid and other unidentified substances

PROPERTIES: Astringent, febrifuge

DOSE: 3–9 grams in decoction or 10–30 drops of the tincture

USED FOR: Excessive menstrual bleeding, diarrhea, wounds, bleeding and injuries

NOTES: Lady's mantle is used for excessive menstrual bleeding, leucorrhea, diarrhea, enteritis and as a wash or poultice for wounds.

Lady's slipper

Cypripedium calceoulus var. *pubescens*

COMMON NAME: Nerveroot

FAMILY: Orchidaceae

PART USED: Root

ENERGY AND FLAVORS: Bitter, pungent, neutral

SYSTEMS AFFECTED: Heart, liver, nerves

BIOCHEMICAL CONSTITUENTS: Volatile oil, volatile acid, tannic and gallic acids, resins and salts

PROPERTIES: Nervine, sedative, antispasmodic

DOSE: 3–9 grams; of the tincture, 10–30 drops

USED FOR: Nervousness

NOTES: One of the purest nervines used for anxiety, stress, insomnia, neurosis, restlessness, tremors, epilepsy and palpitations. It is also useful for depression. It is now considered an endangered species and should not be used commercially until it can be cultivated.

Larkspur

Consolida regalis (Delphinium consolida)

FAMILY: Ranunculaceae

PART USED: Seeds

ENERGY AND FLAVORS: Acrid poison

SYSTEMS AFFECTED: Primarily used externally

BIOCHEMICAL CONSTITUENTS: Poisonous diterpene alkaloids similar to those found in aconite

PROPERTIES: Parasiticide, insecticide

USED EXTERNALLY FOR: Lice, crabs and nits

NOTES: A tincture of larkspur is used as a treatment for nits and lice on the skin and hair. It should never be taken internally as it is a dangerous poison.

Lavender

Lavandula angustifolia, L. officinalis

COMMON NAMES: Garden lavender

FAMILY: Labiatae

PART USED: Flowers

ENERGY AND FLAVORS: Spicy, fragrant, mildly bitter, cool

SYSTEMS AFFECTED: Lungs, liver

BIOCHEMICAL CONSTITUENTS: Volatile oil including linalool, lavandulyl acetate, borneol, camphor, limonene, cadinene, coumarins, ursolic acid, flavonoids (luteolin)

PROPERTIES: Aromatic, carminative, antispasmodic, antidepressant

DOSE: Standard infusion or 10–30 drops of the tincture

NOTES: Lavender is extensively used in perfumery. Spike lavender, which contains higher amounts of camphor and cineole, is used as an insect and moth repellant. It is usually placed in drawers to protect clothing from attack by moths.

Its use as a nervine and antidepressant is in keeping with the general tendency of plants with blue or purplish flowers to have cooling and nervine properties. A good formula for emotional upset and nervous depression is as follows: equal parts lavender flowers, lemon balm, skullcap, camomile and half part each of licorice and ginger roots. Steep one ounce in a pint of boiling water, covered, twenty minutes and take one cup two or three times daily or as needed.

Lemon balm

Melissa officinalis

COMMON NAMES: Melissa, Balm

FAMILY: Labiatae

PART USED: Leaves

ENERGY AND FLAVORS: Sour, spicy, cool

SYSTEMS AFFECTED: Lungs, liver

BIOCHEMICAL CONSTITUENTS: Essential oil, bitter principle, acids, tannin

PROPERTIES: Diaphoretic, calmative, antispasmodic, carminative, emmenagogue, stomachic

DOSE: Steep one ounce in a pint of boiling water, covered, and sweetened to taste if desired; take freely as needed

USED FOR: Fevers, depression and melancholy, nervous tension, helping digestion

EXTERNALLY FOR: Herpes simplex

NOTES: The best application of lemon balm is as a calming diaphoretic for the treatment of fevers. Because of its gentle properties and pleasant flavor, it is most suitable for children and those who tend to be sensitive to the strong bitter flavors of most herbs. Since it removes surface tension from the body, it is effective as a treatment for nervous tension and depression. Lemon balm can also be used like other mints, for upset stomach and gas.

Most recently an external ointment made with lemon balm leaves has demonstrated a high degree of effectiveness in relieving the symptoms of herpes simplex.

Lily of the valley
Convallaria majalis
COMMON NAME: May lily
FAMILY: Liliaceae
PARTS USED: Leaves and whole plant
ENERGY AND FLAVORS: Sweet, bitter, neutral, mildly toxic
SYSTEMS AFFECTED: Heart, kidney
BIOCHEMICAL CONSTITUENTS: Cardiac glycosides, saponins, convallarin and convallaric acid, asparagin, chelidonic acid and various other organic acids
PROPERTIES: Cardiac tonic, diuretic, antispasmodic
DOSE: 150 milligrams of the dried leaf or 1–3 drops of the tincture
Lily of the valley is classed as a poison and should not be used without professional guidance.
NOTES: Lily of the valley has properties similar but milder and much less accumulative than digitalis. One of the problems in using digitalis (foxglove) is determining the correct dose since it is accumulative and potentially fatal if taken in overdose. It is a good practice, according to herbalist Ed Smith, to treat congestive heart failure first for one or two days with digitalis and then to use the safer lily-of-the-valley extract for ongoing maintenance. Of course, at this stage, it is likely to be a serious disease that one should not treat oneself or without professional guidance. Nevertheless, this advice is offered for consideration for those who are licensed medical professionals.

Linden flowers
Tilia platyphyllos
COMMON NAME: Lime flowers
FAMILY: Tiliaceae
PART USED: Flowers
ENERGY AND FLAVORS: Cool, energy
SYSTEMS AFFECTED: Liver, nerves, digestion

BIOCHEMICAL CONSTITUENTS: Volatile oil, flavonoids including hesperidin, quercitin, astralagin and others; mucilage, phenolic acids, tannins

PROPERTIES: Nervine, hypotensive, calming tonic

DOSE: Standard infusion of one ounce steeped in a pint of boiling water for 10–20 minutes; take as often as desired

USED FOR: Colds, influenza, fevers, headaches, hypertension

NOTES: In Europe, linden flowers are commonly used as an herbal beverage tea second only to camomile, with which it combines very well. This is because of both its fine aroma and flavor, especially when sweetened with a little honey. The simple combination of equal parts camomile and linden flowers is an ideal home remedy for the entire family for the treatment of influenzas, colds, common headaches and menstrual discomfort. The flavor is rather pleasant and thus it will readily be taken by those who are adverse to bitter-tasting teas.

In one study (described by Rudoph Weiss, *Herbal Medicine*) conducted by two pediatricians (Traismann and Hardy) at the University of Chicago, fifty-five children with influenza symptoms were treated with bed rest and at most one or two aspirins a day. Thirty-seven were, in addition to this, given sulphonamides, and still another sixty-seven had only antibiotics. The two pediatricians conducting the study were surprised that the children taking only linden blossom tea and bed rest recovered most quickly with the fewest complications (middle ear infections). Those given chemotherapy and antibiotics took longer with more complications. Linden blossom tea was ten times more effective on the average.

One of the best diaphoretic combinations for colds, flus and fevers is equal parts linden blossoms, camomile and elder blossoms. One could add or substitute red clover blossoms or lemon balm for any one of these if desired.

Lobelia
Lobelia inflata

COMMON NAMES: Indian tobacco, Pukeweed

FAMILY: Lobeliaceae

PARTS USED: Leaf and seeds

ENERGY AND FLAVORS: Bitter, neutral

SYSTEMS AFFECTED: Liver, nerves

BIOCHEMICAL CONSTITUENTS: Various alkaloids including lobeline, which has similar effects to nicotine, making it useful in antismoking regimes

PROPERTIES: Expectorant, stimulant, antispasmodic, emetic
DOSE: 3–15 grams; of the tincture, 5–15 drops
USED FOR: Asthma, spasmodic coughs, spasms and tetany, food poisoning (vomit), catalyst for other herbs in formula
NOTES: Lobelia is primarily employed for asthma, bronchitis, spasmodic coughs and upper-respiratory complaints. It is also useful for spasmodic neurological problems and is one of the fastest-acting herbal antispasmodics known. Thus many old-time herbalists commonly added it in small amounts to serve as a catalyst preparing the body to better accept and utilize the major ingredients in a formula.

An aura of controversy has always surrounded the possibility of lobelia toxicity. In my own experience, I have found no problem in its use, which corroborates the experience of the late Dr. Christopher and hundreds of herbalists and doctors before him.

Lobelia is one of the best herbs to use as an emetic and can be useful during the height of an asthmatic attack. The best method I have found is to use acid tincture of lobelia made with apple-cider vinegar. Begin by drinking a large volume of lukewarm mint tea and follow by taking one teaspoon of lobelia tincture every ten minutes for three or four times or until emesis ensues. The lobelia will promote vomiting and leave the body perfectly relaxed.

Externally, it can be applied to bruises, sprains, insect bites, tumors and cancers.

Loquat

Eriobotrya japonica
FAMILY: Rosaceae
PARTS USED: Leaves, fruit
ENERGY AND FLAVORS: Bitter, neutral
SYSTEMS AFFECTED: Lungs, stomach
BIOCHEMICAL CONSTITUENTS: Amygdalin, nerolidol, farnesol
PROPERTIES: Antitussive, expectorant, antiinflammatory
DOSE: 6–15 grams in cold-water infusion
LOQUAT FRUIT IS USED FOR: Nutrient
LOQUAT LEAVES ARE USED FOR: Coughs, upper-respiratory problems
NOTES: The leaves are used for coughs, lung and bronchioles inflammation, mucus and phlegm in the lungs, hiccoughs, vomiting and belching. Loquat is readily available as it grows in gardens throughout the country. Generally speaking, amygdalin, the active constituent of

loquat leaves, is found in apricot kernel and wild cherry bark, two other similar herbs used to quiet and lower the cough reflux. One possible error in their use, both in traditional Chinese medicine and by many in the West, is to boil or cook. It has been demonstrated that the active constituents of these plants are better extracted in a cool-water infusion. Soak the loquat leaves, apricot seeds, or wild cherry bark overnight in cool water. The active ingredients leach out and will yield an almondlike scent and flavor, which is the amygdalin. This can then be lightly warmed or mixed with honey or brown-sugar syrup.

Malva

Malva sylvestris and other species

COMMON NAMES: Cheeses, Marshmallow root (*Althea officinalis*), Hollyhock (*Athea rosea*)

FAMILY: Malvaceae

PARTS USED: Leaves, flowers and root

ENERGY AND FLAVORS: Cool energy, sweetish, bland taste

SYSTEMS AFFECTED: Lungs, stomach

BIOCHEMICAL CONSTITUENTS: Mucilage, anthocyanidins, starch, vitamin A, and other nutrients

PROPERTIES: Demulcent, nutritive, alterative, diuretic, vulnerary, mild laxative

DOSE: Two ounces covered and steeped in a quart of boiled, hot water

USED FOR: Inflammations, irritations, ulcers and sores, urinary and gall stones

NOTES: Malva and hollyhock have similar properties, with marshmallow root having by far the greater amount of starchy mucilage, which is the primary therapeutic ingredient of the plants (along with chlorophyll and vitamin A). Malva, being milder, is more suitable as a potherb and is commonly used by people in countries where it grows. The tender leaves can be lightly steamed and served as a spring potherb.

These plants all have soothing, demulcent, antiinflammatory properties that relieve irritations and promote healing when applied either internally, or externally in the form of a poultice. They are used for ulcers, intractable sores (such as bedsores), stomach disorders and to soothe the pain of urinary and gall stones. Externally, make a poultice using the moist ground or pulverized root with a small amount of cayenne as a catalyst to heal blood poisoning, gangrene, septic wounds, intractable sores, burns and bruises. This should first be lightly steamed and applied warm and moist and changed three times daily. It is very effective when used along with frequent internal doses of echinacea.

Marshmallow root is generally combined with other diuretic herbs such as parsley root, gravel root and juniper berries to aid in relieving the pain of, and breaking down and expelling, urinary stones and gravel. It is also combined with laxative herbs for chronic constipation. Finally, it is used for irritations associated with diarrhea and dysentery.

Mayapple

Podophyllum peltatum

COMMON NAMES: Mandrake, Devil's-apple

FAMILY: Berberidaceae

PARTS USED: Dried rhizome and resinous extract

SYSTEMS AFFECTED: Liver, colon

BIOCHEMICAL CONSTITUENTS: A neutral crystalline substance, podophyllo-toxins, an amorphous resin, picropodophyllim, quercitin, starch, sugar, fat and yellow coloring matter

PROPERTIES: Cathartic laxative, hepatic tonic, cholagogue, alterative, emetic, stimulant, counterirritant

DOSE: 10–30 grains of the powdered root or 1–10 drops of the tincture, once or twice daily; in formulas, 1–3 grams

USED FOR: Liver congestion, constipation, externally for warts

Avoid use during pregnancy. Mayapple is a poisonous plant that should be used only under supervision of a qualified health care provider.

NOTES: Mayapple is a powerful glandular stimulant that should be taken in small doses and with great respect for its potency. It is excellent for the treatment of chronic liver diseases, skin eruptions, bile imbalances and obstructions in digestion and elimination. It is best taken in small doses in combination with such supporting herbs as Oregon grape or barberry root, ginger and licorice.

Externally, the concentrated tincture (obtained by gently cooking down the tea and adding 20% alcohol to preserve it) is applied topically to remove warts. A prescription drug, podophyllin, is the resinous black extract and is commonly prescribed for venereal warts.

Care should be taken to apply this only to the wart and to avoid contact with the surrounding skin. Large doses, even externally applied, are potentially toxic.

Melilot
Melilotus officinalis
COMMON NAMES: Sweet melilot, Common melilot, Ribbed melilot
FAMILY: Leguminosae
PARTS USED: Aerial portions
ENERGY AND FLAVORS: Cool, sweet
SYSTEMS AFFECTED: Veins and circulatory system
BIOCHEMICAL CONSTITUENTS: Coumarin and flavones
PROPERTIES: Antirheumatic, antispasmodic, analgesic, aromatic, carminative

Because of the blood-thinning properties of its coumarin constituents, melilot directs its energy to the veins and can be used to enhance circulation and relieve varicose veins and thrombophlebitis. It also helps lymphatic circulation and can be used to relieve lymphedema. Finally, it is a very effective adjuvant with other herbs, such as black cohosh, sarsaparilla, and sassafras for arthritic and rheumatic problems. Do not take it if you have anemia or are using prescription blood thinners.

DOSE: Infuse 1–2 teaspoons in 1 cup of boiling water for 20 minutes. Take 3 cups daily.
USED FOR: Rheumatic problems, improving circulation, promoting lymphatic drainage

Milk thistle
Silybum marianum, Carduus marianus
COMMON NAME: St.-Mary's-thistle
FAMILY: Compositae
PARTS USED: Seeds and aerial portions
ENERGY AND FLAVORS: Bitter, sweet, cool energy
SYSTEMS AFFECTED: Liver, spleen
BIOCHEMICAL CONSTITUENTS: Flavolignans that are collectively known as silymarin.
PROPERTIES: Hepatoprotective, bitter tonic, demulcent, antidepressant
DOSE: 420 milligrams daily
NOTES: An extract of the seeds of milk thistle has been shown to be conclusively liver protective and regenerative even against one of the

most virulent liver toxins known, the death cap mushroom (*Amanita phalloides*). In its early stages of growth, this mushroom resembles the common agaricus and is mistakenly eaten. The result is usually fatal, especially since the fatal condition seems to develop slowly over a few days. Pretreatment of animals with silymarin and silybin gives 100% protection against this poison.

Milk thistle is also effective against chronic liver cirrhosis, necroses and hepatitis A and B. It is hypolipidaemic and lowers fat deposits in the liver of animals.

Motherwort

Leonurus cardiaca
COMMON NAME: Lion's-tail
FAMILY: Labiatae
PART USED: Leaves
ENERGY AND FLAVORS: Bitter, spicy, slightly cold
SYSTEMS AFFECTED: Pericardium, liver
BIOCHEMICAL CONSTITUENTS: Iridoids, leonurin, bitter principle and bitter glycosides, alkaloids, flavonoids, rutin, tannin, essential oil, resin, organic acids
PROPERTIES: Emmenagogue, cardiac tonic, antispasmodic, nervine, diuretic, carminative
DOSE: Standard infusion of one ounce to a pint of boiling water or 10–30 drops of the tincture three times daily
USED FOR: Suppressed menstruation, promote blood circulation, heart problems and arteriosclerosis, nervousness and insomnia
NOTES: Motherwort is useful for suppressed menstruation and other female disorders. For blood congestion and painful menstruation, one can combine equal parts motherwort, tang kuei, calendula and cramp bark.

It is also a good heart tonic. It promotes blood circulation, helps to remove arteriosclerosis and dissolve blood clots, and resultant symptoms of heart dysfunction including angina, palpitations and heart neuralgia.

Since it also has nervine properties, it is good for treating various neurotic conditions as well as hysteria, convulsions and insomnia.

Its emmenagogic or menses promoting powers made it historically useful to ancient Chinese courtesans, who called it IMU. They would take it on a daily basis to prevent pregnancy and to protect themselves against venereal disease.

Avoid internal use during pregnancy.

Mugwort

Artemisia vulgaris

COMMON NAME: Moxa

FAMILY: Compositae

PART USED: Leaves

ENERGY AND FLAVORS: Bitter, acrid, slightly warm

SYSTEMS AFFECTED: Spleen, liver, kidney

BIOCHEMICAL CONSTITUENTS: Essential oil, cineole, thujone, bitter principle

PROPERTIES: Cholagogue, vermifuge, emmenagogue, hemostatic, antispasmodic, diaphoretic, mild narcotic, bitter tonic

DOSE: 3–9 grams in infusion or 5–20 drops of the tincture

USED FOR: Liver, stomach and intestinal problems, worms, promote menses, calm nervousness, moxa, for ritual purification

NOTES: Mugwort is an excellent nervine for uncontrollable shaking, nervousness and insomnia. It may be taken as a tea, using an ounce of the herb to a pint of water steeped twenty minutes. The dose is one tablespoon three times daily. Mugwort can also be smoked, filling the lungs three to six times.

The tea or alcoholic tincture is used for treating liver and stomach disorders, and for this purpose it is diluted three times to help overcome the strong bitter taste. (It may be taken hot to induce sweating.) The tea was used by the Native Americans for colds and flus, bronchitis and fevers.

Mugwort has strong emmenagogic properties and can be used to help induce menses. As such, it can be combined with other herbs such as cramp bark for the treatment of menstrual cramps. It should be avoided during pregnancy.

The Chinese dry and render into a cottony mass a species of mugwort that is then burned directly on the skin in a therapeutic technique called moxabustion. Mugwort is ideally suited for this because of its cottonlike consistency and also because its volatile oils help promote blood circulation, relax the underlying nerves and burn quickly at a low temperature. Usually anywhere from three or more small red-bean-sized cones are rolled into a pyramid shape and lit with an incense stick and allowed to burn down to the skin. This powerfully stimulates the immune system and associated meridians or nervous system depending upon the acupuncture point selected. It is specifically indicated for all conditions associated with coldness and deficiency and as such has a better effect than the use of needles. A common alternative to the direct burning on the skin is to roll the moxa into a cigar shape and lighting one end, pass it in a clockwise motion over a specific point or area until it becomes hot. This is repeated several times and is effective in removing chronic cold spasms and pains including the pains of injuries.

The ash of mugwort or wormwood can be applied topically or drunk internally to stop hemorrhage and bleeding.

The crumpled dried leaves are ritualistically burned in a large sea-shell by Native Americans to "smudge" or purify bad spirits.

Wormwood (*Artemisia absinthium*) has similar properties and the tincture can be taken three times daily when traveling to tropical countries to prevent malaria. It can also be taken as a bitter stomachic, like mugwort, and used for stomach and intestinal complaints including worms and parasites.

Avoid internal use during pregnancy.

Muira puama
Dulaciainopiflora, Liriosma ovata
COMMON NAMES: Marapuama, Potentwood
FAMILY: Oleceae
PARTS USED: Roots, bark, wood, balsam
ENERGY AND FLAVORS: Warm, astringent, spicy
SYSTEMS AFFECTED: Kidneys
BIOCHEMICAL CONSTITUENTS: Various alkaloids and sterols
PROPERTIES: Stimulant; mild aphrodisiac especially for women, but also
   useful for impotence and diarrhea
DOSE: 10–30 drops of the fluid extract, two or three times daily or 1
   hour before lovemaking
USED FOR: Aphrodisiac, impotence, diarrhea

Mulberry
Morus alba
COMMON NAME: White mulberry
FAMILY: Moraceae

PARTS USED: Fruit, leaves, twigs, root bark

ENERGY AND FLAVOR:

OF FRUIT: Sweet, slightly cool

OF LEAVES: Bitter, sweet, cool

OF TWIGS: Bitter, neutral

OF ROOT BARK: Sweet, cold

SYSTEMS AFFECTED:

BY FRUIT: Kidney-adrenals, liver, heart

BY LEAVES: Lungs, liver

BY TWIGS: Liver

BY ROOT BARK: Lungs

BIOCHEMICAL CONSTITUENTS: The fruit contains 27% saccharides, 3% citric acid, vitamin C; the leaves contain carotene, succinic acid, adenine, choline, amylase; the root bark contains flavonoid (morusin, mulberrin, mulberrochromene, kuwanone-A, -B, cyclomorusin), coumarin (scopoletin, umbelliferone), triterpenoid, tannin.

NOTES: Mulberry fruit is a Yin and blood tonic with demulcent nutritive properties. It is used for symptoms of hypersensitivity, nervousness, anemia, dizziness, tinnitus caused by weakness and deficiency, hypertension, dry constipation. It is contrindicated for someone with a tendency towards diarrhea. Dose, 15–30 grams.

Mulberry root bark is an expectorant, antitussive and is used primarily to clear inflammation of the lungs. It helps stop coughs, reduces and then helps bring up phlegm, and lowers hypertension. It is contraindicated for someone whose cough is caused by coldness. Dose, 9–18 grams in decoction.

Mulberry leaf is a cooling and calming diaphoretic and is used for feverish colds, headache, sore throat, acute conjunctivitis and vomiting of blood. It is contraindicated for someone with a cold, weak condition of the lungs with low vital energy. Dose, 5–10 grams.

Mulberry branch is primarily used as an antirheumatic and antispasmodic for the treatment of arthritic and rheumatic problems as well as hypertension. Dose, 9–15 grams.

Even the mistletoe growing on the mulberry tree has positive therapeutic properties not unlike European mistletoe (*Viscum album*). Both are used for hypertension and are classified as being antispasmodic and antirheumatic. Both have analgesic and anticarcinogenic properties. They are used for hypertension and to relieve rheumatic pains and spasms especially of the upper part of the body. Dose, 9–15 grams.

Mullein

Verbascum thapsus

FAMILY: Scrophulariaceae

PARTS USED: Leaf, flower, root

SYSTEMS AFFECTED: Lungs, stomach

BIOCHEMICAL CONSTITUENTS: Mucilage, flavonoids, rutin, saponins, aucubin, traces of essential oil

PROPERTIES: Expectorant, demulcent, antispasmodic, antitussive, astringent, anodyne, vulnerary

DOSE: Standard infusion or 3–9 grams of the leaves; of the tincture, 10–30 drops

USED FOR: Lung and bronchial congestion, spasmodic coughs, sore, irritated throat, flowers for earaches, lymphatic congestion

NOTES: Mullein may be smoked for the treatment of lung and bronchial congestion and coughs. For the same purpose, a tea is made combining yerba santa, wild cherry bark, licorice root and elecampane.

Mullein flower oil is made by macerating the flowers of mullein in olive oil. This is press-strained through a cloth and a few drops inserted in each ear with a wad of cotton each night for earaches.

The root can be made into a tea and used for lymphatic congestion, cramps and diarrhea.

Myrobalans

COMMON NAMES: Chebulic M. "Haritaki," Emblic M. "Amlaki," Berelic M. "Bishitaki"

PART USED: Fruits

Chebulic Myrobalan

Terminali chebula

COMMON NAMES: Haritaki, haridra

FAMILY: Combretaceae

ENERGY AND FLAVORS: Bitter, sour, sweet, pungent, astringent, hot energy

SYSTEMS AFFECTED: Colon, lungs, liver, uterus

BIOCHEMICAL CONSTITUENTS: Anthraquinone glycoside called sennoside, tannins, ellagic and gallic acids, chebulinic acid, fixed oil

PROPERTIES: Laxative, astringent, vermifuge

NOTES: Myrobalan is a purifying and bowel cleansing herb-fruit of India. It is regarded as sacred by the Tibetans, who depict the image of the Medicine Buddha holding the large seeds in one hand. The Tibetans in fact called it "the king of medicines" for reasons that we shall see. It is also considered sacred to the Indian god Shiva, the god of destruction and purification.

Chebulic myrobalan is one of the three important ingredients of triphala and the one with the greatest laxative action. It is considered to be a tonic, non-habit-forming laxative, especially when combined with the other two ingredients of triphala. Thus triphala is ideally suited for chronic constipation and will clense the entire digestive tract without habit-forming dependency or creating deficiencies.

Chebulic myrobalan is effective for the humoral sphere of air. Thus, its tonic properties are that it promotes longevity, rejuvenates, stimulates enzymatic action and helps transform arteriosclerosis. Chinese medicine calls it ho-tzu and classifies it as having a bitter, sour and spicy taste with a warm energy. The Chinese use it for intestinal problems, including worms and parasites, to strengthen the lungs, cure chronic cough, chronic diarrhea, dysentery, prolapsed rectum, gas as well as female leucorrhea, seminal emission and excessive perspiration.

It was formerly used in Western medicine and described in *Tabernaemontanus,* an early-sixteenth-century herbal with woodcut illustrations of plants, which claimed it had gentle purgative properties. It further benefited the heart, sharpened the senses, promoted appetite, cleared the skin, strengthened the nerves and eliminated melancholy and depression.

Thus we see how this remarkable herb-fruit, one of the three of triphala, has both eliminative as well as tonic properties.

The other two, also members of the myrobalan group, include amla, which controls *pitta* or fire, and *baheera* or beleric, which controls water or phlegm. Thus triphala is considered both a tonic and elminator of the three traditional "humors" of Indian Ayurvedic medicine and is used as a common household item at least on a weekly basis by most traditional Indian families.

Emblic myrobalan
Phyllanthus emblica
COMMON NAMES: Amla or amlaki

FAMILY: Euphorbiaceae
ENERGY AND FLAVOR: Sour, astringent, sweet, pungent, bitter, cool energy
SYSTEMS AFFECTED: Lungs, liver, stomach, heart, pancreas, urinary tract
NOTES: Amla (emblic myrobalan) is called Indian gooseberry and is antiinflammatory. One small amla fruit has approximately twenty times the vitamin C of an orange. While this makes it one of the highest-concentrated sources of this important vitamin known, it is of even greater importance to realize that the vitamin C content of amlas are thermostable because they are bound up with certain tannins that make it nearly impervious to dissolution after drying, aging or subjection to heat. Amla is very sour and is one of the primary tonic herb foods of India. Besides its inclusion in triphala, it is also used as the primary tonic ingredient in chyavanprash, a deliciously pastelike mixture of 50% amla fruits together with over forty-four other herbs and spices, raw brown sugar, honey and ghee.

Amla has mild laxative and rejuvenating powers and is used both as a nourishing health food and tonic.

It is good for failing eyesight and for thinning hair (boiled with sesame oil and gotu kola, which is greasy, or with coconut oil, which is not greasy). In addition, it is used for skin diseases, hemorrhoids, diabetes, heart disease, anemia, hemorrhage, diarrhea, jaundice, bronchitis and asthma.

Western herbalism formerly used it to purify the stomach and intestinal tract of foul phlegm and mucus and as a stomach tonic. It was also used to strengthen the brain, heart, nerves and lungs and to improve appetite, reduce inflammation and quench thirst. *Tabernaemontanus* describes that various types of jams were made from this fruit with the addition of various spices such as cinnamon, cardamom, nutmeg, pepper and others (this was probably a variation of the chyavanprash formula).

Beleric myrobalan

Terminalia bellerica
COMMON NAME: Bhibitaki
FAMILY: Combretaceae
ENERGY AND FLAVORS: Astringent, warm energy
SYSTEMS AFFECTED: Lungs, heart, liver
DOSE: 3–9 grams of the powder
CHEBULIC MYROBALAN IS USED FOR: Chronic constipation

EMBLIC MYROBALAN IS USED FOR: Inflammation and tonification

BELERIC MYROBALAN IS USED FOR: Mucus and lymphatic congestion

NOTES: Beleric myrobalan is the third fruit of triphala and it is particularly useful for eliminating mucus. It is also useful for bronchitis, asthma, vomiting (especially morning sickness during pregnancy), allergies, constipation and colicky pains. It also benefits the eyes and hair and like the previous two, is useful for regulating bowels, digestion and reducing weight.

The term *myrobalan* refers to the use of these fruits in tanning.

Myrrh

Commiphora myrrha

COMMON NAME: Guggul

FAMILY: Burseraceae

PART USED: Gum resin

ENERGY AND FLAVORS: Bitter, spicy, neutral

SYSTEMS AFFECTED: Heart, liver, spleen

BIOCHEMICAL CONSTITUENTS: Essential oil, resins, gum; guggul made from the prepared gum resin has steroid activity useful for arthritic and rheumatic problems

PROPERTIES: Antiseptic, stimulant, emmenagogue, astringent, carminative, expectorant, antispasmodic

DOSE: 1–15 grains of the powder; in formulas, 3–12 grams

USED FOR: antiseptic, menstrual congestion, pains, gas, mouthwash, with echinacea for infections

NOTES: Myrrh is one of the best antiseptics known and is commonly applied as a disinfectant to wounds. When combined with goldenseal, it can be made into a healing antiseptic salve useful for the treatment of hemorrhoids, bedsores and wounds. A tincture of myrrh diluted with water is excellent as a mouthwash and for spongy gums, pyorrhea, sore throat and other ailments requiring an antiseptic astringent.

Internally, myrrh has a variety of uses including the treatment of indigestion and gas, suppressed and painful menses, arthritis and rheumatic complaints, chronic catarrh (phlegm) and bronchial congestion, and the treatment of ulcers. It also combines well with echinacea root, goldenseal, chapparal and garlic as an antibiotic and antiviral agent against most acute inflammatory conditions.

In India, the gum of a particular species is purified by cooking it in triphala (a special detoxifying combination of fruits). This is cooked down into a thick black substance that is dried and called guggul. It is taken for arteriosclerosis, arthritic and rheumatic problems and to open the channels of blood and nerve conduction. The average dose is two or three mung-bean-sized pills three times daily.

Generally, because of its emmenagogic properties, myrrh should be avoided during pregnancy. Further, because resins can be hard on the kidneys if taken over a prolonged period—longer than a couple of weeks—it should not be taken continuously unless properly balanced with other demulcent herbs. This is not true of the purified guggul, however.

Neem tree
Azadirachta indica
COMMON NAMES: Azedarach, Nim, Margosa, Melia A.
FAMILY: Meliaceae
PARTS USED: Bark, leaves and seeds
ENERGY AND FLAVOR: Bitter, astringent
SYSTEMS AFFECTED: Skin, lungs, colon
BIOCHEMICAL CONSTITUENTS: Terpenoids such as the azadirachtins, triterpenoid bitters, tannins, flavonoids, etc.
PROPERTIES: Antiinflammatory, antipyretic, anthelmintic, astringent
DOSE: Standard decoction of the leaves or bark; of the tincture, 10–30 drops
GOOD FOR: Inflammations, fevers, skin diseases, gum disease, as an agricultural spray against insects
NOTES: Neem seed oil is used in India as a treatment for a wide variety of skin diseases. An extract of the leaves and bark has powerful antibacterial and antiviral activity with little or no toxicity. It is also taken internally to eliminate worms. The branches of the tree are chewed and used to clean the teeth and cure and prevent gum inflammation. An extract of the leaves and bark is used in agriculture as one of the most effective natural substances to control insects and disease. When sprayed directly onto the plants and ground, the nontoxic protective property seems to become systemic in the plant and continues its effects for some time after.

Nettles
Urtica urens and other species
COMMON NAME: Stinging nettle

FAMILY: Urticaceae

PART USED: Leaves

ENERGY AND FLAVORS: Bland, slightly bitter, cool

SYSTEMS AFFECTED: Small intestines, bladder, lungs

BIOCHEMICAL CONSTITUENTS: High amounts of chlorophyll, indoles including histamine and serotonic, acetylcholine, vitamin C, A and other important vitamins, silicon, potassium, protein and fiber

PROPERTIES: Diuretic, astringent, tonic, hemostatic, galactagogue, expectorant, nutritive

DOSE: Standard infusion; of the tincture, 10–30 drops

NOTES: The young nettle leaves can be steamed as a potherb. Taken over a long period, nettles is a tonic that will benefit the whole body, especially the lungs, stomach and urinary tract. The high concentration of nutrients in nettles makes it ideal for anemia. Also, by sprinkling the powder on a wound, it helps to stop bleeding.

Another treatment for internal, as well as external, bleeding is to heat nettles over a low heat for thirty minutes and squeeze them through a cloth; a tablespoonful of this juice is taken every hour to stop bleeding. Applied to the scalp, nettles help stimulate hair growth.

Nettles tea is useful for asthma, chronic and acute urinary complaints, urinary stones, nephritis and cystitis. It is also taken for diarrhea, dysentery, hemorrhoids and chronic arthritic and rheumatic problems.

The leaves when lightly touched will sting and cause a mild to severe rash; gloves are advised when picking. The rash is treated by rubbing the freshly bruised leaves of yellow dock or plantain over the affected area. These are often found growing nearby. One of the symptomatic treatments to relieve arthritic pains is to sting oneself deliberately over the affected area with a freshly picked nettle branch.

For bleeding such as endometriosis, or uterine bleeding, combine equal parts nettles leaf, agrimony, bayberry and cinnamon barks. Steep in boiling water for twenty minutes and take a cupful every hour, tapering off as bleeding subsides.

A clinical study of nettle roots has found them to be highly effective for the treatment of enlarged prostate. The root contains high amounts of sterols, especially sitosterol and isolectins, which stimulate the production of white blood cells that counteract infections and inflammations.

Nigella

Nigella sativa L.

COMMON NAMES: Black cumin, Love-in-the-mist, Fitches (biblical: ". . . For the fitches are not thrashed with a threshing instrument . . . but the fitches are beaten out with a staff . . ." Isaiah 28)

PARTS USED: Seeds

ENERGY AND FLAVORS: Hot, spicy

SYSTEMS AFFECTED: Lungs, stomach, spleen

BIOCHEMICAL CONSTITUENTS: Alanine, arginine, ascorbic acid, asparagine, campesterol, caryone, cymene, cystine, dehydroascorbic acid, eicosodienaic acid, glucose, glutamic acid, glycine, iron, isoleucine, leucine, D-limonene, linoleic acid, linolenic acid, lipase, lysine, methionine, myristic acid, nigellin, nigellone, oleic acid, palmitic acid, phenylalanine, phytosterols, potassium, beta-sitosterol, alpha-spinaster, stearic acid, stigmasterol, tannin, threonine, thymohydroquinone, thymoquinone, tryptophan, tyrosine

PROPERTIES: Stimulant, aromatic, carminative, digestive, diuretic, emmenagogue, excitant, galactagogue, purgative, resolvent, stimulant, stomachic, sudorific, tonic, and vermifuge

NOTES: The common name love-in-the-mist aptly describes the poetry of this exquisite plant. In the garden, one easily imagines etheric spirits flitting about among its evanescent bluish white blossoms. Even the seed pods, which are so often used in dried-flower arrangements, suggest an otherworldly sense of exotic enchantment. Is it possible that such a delicately beautiful herb would have such potent medicinal properties and be so hardy as to easily reseed itself in our gardens year after year?

Nigella holds an exalted position among herbalists in the Middle East and to a somewhat lesser extent in India and other Eastern lands. What information I have about nigella I owe to herbalist and plant scientist Jim Duke who presented it in his book *Medicinal Plants of the Bible*. In it he describes black cumin as a Muslim miracle herb; which an Arab proverb says that "in the black seed is the medicine for every disease except death."

A Turkish colleague of mine reports that the herb's seeds are widely cultivated and traded in ton lots within his country throughout the Midle East, northern Africa, and India. The seeds are used as a condiment in bread, cakes, and various confections; used like pepper; or combined with pepper, such as cayenne, in sauces. The Ethiopians add nigella, along with other spices, to flavor local alcoholic beverages. Still another use is to sprinkle it on woolen garments as a moth repellant.

The major uses to which I have put the herb are in treating upper respiratory conditions, allergies, coughs, colds, bronchitis, fevers, flu, asthma, and emphysema, for which it is effective. Simply collect the abundance of seeds from the pods, grind them to a paste, and mix the paste with melted honey to a *hahlava* (a Middle Eastern confection usually made with toasted sesame seeds and honey). Jim Duke confirms nigella's folk use for these and a wide variety of other diseases and conditions, including bilious ailments, calluses, cancer, colic, corns, eruptions, headache, jaundice, mymecia, orchitis, puerperal fever, sclerosis, snakebite, stomachache, swellings, tumors of the abdomen and eyes, and warts. In Algeria, the roasted seeds are combined with butter for cough and honey and taken for colic.

For upper respiratory conditions, at least a few of its constituents have shown an antihistamine-like action, which explains its positive effects on such diseases as asthma and bronchitis, and on cough. The oils of the seed increase milk flow, which explains its folk use as a galactagogue. In large quantities, however, the seeds have also been used to induce abortion.

It is unusual for a hot, spicy herb to have a positive effect on liver diseases but the Lebanese use it this way. Of course, one of its most obvious uses is for diarrhea and dysentery in combination with astringents. The seeds can be ground to a powder, mixed with a little flour to bind the paste, and applied directly to abscesses, on the forehead for headache, to nasal ulcers, for orchitis, and for rheumatism. The seeds also are a rich source of sterols, especially beta-sitosterol, which is known to have anticarcinogenic activity. This substantiates its folk use for indurations and/or tumors of the abdomen, eyes, and liver.

In India, nigella seeds are combined with various purgatives to allay the gripes and colic and also help kill and expel parasites. Middle Eastern Unani medicine affirms its abortifacient properties; it is also used as a diuretic to relieve ascites, for coughs, eye sores, hydrophobia, jaundice, paralysis, piles, and tertian fever.

Do not take nigella during pregnancy.

Night-blooming cereus

Selenicereus grandiflorus (Cereus grandiflorus), (Cactus grandiflorus)
COMMON NAME: Cactus
FAMILY: Cactaceae
PARTS USED: Fluid extract made from flowers and green stems
SYSTEMS AFFECTED: Heart, lungs, nervous system
BIOCHEMICAL CONSTITUENTS: Unavailable
PROPERTIES: Sedative, diuretic, cardiac tonic
DOSE: 5–10 drops; no toxicity has been observed
USED FOR: Heart problems
NOTES: Night-blooming cereus is used for heart weakness, palpitations, tachycardia, angina, carditis, pericarditis, arrhythmia, valvular disease, mitral regurgitation, interstitial pneumonia, hypertrophy, and dyspnea. Cactus is specifically indicated for irregular, feeble pulse accompanied by shortness of breath and a sensation of tightness and constriction around the chest. In addition, it can be employed for neurological conditions associated with hypersensitivity and for a variety of other problems ranging from chronic and acute headaches to numbness of the extremities, cough, PMS, and Raynaud's disease.

A good combination for most heart problems is equal parts night-blooming cereus, hawthorn berry, lily of the valley, motherwort, *Salvia milthiorrhiza,* and *tienchi* ginseng. This combination should be taken as a tea, powder, or a tincture. The latter is made by macerating the crushed or powdered ingredients in vodka, gin, or brandy.

Noni

Morinda citrifolia
COMMON NAMES: Indian mulberry, Nono, Painkiller tree, Polynesian bush fruit
FAMILY: Rubiaceae
PARTS USED: Bark, leaves, flowers, fruit, seeds
ENERGY AND FLAVORS: Sour, sweet, bitter
BIOCHEMICAL CONSTITUENTS: Various terpene compounds, L-asperuloside, aucubin, glucose, caproic and caprylic acids, vitamin C. The leaf contains anthraquinones, glycosides, phenolic compounds, resins, B-sitosterol, ursolic acid; the flower contains acacetin 7-0-D; the fruit contains caproic and caprylic acids, essential oil, B-D-glucopyranose pentaacetate 2, asperuloside tetraacetate, glucose, ascorbic acid; the root and its bark contain alizarin, anthraquinones (morindone), car-

bonate, rubicholric acid, chrysophanol, soranjidol, chlororubin, phosphate, magnesium ferric iron, sodium glycosides, morindadiol, morindine, resins, rubiadin, sterols.

Ralph Heinicke, Ph.D., a biochemist, discovered that noni fruit contains an alkaloid precursor to a vital compound called xeronine. Xeronine is an alkaloid that the body produces to activate enzymes and generally energize the body. It has never previously been found because it is immediately used and broken down by the body. However, without it we would die, since it is basic to the utilization of proteins. Lack of it, therefore, can give rise to many diseases. Noni is considered the best source of proxeronine available.

PROPERTIES: Antibacterial, antimicrobial, alterative, tonic, antiparasitic, emmenagogic, stomachic, anticancer, antiinflammatory, antiarthritic, immune tonic, antioxidant, analgesic, antihypertensive.

Noni is considered the major medicinal herb of the South Pacific. When the fruit is ripe, one will often find traditional Hawaiians picking the fruits. The leaf and leaf juice is good for various inflammations and fevers. It can be used for just about every acute and chronic disease, including such chronic respiratory conditions as tuberculosis, influenza, asthma, coughs, colds, sinusitis, and sore throat. It is also effective for digestive problems, including diarrhea, constipation, indigestion, gastric ulcers, intestinal parasites. It is also used for skin and gum diseases, including wounds, cuts, abscesses, boils, acne, burns, gingivitis, and thrush. Noni uses extend to the urinary system for bladder and kidney infections, to the cardiovascular system for hypertension, and to the endocrine system for the treatment of diabetes. In fact, because of its ability to stimulate production of xeronine, Noni has been used for practically any and every condition one can think of.

Noni fruit juice extract is the most commonly available form. The best-quality noni supplements are made from the unripened green fruit. Noni should be taken on an empty stomach before meals, since stomach acids and enzymes tend to destroy the specific enzyme that liberates the xeronine compound.

CONTRAINDICATIONS: Avoid using it during pregnancy or while nursing a baby.

DOSE: Currently noni is available in juice, dried, encapsulated, and oil forms. Follow the dose indicated on the package.

USED FOR: Tonic for various systems of the body, the immune system, chronic respiratory conditions, hypertension, diabetes, digestive weakness, diarrhea, constipation, gum disease, infections—including urinary tract infections

Oak

Quercus species
FAMILY: Fagaceae
PARTS USED: Bark, acorns
ENERGY AND FLAVORS: Astringent, bitter, neutral
SYSTEMS AFFECTED: Spleen, stomach, intestines
BIOCHEMICAL CONSTITUENTS: Up to 15–20% tannins
PROPERTIES: Bark and gall are astringent, antiseptic, hemostatic
DOSE: One teaspoon of the bark simmered in a cup of boiling water twenty minutes; is one cup three times daily
NOTES: Oak bark is used to treat diarrhea, dysentery and bleeding. For external use the bark or leaves are boiled or steamed and applied to relieve bruises, injuries, varicosities, swollen tissues and bleeding.

Oats

Avena sativa
COMMON NAME: Oat groats
FAMILY: Gramineae
PART USED: Seeds
ENERGY AND FLAVORS: Sweet, neutral to warm energy
SYSTEMS AFFECTED: Stomach, spleen, lungs
BIOCHEMICAL CONSTITUENTS: Proteins, avenins, glycosides, fixed oil, vitamin E, starch, etc.
PROPERTIES: Antidepressant, tonic against depression and debility
DOSE: 10–30 drops of the tincture
USED FOR: Debility, depression
NOTES: Oats are used as a tonic to increase strength of mind, spirit and body. They are useful against depression, menopause and symptoms of drug withdrawal. Avena is a specific nerve tonic, stimulant, and antispasmodic. One of its more recent uses is as a sexual tonic for both men and women. It is available in Planetary Formula's line as Avena Sativa for Men and Avena Sativa for Women. The whole fresh oat picked while still green and milky, with the outer husk, should be used. These are then rendered into a juice using 25% alcohol to

preserve it. Of course, eating oats is also beneficial; recent studies have revealed that oat bran is effective in removing cholesterol.

Olive
Olea europa
FAMILY: Oleaceae
PARTS USED: Oil and leaves
ENERGY AND FLAVORS: Oil is sweet, leaves are bitter
SYSTEMS AFFECTED: Large intestine, liver, gallbladder
BIOCHEMICAL CONSTITUENTS: Approximately 75% oleic acid glycerides, with lesser amounts of linoleic, palmitic, and stearic acid glycerides
PROPERTIES: Oil—nutritive, emollient, mild aperient; leaves—astringent, antiseptic, antihypertensive, antiinflammatory

The oil can be applied externally as a liniment for dry skin and hair to help counteract dandruff. Internally, 1 tablespoon of the oil once or twice daily is a mild laxative. The leaves are can be used internally as a tea for minor feverish conditions, nervous tension, and most commonly to lower blood pressure.
DOSE: Simmer 1 tablespoon of the leaves in 1 cup of boiling water. Take 2 cups daily.
OIL USED FOR: A nutritive, relieving abrasions, a mild laxative
LEAVES USED FOR: Lowering blood pressure, treating inflammation, viruses and fevers

Oregon grape root
Mahonia aquifolium and *M. repens* (*Berberis aquifolium*)
FAMILY: Berberidaceae
PARTS USED: Rhizome and root
ENERGY AND FLAVORS: Cool energy, bitter taste while the berry is sour
SYSTEMS AFFECTED: Liver and gallbladder
BIOCHEMICAL CONSTITUENTS: Berberine alkaloid
PROPERTIES: Cholagogue, alterative, antiinflammatory
DOSE: Standard decoction or 10–30 drops of the tincture three times daily
USED FOR: Liver problems, menstrual irregularities, skin diseases, arthritis, cancer
NOTES: The yellow rhizome is used as a gentle hepatic-biliary stimulant. By enhancing the flow of bile through the liver and gallbladder, the

entire function of the liver is improved. Thus the blood is purified of toxins.

For this reason, Oregon grape root can be used for all liver diseases including hepatitis and gallstones. It is also used for skin diseases, bronchial congestion, arthritis, cancers, tumors and other serious diseases. Since they grow together, a tradition from the mountains of the Pacific Northwest is to combine equal amounts of Oregon grape root and pipsissewa together for the treatment of many acute and chronic diseases including hepatitis, jaundice, arthritis, cancer and heart problems. For liver problems including jaundice and hepatitis, combine equal parts Oregon grape root and dandelion root with a quarter part fennel seed for flavoring. Drink at least three cups daily during the acute crises. Eat very simple, bland, moist foods such as porridge, soups or steamed vegetables.

It's an effective treatment when combined with other herbs such as tang kuei or chaste berry for PMS in women. A good formula is to combine equal parts Oregon grape root, tang kuei, cramp bark, chaste berries and a half part ginger; take as a tea two times daily a week before menses.

Oregon grape root can be considered the Pacific Northwestern counterpart of barberry, which grows in the Northeast. For that matter, there are similar species and varieties that grow in many areas throughout the world. The Eclectics found all species of berberis and berberine-containing herbs, such as goldenseal to be a specific tonic for chronic affections of the mucous membranes. Oregon grape root is therefore effective for any abnormal discharges, including phlegm and catarrh, leucorrhea, and spermatorrhea.

Having a cool energy, it should not be taken over a prolonged time by those suffering from a generally cold and deficient constitution with symptoms of anemia and hypothyroid.

Papaya

Carica papaya
COMMON NAME: Pawpaw
FAMILY: Caricaceae
PARTS USED: Fruit, seeds, leaf
ENERGY AND FLAVORS: Cool energy, sweet flavor
SYSTEMS AFFECTED: Spleen, stomach
BIOCHEMICAL CONSTITUENTS: Proteolytic enzymes, mainly papain and

chymopapain which specifically aid in the digestion of protein. The seeds contain carpasemine and benzylsenevol.

PROPERTIES AND USES: The fruit is digestive. Papain, a derivative of the fruit, is used to tenderize meat. The seeds are taken as an anthelmintic to destroy worms and are an abortifacient. The leaves are diuretic.

DOSE: Either the fruit as described or a specific indication of papain derivative

FRUIT IS USED FOR: Promoting digestion

SEEDS ARE USED FOR: Worms and internal parasites

Parsley

Petroselinum sativum

FAMILY: Umbelliferae

PARTS USED: Leaves, seeds, fruit, root

ENERGY AND FLAVORS: Root is sweet, bland, neutral; the leaves are spicy

SYSTEMS AFFECTED: Lung, stomach, bladder, liver

BIOCHEMICAL CONSTITUENTS: Volatile oil, apiin, bergapten, isoimperatorin, mucilage in the root, sugar. The seeds are stronger in essential oil and include apiole, myristicin, pinene and other terpenes, flavone glycosides, furanocumarin, fatty oil, petroselinic acid; the leaves are similar but weaker in the above constituents.

PROPERTIES: Diuretic, carminative, aperient, antispasmodic, antiseptic, expectorant, antirheumatic, sedative, emmenagogue (the seeds)

DOSE: Standard infusion or 10–30 drops of the tincture

USED FOR: Urinary inflammations

NOTES: The leaves and root are used for urinary tract infections, with the root particularly helping to dissolve and expel stones and gravel. All parts are good for digestive weakness and bronchial and lung congestion. The seeds are particularly beneficial for rheumatic complaints.

A good diuretic formula useful for helping to dissolve and eliminate urinary stones is equal parts parsley root, gravel root, half part each marshmallow root and ginger.

Passionflower

Passiflora incarnata

FAMILY: Passifloraceae

PARTS USED: Leaves; fruit is eaten as a food

ENERGY AND FLAVORS: Leaves are bitter, cool; fruit is sour, sweet and cool

SYSTEMS AFFECTED: Heart, liver

BIOCHEMICAL CONSTITUENTS: The leaves contain various harmine alkaloids, flavonoids, sterols, gums and sugars

PROPERTIES: Mild sedative, hypnotic, antispasmodic, anodyne, hypotensive

DOSE: Standard infusion of the leaves; of the tincture, 10–30 drops

USED FOR: Insomnia, nervous disorders

NOTES: Passionflower leaves are used for insomnia and various neurologic disorders including Parkinson's, epilepsy, hysteria, neuralgia, shingles, anxiety and hypertension.

For nervousness and insomonia combine equal parts passionflower, skullcap, wood betony, valerian and half part each of licorice and ginger.

Pau d'arco

Tabebuia heptaphylla, T. impetiginosa and other species

COMMON NAMES: Tabebuia, Lapacho, Purple lapacho

FAMILY: Bignoniaceae

PART USED: Inner bark of the tree

ENERGY AND FLAVORS: Cool energy, bitter flavor

SYSTEMS AFFECTED: Blood, liver, lungs

BIOCHEMICAL CONSTITUENTS: Quinones, principally lapachol. Lapachol and its derivatives have shown in vivo effects against various cancers. It is also good as a protective antibacterial.

PROPERTIES: Alterative, antifungal, hypotensive, antidiabetic, bitter tonic, digestive, antibacterial, antitumor

DOSE: A tea of the sifted inner-bark pieces is made by simmering one ounce in a pint of boiling water. One cup is taken three to four times daily for acute conditions; for chronic conditions a half cup is taken three or four times daily. Of the tincture, 25–40 drops is taken three or more times daily.

USED FOR: Slowing and inhibiting the growth of cancers and tumors, for skin diseases

NOTES: Pau d'arco is the name of a tree found growing in the forests of Brazil. Lapacho is a name given to the same tree, which some believe to grow in more abundance and potency, in Argentina.

History records its use by the Calaway tribe, descendants of the Incas, for the treatment of cancer and a wide range of other diseases. Its healing power was brought to the attention of the scientific community by Dr. Theodore Meyer and Prats Ruiz of Argentina. According to Dr. Paulo Martin, a medical researcher for the Brazilian government, "Dr. Meyer learned of purple lapacho from the Callaway, using it on his patients and reporting complete cures for five leukemia victims."

In 1960, its use was taken up by the Municipal Hospital of Santo André where medical doctors used a brew of the bark on terminal cancer patients. They reported that within thirty days of treatment using this herb, most patients no longer exhibited pain and many found their tumors also gone or greatly diminished.

Reportedly since that time the bark has routinely been used at the Municipal Hospital of Santo André to treat leukemia as well as many other diseases suspected to be caused by viruses. Both herb stores and regular pharmacies in Brazil now sell this bark.

Lapacho seems to first eliminate the pain caused by the disease and then multiply the numbers of red corpuscles. Thus the range of its curative action is phenomenal. It is good for ulcers, diabetes, rheumatism, osteomyelitis, leukemia, various cancers, ringworm, bronchitis and other respiratory problems, gonorrhea, hemorrhages, cystitis, colitis, gastritis, Parkinson's disease, arteriosclerosis, Hodgkin's disease, lupus, polyps, prostatitis, leucorrhea, inflammations of the genital urinary tract and anemia.

Both Drs. James Duke of the National Institutes of Health and Dr. Norman Farnsworth of the University of Illinois agree that lapacho contains active substances found to be effective against cancers.

The quality of the bark can influence its effectiveness. The most potent part of the tree is the inner bark, which must be aged after harvesting to maximize its effectiveness. Many companies, however, try to sell the outer bark or harvest it from immature trees.

Pennyroyal
Mentha pulegium

COMMON NAMES: European pennyroyal; American species is *Hedeoma pulegioides*

FAMILY: Labiatae

PART USED: Leaves

ENERGY AND FLAVORS: Spicy, bitter, warm energy

SYSTEMS AFFECTED: Liver, lungs, female reproductive organs

PROPERTIES: Diaphoretic, emmenagogue, carminative, antispasmodic, mild sedative

PRECAUTIONS: Not for use during pregnancy

DOSE: Standard influsion

USED FOR: Colds, flus and fevers

OIL USED AS: Mosquito repellent

NOTES: Used to promote perspiration in colds and flus, and promote menses. A good combination for the first stages of colds and flus is to combine equal parts pennyroyal, elder flowers and yarrow. Steep one ounce of the mixture in a pint of boiling water, covered. To incude sweating, take one to two cups before retiring.

It is also useful for gas, nausea and nervous tension. The oil is applied externally to repel flying insects and should not be taken internally.

Peony
Peonia officinalis

PART USED: Root

ENERGY AND FLAVORS: Slightly cold, sour, bitter

SYSTEMS AFFECTED: Liver, spleen

BIOCHEMICAL CONSTITUENTS: Paeoniflorin, paeonol, paeonin, benzoic acid, tannin

PROPERTIES: Antispasmodic and soothing to the nervous system.

Peony is widely used in Traditional Chinese herbal medicine and was formerly in use by Western herbalists as a major remedy for chorea, epilepsy (TCM, internal liver wind), and childhood convulsions. It is also effective for spasmodic coughs and whooping cough. Wild peony is also used as an emmenagogic circulatory stimulant.

DOSE: Of the tincture, 1–30 drops, of the whole herb, 9–18 grams in decoction

USED FOR: Regulating menstruation, calming the nerves, epilepsy and chorea, spasmodic coughs

Pipsissewa
Chimaphila umbellata

COMMON NAMES: Prince's pine, ground holly

FAMILY: Pyrolaceae

PART USED: Leaves

ENERGY AND FLAVOR: Bitter, astringent, cool

SYSTEMS AFFECTED: Heart, bladder, small intestine, spleen

BIOCHEMICAL CONSTITUENTS: Quinones including the hydroquinones ar-

butin and isohomoarbutin; naphthaquinones, chimaphilin and reni-
folin; flavonoids, methylsalicylate, tannins, etc.

PROPERTIES: Diuretic, astringent, alterative, aperient, bitter tonic

DOSE: Standard infusion or 3–9 grams

USED FOR: Urinary tract infections, arthritis and rheumatic complaints

NOTES: Pipsissewa has similar but gentler properties than uva ursi in
that it contains fewer tannins and similarly disinfects the urinary
tract. It is also used as a treatment for arthritis and rheumatic conditions. For urinary inflammations combine two parts pipsissewa with
one part uva ursi, half part marshmallow root and quarter part ginger.
For arthritic and rheumatic problems combine equal parts pipsissewa, Oregon grape root, sarsaparilla, angelica root, prickly ash and
half part licorice root. Take as a decoction, one cup two or three
times daily.

Plantain

Plantago species

COMMON NAMES: Englishman's foot, Ribwort, Greater plantain

FAMILY: Plantaginaceae

PARTS USED: Leaves and seeds

ENERGY AND FLAVORS: Bland, somewhat bitter, cool

SYSTEMS AFFECTED: Bladder, small intestine, gallbladder

BIOCHEMICAL CONSTITUENTS: There are two general species: a narrow-
leaved variety called *P. lanceolata* and a broad-leaved variety called *P.
major*. Generally the broad-leaved variety is preferred, but the nar-
row-leaved species seems to work just as well. Plantain is one of the
most common plants in the world.

Contains iridoids, aucubin, flavonoids, mucilage, tannins.

PROPERTIES: Diuretic, alterative, antiinflammatory, aperient

DOSE: Standard influsion

USED FOR: Urinary tract infections, hepatitis, stings, bites and wounds

NOTES: Plantain is useful for urinary tract infections; the aucubin helps
the secretion of uric acid from the kidneys. The apigenin and baical-
ein are antiinflammatory and antiallergenic. It is good internally for
all inflammations including hepatitis and bacillary dysentery. The
leaves are applied externally to antidote bites and stings of venomous
insects and animals. For more serious cases, a poultice of the leaves
is applied and an extract of tea or tincture is taken internally every
half hour until symptoms subside. Its astringent properties make it

useful to stop bleeding and to promote the healing of wounds and injuries.

Pleurisy root

Asclepias tuberosa

COMMON NAME: Butterfly weed

FAMILY: Asclepiadaceae

PART USED: Root

ENERGY AND FLAVORS: Bitter, acrid, cool

SYSTEMS AFFECTED: Bronchioles, lungs and colon

PROPERTIES: Diaphoretic, expectorant, carminative, diuretic, cardiac tonic

DOSE: Standard infusion or 3–9 grams; of the tincture, 5–40 drops every three hours as required.

USED FOR: Pleurisy, lung and bronchial congestion, colds and flus

NOTES: Pleurisy root is useful in treating pleurisy and pains accompanying breathing. It is also used to help treat the common cold, flu, fevers and various other pulmonary problems.

For lung and bronchioles problems combine equal parts pleurisy root, elecampane root, mullein herb and yerba santa. Take three cups daily.

Poke

Phytolacca americana (P. decandra)

COMMON NAME: Pokeweed

FAMILY: Phytolaccaeae

PARTS USED: Root and berries

ENERGY AND FLAVORS: Bitter, cold, toxic

SYSTEMS AFFECTED: Lung, spleen, kidneys

BIOCHEMICAL CONSTITUENTS: Saponin, formic acid, tannin, fatty oil, resin, sugar

PROPERTIES: Alterative, antirheumatic, antiinflammatory, emetic, cathartic

DOSE: Of the tea, simmer one teaspoon of the powdered or cut and dried root in a cup of water, take one mouthful several times throughout the day; of the tincture, take only 1–5 drops

USED FOR: Blood and lymphatic purification, swollen glands, arthritis and rheumatism

NOTES: Poke root is used as an antibacterial, antiviral and antiinflammatory for a great many complaints. Highly regarded by herbalists for its effects upon the glandular system, it is prescribed for a variety of ailments, from swollen and inflamed glands to breast cysts and tumors. It is also widely used in folk practice as an antiinflammatory for arthritic and rheumatic complaints. The berries are milder in action and are used by homeopathic practitioners to help in weight loss.

For all of the above symptoms a good formula to use is equal parts dried poke root, sarsaparilla root, dandelion root, burdock root and spikenard (*Aralia racemosa*), ginger, and half part licorice root. Make into a standard decoction and take two or three cups daily.

Some people seem to exhibit greater sensitivity and toxic reactions to poke so the dose should be administered carefully. Characteristically these toxic reactions involve various gastrointestinal symptoms that, in a few instances, can prove fatal. It is wise to begin with a small dose and then gradually increase as tolerance permits. Further, I have found that the dried root, especially used in combination with other alteratives, generally exhibits no toxic properties.

Poppy

Papaver species

Various other species including: Opium poppy (*P. somniferum*), Red poppy (*P. rhoeas*), California poppy (*Eschscholtzia californica*)

FAMILY: Papaveraceae

PART USED: Latex exudes from the opium poppy, the flowers of the red poppy, and the whole plant of the California poppy

ENERGY AND FLAVOR: Bitter flavor, cool energy

SYSTEMS AFFECTED: Liver and nervous system

BIOCHEMICAL CONSTITUENTS: All contain a number of alkaloids with sedative and hypnotic properties including isoquinolones, which include papaverine and narcotine. The opium poppy contains morphine and codeine types while the California poppy is more gentle and contains flavone glycocides that are not considered narcotic.

PROPERTIES: Generally sedative, narcotic, analgesic antidiarrheal, antitussive and diaphoretic.

GOOD FOR: Pain, insomnia, nervousness, coughs, diarrhea

NOTES: Poppy is used for the relief of pain, as a sedative for insomnia; to help with anxiety; to inhibit the cough reflex; to allay diarrhea.

Prickly ash

Zanthoxylum americanum (Northern), *Z. clava-herculis* (Southern)

COMMON NAME: Toothache tree

FAMILY: Rutaceae

PARTS USED: Bark and berries

ENERGY AND FLAVOR: Spicy, warm and diffusing

SYSTEMS AFFECTED: Blood and lymphatic circulation, spleen, stomach, kidney

BIOCHEMICAL CONSTITUENTS: Alkaloids, fagarine, coumarins, resin, tannin and volatile oil

PROPERTIES: Stimulant, antirheumatic alternative, diaphoretic, carminative, antidiarrheal, antipyretic, emmenagogue, rubefacient

DOSE: Standard decoction

USED FOR: Sluggish circulation, arthritis and rheumatic problems, toothache and gum problems

NOTES: A stimulant of blood and lymphatic circulation, prickly ash is used for arthritic and rheumatic complaints, lethargy and wounds that are slow to heal. In addition, it is also a blood purifier and useful for treating skin diseases and accumulations in the joints.

Prickly ash is very warming to the stomach and is thus useful for weak digestion, colic and cramps.

External it can be applied as a poultice or fomentation to help dry and heal wounds. The powder of the bark can be chewed or brushed on the gums to relieve toothache, and to treat pyorrhea or receding gums.

A good combination for treating arthritis is equal parts prickly ash bark, guiacum, sarsaparilla, black cohosh and sassafras. This is made into a tea using an ounce of the combination to a pint of water. Three cups are taken daily. Positive results are usually evident within the first two weeks; for more permanent results one may have to take it for two to three months or more.

For pyorrhea and receding gums make a tooth powder using varying amounts prickly ash bark, bayberry bark, finely powdered myrrh, cinnamon and echinacea root. Brush the teeth and gums twice daily with this.

Privet fruit

Ligustrum lucidum

COMMON NAME: Ligustrum

FAMILY: Oleaceae

PART USED: Fruit

ENERGY AND FLAVOR: Sweet, bitter and neutral

SYSTEMS AFFECTED: Liver and kidney-adrenals

BIOCHEMICAL CONSTITUENTS: Oleanolic acid, ursolic acid, mannitol, glucose, fatty oil

PROPERTIES: Yin and blood tonic, demulcent, nutritive tonic

DOSE: 9–15 grams in decoction

USED FOR: Individuals who are burnt-out, premature graying or loss of vision, weakness of lower back and joints

NOTES: Privet is a common plant that grows quickly and appears as a common hedge in many yards and gardens, but few realize the tremendous health benefits of the small fruits that it yields so abundantly.

It is used to replenish the vital essence of the kidney-adrenals and liver, which in turn tends to darken the hair, restore failing eyesight, strengthen the back, waist and knees. It is also used for lumbago, vertigo, hypernervous sensitivity, retinitis and cataract.

Since it has a moist nature, it is contraindicated for diarrhea or loose stools, individuals with coldness and a loss of vitality and drive (Yang energy).

Psyllium

Plantago ovata, P. arenaria (P. psyllium, P. indica)

COMMON NAME: Isapghul

FAMILY: Plantaginaceae

PARTS USED: Seeds and husk of the seeds

ENERGY AND FLAVOR: Sweet, neutral to cool

SYSTEMS AFFECTED: Colon, spleen, stomach

BIOCHEMICAL CONSTITUENTS: Mucilage, polysaccharides, monoterpene alkaloids, aucubine, protein, enzymes and fat

PROPERTIES: Lubricating bulk laxative

DOSE: One teaspoon boiled down from a half quart of the seeds; of the powdered husks, simply stir into a cup of water or fruit juice each evening.

USED FOR: Dry constipation

NOTES: Psyllium is used for acute and chronic constipation for which the husk is most effective. The whole-seed meal can be applied to the surface of the skin to help relieve and heal skin irritations.

For dry constipation, combine two parts psyllium seed husks together with equal parts flax and chia seeds. Soak three or four tablespoons with warm water or a cherry juice. Take in the evening before retiring.

Pygeum

Pygeum africanum

PARTS USED: Trunk bark

ENERGY AND FLAVORS: Cool, bitter

SYSTEMS AFFECTED: Prostate, kidneys

BIOCHEMICAL CONSTITUENTS: Ferulic acid esters, as well as beta-sitosterol and beta-sitosterone, which serve as hormone precursors

PROPERTIES: Antiinflammatory

Pygeum is specifically useful for benign prostatic hyperplasia, prostatitis, urinary tract infections, and male infertility and impotence.

DOSE: Simmer 1 ounce in 1 pint of boiling water for 20 minutes. Cool and take 1 cupful three times daily. It is most commonly found in various herbal preparations along with saw palmetto berries (Planetary Formula's Saw Palmetto Classic).

USED FOR: Enlarged prostate (noncancerous), prostatitis, urinary tract infections, impotence

Raspberry leaf

Rubus idaeus

FAMILY: Rosaceae

PARTS USED: Leaves, fruit

ENERGY AND FLAVORS: Mild, bitter, cool

SYSTEMS AFFECTED: Spleen, liver, kidneys, reproductive organs

BIOCHEMICAL CONSTITUENTS: Flavonoids, glycosides of kaempferol and quercitnin, tannin; the fruits contain 1–2% organic acids of which 90% is citric acid, vitamin C, pectins and sugar

PROPERTIES: Hemostatic, astringent, mild alterative, parturient

DOSE: Standard infusion, two or three cups daily

USED FOR: Pregnancy and delivery, menstrual irregularities, leucorrhea, fevers

NOTES: For centuries, raspberry leaves have been taken by women throughout pregnancy to facilitate delivery and prevent miscarriage. Its uterine relaxant effects have been demonstrated on animals in

numerous studies. They are also used for most other menstrual irregularities, especially to control frequent or excessive bleeding. It is
used as well to reduce fevers and generally help stop bleeding.

The fruit is a nutritive tonic, especially good for strengthening the
blood.

As good prenatal care to tone up and prepare the uterus for childbirth, combine equal parts raspberry leaves and squawvine. Steep a
teaspoon in a cup of hot water and drink one cup two or three times
daily. If there is a threatened miscarriage, add false unicorn root and
cramp bark to the combination in equal parts.

Red clover
Trifolium pratense
FAMILY: Leguminosae
PART USED: Blossoms
ENERGY AND FLAVORS: Sweet, salty, cool
SYSTEMS AFFECTED: Blood, liver, heart, lungs
BIOCHEMICAL CONSTITUENTS: Isoflavones, flavonoids, coumarins, resins,
   minerals, vitamins, etc.
PROPERTIES: Alterative, antispasmodic, expectorant, antitumor
DOSE: Standard infusion or 6–15 grams; of the tincture, 10–30 drops
USED FOR: Cancer and tumors, skin diseases, fevers, colds, coughs
NOTES: Red clover is used for the treatment of tumors and cancers of
   various types. The coumarins tend to have mild blood-thinning
   properties, which make it useful for many chronic degenerative complaints. Red clover is effective for skin complaints, eruptions, psoriasis and eczema. Its antispasmodic and expectorant properties make
   the blossom useful for coughs, colds and other diseases associated
   with mucous congestion.

For the treatment of cancer and tumors combine equal parts red
clover blossoms, chaparral, poke root, burdock root, dandelion root,
stillingia root, Oregon grape or barberry root, echinacea root, sarsaparilla root, sassafras and devil's club, and then make a tea using one
ounce of the combination simmered in a pint of boiling distilled
water for twenty minutes. Take three or four cups daily with six "00"
capsules of powdered kelp. One should, however, consider seeking
professional advice about the treatment of such serious life-threaten-
ing diseases.

Rhubarb

Rheum palmatum, R. officinale and other species

COMMON NAMES: Chinese rhubarb, Da huang, Garden rhubarb, Turkey rhubarb

FAMILY: Polygonaceae

PART USED: Rhizome

ENERGY AND FLAVORS: Cold, bitter

SYSTEMS AFFECTED: Intestines, spleen, liver, pericardium

BIOCHEMICAL CONSTITUENTS: Anthraquinones derivatives, chrysophanol, physcion, sennidin, rheidine, palmidine, tannins, glucogallin, terarin, catechin, gallic acid, flavone, starch, pectin, phytosterol

PROPERTIES: Purgative, aperient, astringent (in smaller doses), alterative, antibiotic, anthelmintic, vulnerary

DOSE: Standard infusion of one teaspoon per cup of water, or in formula, 3–9 grams as needed

GOOD FOR: Constipation, worms, dysentery, diarrhea, dysmenorrhea, amenorrhea

NOTES: Rhubarb is used for constipation, and in smaller doses, for diarrhea and dysentery. In small doses it is an aid to digestion, being tonic to the stomach and small intestines. When chewed, it stimulates salivation.

Rhubarb also promotes blood circulation in the pelvic cavity and is, therefore, useful as a treatment for dysmenorrhea, especially when there is heavy clotting. Generally, it is good to combine laxative herbs with a smaller amount of a warming, antispasmodic stimulant such as ginger to prevent griping pains in the abdomen.

For occasional constipation, use three to nine grams dried rhubarb root combined with two grams ginger root and one gram licorice.

For diarrhea, burn dried rhubarb root in an iron skillet until black, grind to a powder, bottle and cork. Take 10 to 20 grams in water 3 to 6 times daily.

Rice

Oryza sativa

COMMON NAME: Brown rice, various varieties

FAMILY: Gramineae

PART USED: Seeds

ENERGY AND FLAVOR: Neutral, sweet

SYSTEMS AFFECTED: Spleen, pancreas, stomach, intestines

BIOCHEMICAL CONSTITUENTS: Glucose, starch, fixed oil, vitamins, etc.
PROPERTIES: Nutritive, stomachic, demulcent, antiallergenic
DOSE: As required
NOTES: Sprouted rice is high in digestive enzymes and thus helpful in promoting digestion. Since enzymes usually have to be fresh to be effective by Western standards, it remains a mystery why the dry sprouted rice sold in Chinese pharmacies is effective for digestive weakness.

Because it is considered one of the most balanced grains, one's ability to digest it can be an important barometer of general health and well-being. Nevertheless, for many, digestive fire seems to diminish with age, and some may have difficulty digesting brown rice. In this case, the East Indian basmati rice is an acceptable substitute.

Rice congee is made by slowly cooking one part brown rice to 7–10 parts water, for 6–12 hours. This makes an easily digested porridge that can usually be eaten even when all else fails. Various other tonic foods are herbs such as astragalus, ginseng, codonopsis, tang kuei, jujube dates and lycii berries can be added to the rice to make a superior tonic for all ages. This can be served once or twice daily or at least once a week, as needed.

Dry-roasted brown rice cooked in the normal water ratio of two to one is more Yang and thus is useful for the treatment of diarrhea. Eating one or two tablespoons of dry-roasted, uncooked rice each morning is effective in preventing and eliminating worms.

Rosemary

Rosmarinus officinalis
FAMILY: Labiatae
PART USED: Leaves
ENERGY AND FLAVORS: Spicy, cool
SYSTEMS AFFECTED: Liver, stomach, spleen-pancreas
BIOCHEMICAL CONSTITUENTS: Volatile oil including borneol, camphene, camphor, cineole, limonene linalool; flavonoids, ursolic acid, oleanolic acid, etc.
PROPERTIES: Antipyretic, antiinflammatory, stomachic, nervine, diaphoretic, astringent, anodyne, antiseptic
DOSE: One teaspoon steeped in a cup of boiling water
USED FOR: Headaches, indigestion, colds, inflammation of the joints, for scalp and hair

NOTES: Rosemary is useful for dyspepsia or digestive upset, headaches, common cold and as a hair strengthener. A simple cup of rosemary tea is as effective as aspirin for headaches and other inflammatory symptoms including the relief of arthritic pains.

Combine equal parts powders of rosemary, wintergreen, willow bark, poplar bark and licorice root, take two "00" capsules of this combination as needed for headaches and the symptomatic relief of fevers and most minor aches and pains. While this can be used as an alternative to most drug analgesics such as aspirin, it is wise to determine and address the underlying cause of the problem.

Rue

Ruta graveolens
COMMON NAME: Garden rue
FAMILY: Rutaceae
PART USED: Aerial portions
ENERGY AND FLAVORS: Bitter, pungent, warm
SYSTEMS AFFECTED: Liver, spleen, nerves, tendons, uterus, circulation
BIOCHEMICAL CONSTITUENTS: Volatile oil, flavonoids, rutin, hypericin, tannin, pectin, choline
PROPERTIES: Antispasmodic, emmenagogue, stimulant, rubefacient
DOSE: One teaspoon of the leaves in infusion, 10–15 drops of the tincture, externally as needed. Any possible allergic reaction to rue can be antidoted by applying goldenseal either internally or externally.
USED FOR: Spasms, neuralgias and cramps, menstrual cramps, earaches
NOTES: Rue is used in the treatment of nervous spasms, neuralgia, trauma, cramps, and to relax strained muscles and tendons. As such it is applied externally as alcoholic tincture or oil of rue. It is also taken internally as well but should be used moderately. A few drops of rue oil (made by macerating the herb in olive oil) can be applied to a wad of cotton to treat earaches in children or adults.

The Chinese use tincture of rue for sedation, relieving rheumatic pains, increasing local circulation and reducing swelling.

Given in small doses of one-half to one teaspoon at a time, the tincture helps relieve menstrual cramps and promotes blood circulation through the female reproduction organs. It should strictly be avoided during pregnancy.

Sarsaparilla
Smilax medica

COMMON NAMES: Also known as *S. officinalis* and includes the American and Mexican varieties; *S. regelii* is Honduran; *S. ornata* is Jamaican, considered to be the best medicinal variety; *S. febrifuga* is Ecuadorian; Indian sarsaparilla, *Hemidesmus indicus,* is an often-found adulterant that is considered inferior to the above varieties.

FAMILY: Liliaceae

PARTS USED: Roots or rhizome

ENERGY AND FLAVORS: Sweet, mild, spicy neutral to cool

SYSTEMS AFFECTED: Liver, stomach, kidneys

BIOCHEMICAL CONSTITUENTS: Saponins, parillin, sarsaponin, glycosides, sitosterol, stigmasterin, essential oil, resin, sugar, fat

PROPERTIES: Alterative, heat clearing, antiinflammatory, antipruritic, diaphoretic, tonic

DOSE: Standard decoction, 6–15 grams; in tincture, 10–30 drops

USED FOR: Skin eruptions, venereal diseases such as syphilis and gonorrhea, liver disorders such as hepatitis, inflammatory conditions

NOTES: Sarsaparilla is used for various kinds of eruptive skin disorders including psoriasis. Also useful for venereal disease including syphilis and gonorrhea, liver disorders such as jaundice and hepatitis and gout. A good alterative for eczema, psoriasis and other skin diseases is the combination of equal parts sarsaparilla root, sassafras, burdock root, yellow dock root, dandelion root and red clover. Make into a strong decoction using one ounce of the combination to a pint of water and take three cups daily. Results will usually be apparent in two to four weeks. However, the diet will have to be adjusted and the herbal formula may need to be taken longer to achieve more lasting results.

Sassafras
Sassafras albidum

COMMON NAMES: *S. varifolium, S. officinale*

FAMILY: Lauraceae

PARTS USED: Root bark and root

ENERGY AND FLAVORS: Spicy, warm

SYSTEMS AFFECTED: Lungs, kidneys

BIOCHEMICAL CONSTITUENTS: Essential oil, safrole, resin and tannin, and
some alkaloids

PROPERTIES: Alterative, diaphoretic, diuretic, carminative, antirheumatic

DOSE: Standard infusion, 3–9 grams, or 10–30 drops of the tincture

USED FOR: Arthritis and rheumatism, acne and various skin eruptions,
colds and flus

NOTES: Sassafras is very effective as a blood-purifying alterative for a
wide variety of skin diseases including acne. It is also commonly used
by the rural folk of Appalachia and the Ozarks as diuretic and treatment for arthritic and rheumatic complaints, pains, ulcers, colds and
flus.

Concern for the carcinogenic properties of safrole, which is present in small concentrations in sassafras root bark, has brought up
another problem as to the possible safety of sassafras as an herb and
recreational beverage in root beers and teas. It must be remembered
that while a particular plant constituent may be toxic when isolated
and concentrated, as part of the dynamic combination of complex
elements in the whole herb it is quite safe. In the case of safrole, it is
characteristically found in many common foods and spices including
sweet basil, nutmeg and black pepper.

The small concentration of safrole in sassafras, together with its
traditional widespread use in rural areas of Southeast North America,
an area notably low in cancer as compared to other areas of the U.S.,
leaves some question as to the equating of the carcinogenic properties
of pure safrole with the use of the whole herb. There seems to be
some research which supports this opinion.

It has been found that whole sassafras when fed to rats and mice
does result in the formation of live tumors. However, when the safrole, which accounts for part of the characteristic aroma and flavor
of sassafras is removed, the rats still develop liver tumors. It would
seem that something in sassafras simply does not agree with the metabolism of rats.

In 1977, however, Swiss toxicologists performed a study giving
sassafras by mouth to human volunteers regularly over an appropriate period of time. They found that safrole was not metabolized
into l'-hydroxysafrole, which is the metabolist responsible for safrole's carcinogenicity.

Furthermore, sassafras is seldom used alone, so that its combination with other herbs tends to lessen the standard dose and offset any

possible side effects. This same formula can be used for arthritic and rheumatic complaints.

Saw palmetto

Serenoa repens

COMMON NAMES: Sabal, Seronoa, Seronna serrulata

FAMILY: Palmaceae

PART USED: Fruit

ENERGY AND FLAVORS: Pungent, sweet, warm

SYSTEMS AFFECTED: Kidney, spleen, liver

BIOCHEMICAL CONSTITUENTS: Essential oil, fatty acids, carotene, polysaccharides, tannin, sitosterol, invert sugar, estrogenic substance

PROPERTIES: Nutritive Yin tonic, diuretic, expectorant, roborant, sedative, endocrine and anabolic agent, aphrodisiac

DOSE: Standard decoction or 3–12 grams three times daily

USED FOR: Wasting diseases, underweight conditions, prostate, urinary tract infections, impotence and frigidity

NOTES: Saw palmetto is used for debilitating and wasting conditions, prostatic enlargement (especially when combined with echinacea and damiana), urinary tract infections, impotence and frigidity.

For enlarged and debilitated prostate, combine equal parts saw palmetto berries, damiana and echinacea. Grind to a powder (saw palmetto is not very appealing to most people) and take two to four "00" capsules three times daily.

Herbal Body-Building Regime

For strengthening and general body building, or to counteract wasting and severe debilitated conditions, eat only cooked food, especially cooked whole grains, black beans, okra, ghee (clarified butter), and incorporate walnuts into the diet regularly. Make an herbal combination of six parts powdered saw palmetto, four parts marshmallow root, three parts tang quai root, two parts American ginseng, one part ginger root. Also boil six slices of astragalus root in two cups of water down to one-half the total volume of liquid, add two eight-ounce glasses of whole, raw cow's milk (goat's milk is also good) and either six slices of raw ginger or two teaspoons of dried ginger; boil for five minutes. Add honey to taste. Drink two glasses of the ginger-astragalus warm milk tonic along with four tablets of the saw palmetto compound and seven freshly shelled walnuts in the morning and evening. For extra body-building power add one organic raw egg with the drink.

Senna

Cassia senna C. angustifoli, C. acutifolia
FAMILY: Leguminosae
PARTS USED: Leaves and pods
ENERGY AND FLAVORS: Bitter, sweet, cold
SYSTEMS AFFECTED: Colon
BIOCHEMICAL CONSTITUENTS: Anthraquinones, flavones, tartaric acid, mucin, salts, essential oil, traces of tannin and resin
PROPERTIES: Laxative, purgative
DOSE: One teaspoon steeped in a cup of boiling water, or 3–9 grams, either of which is taken in the evening before retiring
USED FOR: Constipation
NOTES: Senna is useful for the occasional problem of acute constipation. The leaves are considered to have a stronger laxative effect than the pods. To prevent griping pains in the intestines, it is best when combined with a smaller amount of a warming stimulant and antispasmodic such as ginger or some other suitable herb. Too frequent usage can lead to laxative dependency. As with most purgatives, it is generally not used during pregnancy because of its strong downward energy that seldom will, but possibly could, cause miscarriage.

Shepherd's purse

Capsella bursa-pastoris
FAMILY: Cruciferae
PARTS USED: Entire plant, especially the aerial portions
ENERGY AND FLAVORS: Pungent, sweet, neutral
SYSTEMS AFFECTED: Blood, liver, stomach and uterus
BIOCHEMICAL CONSTITUENTS: Flavonoids, luteolin-7-rutinoside, quercitin-3-rutinoside, plant amino acids, choline, tyramine, diosmin and acetylcholine
PROPERTIES: Hemostatic, antihemorrhagic, diuretic and urinary antiseptic, antipyretic
DOSE: Standard infusion of 5–15 grams; of the tincture, 10–30 drops. Take externally.
USED FOR: Bleeding, endometriosis, cystitis

Notes: The alcoholic extract of fresh shepherd's purse is quite effective for stopping bloody fluxes and hemorrhages. It is specific for chronic menorrhagia and endometriosis with frequent and prolonged menstruation or when the discharge is practically constant and colorless. It is also used by midwives for postpartum bleeding, Finally, it is effective as a treatment for urinary inflammations such as cystitis.

For the symptomatic relief of bleeding and endometriosis, take thirty drops every half hour, tapering off gradually as symptoms subside. If symptoms persist, try to obtain professional advice.

Siberian ginseng
Eleutherococcus senticosus
Family: Araliaceae
Part Used: Bark of the root
Energy and Flavors: Sweetish, acrid, warm
Systems Affected: Adrenals, spleen-pancreas
Biochemical Constituents: Eleutherosides, essential oil, resin, starch, vitamin A
Properties: Adaptogenic energy tonic, antirheumatic, antispasmodic
Dose: 3–15 grams or 10–30 drops of the alcoholic extract once to three times daily
Used for: Low energy, increasing endurance
Notes: Siberian ginseng was thoroughly studied by Dr. I. I. Brekhman and other Russian researchers. It was experimentally given to thousands of athletes, factory workers and others with outstanding results. Among 15,350 workers, incidence of disease was lowered on the average some 37.1%; among athletes and other individuals whose work requires high levels of endurance and stamina, the results were better running times, work-load capacities and quicker recovery rates after exertion.

Only recently have there been successful efforts to cultivate the plant in North America. This is a very welcome development since much of the commercially available powdered or extracted forms have been heavily adulterated with a bogus herb (*Hemedesmus indicus*). There is some possibility, not as yet proven, that our own Pacific Northwestern devil's-club (*Oplopanax horridus*), which has traditionally been used to treat diabetes and other serious diseases by the Northwestern Natives, might possess similar adaptogenic properties.

Skullcap

Scutellaria lateriflora and other species
FAMILY: Labiatae
PART USED: Aerial portions
ENERGY AND FLAVORS: Bitter, cool
BIOCHEMICAL CONSTITUENTS: Volatile oil, scutellarin, bitter glycoside, tannin, fat, bitter principles and sugar
PROPERTIES: Sedative, nervine, antispasmodic
DOSE: Standard infusion or 3–9 grams; of the tincture, 10–30 drops
USED FOR: Nervousness, insomnia, alcohol and drug withdrawal, epilepsy and chorea
NOTES: Skullcap relaxes nervous tension, induces inner calm, and counteracts sleeplessness. In addition it is also used for neurological diseases such as epilepsy and chorea. It is one of the most effective herbs to use to withdraw from alcohol and drugs use; it has considerable detoxification properties that will often prevent or lessen the severity of such withdrawal symptoms as delirium tremens.

A typical mild sedative is a combination of equal parts skullcap, hops and valerian root tea or tincture taken three times daily and especially a half hour before retiring.

For withdrawing from drugs or alcohol, take 15–20 drops of skullcap every hour or two. This will prevent or lessen the severity of withdrawal symptoms.

Slippery elm

Ulmus rubra (U. fulva)
COMMON NAME: Red elm
FAMILY: Ulmaceae
PART USED: Inner bark
ENERGY AND FLAVORS: Sweet, neutral
SYSTEMS AFFECTED: Lungs and stomach
BIOCHEMICAL CONSTITUENTS: Proteins, mucins, amino acids, iodine, bromine and manganese salts
PROPERTIES: Nutritive demulcent, Yin tonic, expectorant, emollient, mild astringent and vulnerary
DOSE: 9–30 grams of the cut and sifted bark
USED FOR: Irritated sore throat, as a nutritive antinauseous food, gastrointestinal ulcers, dryness of the respiratory tract, externally to heal ulcers, sores and wounds

NOTES: Use slippery elm as a tea or mucilage, mixing the powder with a little water and honey to soothe sore and irritated throats, coughs, and dryness of the throat and lungs. It is also an important survival herb food. The famous slippery elm gruel or mucilage can be taken as food and gives strength when needed. It will usually stay down even when all else causes nausea and vomiting.

For those with severe debilitated wasting and chi deficiency, prepare the gruel with the resultant tea of ginseng. A bit of honey, barley malt or cinnamon will, in most cases, be readily accepted both by young infants as well as the aged.

The somewhat standard way to make slippery elm gruel is to gradually mix warm honey water with four to six tablespoons of slippery elm root powder. Do this until the desired consistency is attained. Add a dash of cinnamon and/or cloves for flavoring. Use freely as needed.

To heal ulcers, bedsores and wounds, combine powders using equal parts slippery elm, comfrey root, marshmallow root and echinacea root. Make into a poultice by adding a small amount of hot water to form a paste. This is then directly bandaged onto the affected area. The dressing should be changed at least daily.

Spearmint
Mentha spicata
COMMON NAME: Garden mint
FAMILY: Labiatae
PART USED: Leaves
ENERGY AND FLAVORS: Spicy, bitter, cool
SYSTEMS AFFECTED: Lungs, liver
BIOCHEMICAL CONSTITUENTS: Volatile oil, menthol, menthone, d-limonene, neomenthol, tannins and other ingredients
PROPERTIES: Diaphoretic, aromatic, stomachic, calmative, antispasmodic, mild alterative
DOSE: Standard infusion
USED FOR: Fevers, colds, flu, stomach gas, depression
NOTES: Spearmint is useful for many minor acute ailments including colds, flus, fevers, indigestion, gas, cramps and spasms. Peppermint (*Mentha piperita*) has virtually the same herbal properties except that it may be just a bit more stimulating.

Combined in equal parts with other complementary herbs such as

St.-John's-wort and red rose petals, mint can be used to offset states
of melancholy and depression. For fevers simply combine equal parts
mint leaves and elder flowers, drinking one or two cups as warm as
possible before retiring to bed. This serves as an effective sweat-
inducing agent and consequently will effectively treat the first stages
of colds, flus and fevers. For gas and digestive upset, combine one
teaspoon each of mint leaves and camomile flowers steeped in a cup
of boiling water, covered for 10–20 minutes. Take freely as needed.

Squawvine
Mitchella repens
COMMON NAME: Partridgeberry
FAMILY: Rubiaceae
PART USED: Herb
ENERGY AND FLAVORS: Bitter, cool energy
SYSTEMS AFFECTED: Uterus, liver
BIOCHEMICAL CONSTITUENTS: Not very well-known, probably some alka-
    loids, glycosides, tannins and mucilage
PROPERTIES: Parturient, astringent
DOSE: Standard infusion; 10–30 drops of the tincture
USED FOR: Menstrual irregularities, to prepare the womb for childbirth
NOTES: Squawvine is used for amenorrhea and dysmenorrhea. Also
    used to prepare the womb for childbirth. Combine squawvine with
    two parts raspberry leaves, one part each black and blue cohosh, false
    unicorn and two parts echinacea root for menstrual irregularities and
    vaginal discharge.

Stevia
Stevia rebaudiana
COMMON NAME: Guarani
FAMILY: Compositae
PARTS USED: Leaves
ENERGY AND FLAVORS: Cool, sweet
SYSTEMS AFFECTED: Spleen, pancreas
BIOCHEMICAL CONSTITUENTS: Stevia's sweet flavor is due to the presence
    of the complex molecule stevioside. This is a glycoside comprised of
    glucose, sophorose, and steviol.
PROPERTIES: An important South American herb, stevia is anywhere
    from 10 to 30 times sweeter than sugar yet it has only 1 calorie per

ten leaves. The sweetness of the extract in which various forms of stevia are presently sold ranges anywhere from 100 to 300 times that of table sugar. It is the ideal noncaloric sweetener; unlike with sac-charine and other chemical sweeteners, one need not be concerned about its having any carcinogenic properties. It has a long history of use in South America in the treatment of diabetes, and some studies claim that it reduces blood glucose levels. Above all, as an herbal noncaloric sweetener of choice, the extract can be used in cooking and as a sweetener of herbal extracts and teas.

DOSE: Planetary Formulas offers both a stevia powder and a stevia liq-uid extract. Since one needs only 1 to a few drops of stevia to sweeten various foods and drinks, it is particularly useful to have on hand as a sweetener.

USED FOR: Noncaloric sweetener, diabetes, flavoring teas and herbal preparations

St.-John's-wort

Hypericum perforatum
FAMILY: Guttiferae
PART USED: Herb
ENERGY AND FLAVORS: Cool, bitter
SYSTEMS AFFECTED: Liver, nervous system
BIOCHEMICAL CONSTITUENTS: Essential oil, hypericin, flavonoids
PROPERTIES: Sedative, antiinflammatory, astringent, antidepressant
DOSE: Standard infusion or 10–30 drops of the tincture
USED FOR: Nerve pains, neuralgia, depression
NOTES: St.-John's-wort is used to treat pains and diseases of the nervous system, including neuralgia, coccygeal pains, rheumatic and arthritic pains and injuries to the nerves. In controlled studies the hypericins relieved symptoms of anxiety and depression in women probably through a process of monoamineoxidase inhibition.

For the relief of neuralgic pains combine equal parts powders of St.-John's-wort, black cohosh, cramp bark, sassafras and willow bark. Take two "00" size gelatin capsules three to six times daily, tapering off as symptoms subside.

For depression, combine equal parts powders of St.-John's-wort, red rose petals and lemon balm. Take two "00" size gelatin capsules every two hours for no more than three days in succession, tapering off to three times daily as symptoms subside.

Suma

Pfaffia paniculata

COMMON NAMES: Para toda, Brazilian ginseng

FAMILY: Amaranthaceae

PART USED: Root

ENERGY AND FLAVORS: Sweet, mildly acrid, warm

SYSTEMS AFFECTED: Spleen-pancreas, lung

BIOCHEMICAL CONSTITUENTS: Nortriterpenoid saponin in which pfaffic acid was identified as a hydrolysis product. Six saccharide derivatives of the pfaffic acid structural type. Five of the six pfaffosides have been found to inhibit cultured tumor cell melanomas. It also contains sitosterol, stigmasterol and allantoin. Further studies have shown the presence of fairly high concentrations of germanium.

PROPERTIES: Energy tonic, adaptogen, demulcent, nutrient

DOSE: Tonic dosage, 3—6 grams two or three times daily; for treatment of conditions described above, I recommend beginning with approximately 3 grams with warm water every two waking hours or at least four times daily. Gradually increase this dose to 6 grams four times daily. The diet should be all cooked food, predominantly whole grains, beans, a little meat or cooked dairy if desired.

NOTES: As an energy tonic adaptogen, suma is at least equal to that of Siberian ginseng and panax ginseng in its effects. One advantage is that it has traditionally been used as a food, despite its bland, vanilla-like flavor. However, considering its powerful tonic properties, it should be more widely appreciated and used in teas and tonic herb food formulas.

Most of the clinical data and research on the use of suma has been undertaken by Dr. Milton Brazzach, who is head of the pharmaceutical department at São Paulo University. His interest began when his own wife was cured of breast cancer by ingesting the root. Since that time he has documented at least 150 cases where fairly high daily amounts of suma (up to 28 grams throughout the day) were taken over a period of several months to a few years. He has successfully used it on some of the most serious diseases of our times, with the most outstanding results on many varieties of cancer, especially leukemia and Hodgkin's disease, and diabetes.

I have personally prescribed many pounds of suma in my clinic and have corroborated its efficacy for the relief of pains associated with cancer. I have also witnessed it increasing a general sense of well-being in at least one very advanced elderly cancer patient, and achieving impressive results on a young teenage boy with childhood leukemia. My most consistent results to date have been on patients with chronic fatigue syndrome or the so-called Epstein-Barr disease.

I would not hesitate to recommend it to anyone with chronic fatigue or low energy.

Thuja
Thuja occidentalis
FAMILY: Cupressaceae
PARTS USED: Leaves
ENERGY AND FLAVORS: Warm, spicy
SYSTEMS AFFECTED: Lymph, spleen, lungs
BIOCHEMICAL CONSTITUENTS: Thujone (major component), terpenic ketones, tannin, wax, sugars, bitter principle, thujic acid, thujin
PROPERTIES: Diuretic, insecticidal, anthelmintic, antiviral, expectorant, emmenagogue, stimulant, anticarcinogenic.

An infusion can be used as an expectorant for bronchial catarrh. It is also effective as a diuretic for cystitis and amenorrhea. One of its unique virtues is as a topical and internal treatment for warts. According to herbalist Donny Yance, thuja is particularly indicated for cancers of viral origin, including colo-rectal cancer, uterine cancer, and breast and lung cancer. It enhances the immune system by stimulating T-lymphocytes and increasing interleukin-2 production. This makes it particularly useful for increasing tolerance of chemo- and radiotherapy.

CONTRAINDICATIONS: Thujone is toxic in large doses, so this herb should be taken only in small prescribed doses.
DOSE: 10 drops of the tincture three times daily
USED FOR: Warts, bronchial catarrh, lymphatic congestion, clearing intestinal parasites, stopped menstruation, cystitis, cancer

Thyme
Thymus vulgaris
COMMON NAMES: Garden thyme, Common thyme
FAMILY: Labiatae
PARTS USED: Leaves and flowers
ENERGY AND FLAVORS: Spicy and warm
SYSTEMS AFFECTED: Lungs, liver, stomach

BIOCHEMICAL CONSTITUENTS: Essential oil with thymol, cavacrol, cymol, linalool, borneol, bitter principle, tannin, flavonoids, triterpenic acids
PROPERTIES: Carminative, antiseptic, expectorant, antitussive
DOSE: Standard infusion
USED FOR: Cough, colds and flus, indigestion and other stomach problems
NOTES: Thyme is used for acute and chronic respiratory affections, including coughs and colds. It is also useful for gastrointestinal problems such as gas, indigestion and diarrhea. Finally, a tea taken before retiring is effective against nightmares.

For coughs, make a syrup of two parts thyme leaves and equal part elecampagne root, wild cherry bark and yerba santa. Take in teaspoon to tablespoon dose as needed.

Turmeric
Curcuma longa
FAMILY: Zingiberaceae
PART USED: Rhizome
ENERGY AND FLAVORS: Spicy, bitter, warm
SYSTEMS AFFECTED: Heart, liver, lungs, gastrointestinal tract
BIOCHEMICAL CONSTITUENTS: Essential oil, curcumin, 60% turmerones, miscellaneous proteins, sugars, fixed oil, vitamins and other constituents
PROPERTIES: Emmenagogue, aromatic stimulant, cholagogue, alterative, analgesic, astringent, antiseptic
DOSE: 3–9 grams in infusion or mild decoction
USED FOR: Menstrual irregularities, gallstones, hepatitis, digestion and assimilation, externally for bruises and injuries
NOTES: One teaspoon of powdered turmeric root can be taken twice daily to help regulate the menses or to prevent or lessen PMS symptoms. This is because it seems to activate gently the liver function that helps to regulate and balance the hormones. This same treatment is useful in helping to lower blood sugar for the treatment of diabetes.

It is also an important aid in helping to prevent and dissolve gallstones, and in treating hepatitis. It promotes digestion and assimilation and as such is combined with other condiments such as coriander and cumin seeds to form the basis of Indian curry powders.

Turmeric promotes blood circulation and has antiinflammatory properties, which make it particularly useful for the treatment of bruises and injuries. For this, it can be combined with other blood moving and stimulant herbs to make an effective external oil or liniment.

Usnea

Usnea barbata

COMMON NAME: Beard lichen

FAMILY: Usneaceae

PART USED: Whole plant, which is a lichen growing on branches of trees

ENERGY AND FLAVORS: Bitter, cool energy

SYSTEMS AFFECTED: Lungs, skin

BIOCHEMICAL CONSTITUENTS: Usnic acid, mucilage

PROPERTIES: Antibiotic, antifungal, tuberculostatic

DOSE: Internally, use mainly in the tincture, 5–10 drops
    Externally, apply as often as needed

NOTES: Usnea is used both internally and externally for fungus infections and for viral and bacterial infections generally. Excellent to combine with echinacea as a general antibiotic, antifungal, etc. Used externally with thuja leaves and echinacea, it makes an excellent salve for fungal infections.

Uva ursi

Arctostaphylos uva-ursi

COMMON NAME: Bearberry

FAMILY: Ericaceae

PART USED: Leaves

ENERGY AND FLAVORS: Bitter, astringent, cool

SYSTEMS AFFECTED: Heart, bladder, small intestine, liver

BIOCHEMICAL CONSTITUENTS: Arbutin, iridoids, flavonoids, tannins, volatile oil, ursolic, malic and gallic acids

PROPERTIES: Diuretic, urinary antiseptic, astringent

DOSE: Standard infusion or 3–9 grams

USED FOR: Cystitis, nephritis

NOTES: Used for urinary tract inflammations including cystitis, nephritis, urethritis and pyelitis. It is also useful for blood in the urine.

    For cystitis and nephritis, combine one ounce uva ursi leaves with a quarter ounce each of marshmallow root and ginger root. Pour one pint of boiling water over the herbs and cover, letting it stand until it reaches room temperature. Take three cups daily.

Valerian

Valeriana officinalis and other species

FAMILY: Valerianaceae

PART USED: Rhizome

ENERGY AND FLAVORS: Spicy, bitter, warm

SYSTEMS AFFECTED: Liver, heart, nervous system

BIOCHEMICAL CONSTITUENTS: Essential oil, valepotriates, alkaloids including actinidine, valerine, and others, choline, flavonoids, sterols, tannins, and other ingredients

PROPERTIES: Sedative, hypnotic, nervine, antispasmodic, carminative, stimulant, anodyne

DOSE: Standard infusion or ten drops to one teaspoon of the tincture

USED FOR: Insomnia, stress and nervousness, menstrual cramps, pain relief

NOTES: Useful for general nervousness and insomnia, valerian also relieves gas, spasms, pains and general symptoms of stress.

For nervousness and insomnia, combine equal parts valerian root, skullcap, herb, passionflower, cramp bark, black cohosh, ginger and licorice. Make into a tea or powder and take one cup three times daily, ideally with a dose of calcium and magnesium.

Vegetable charcoal

Carbo vegetalis

COMMON NAME: Carbo veg

ENERGY AND FLAVOR: Warm, bitter

USED FOR: Gas, hemorrhage, poison antidote

NOTES: Vegetable charcoal can be made from the carbonized residue of nonpoisonous wood ashes, such as oak bark or bayberry bark. It can also be from vegetables and astringent herbs, such as blackberry or raspberry leaves.

It is specific for passive hemorrhage and excessive secretions. It is also used to symptomatically relieve symptoms of gas and flatulence. Other conditions for which it is used include dyspepsia, chronic bronchitis, excessive expectoration, and cyanosis of the extremities. It has a very broad application homeopathically for patients whose constitution tends to be obese, sluggish, and lazy with coldness and chronic complaints. It is specific for individuals who have never fully recovered from previous illness. As an herbal remedy, it is taken only short term to relieve an acute condition. About 1 teaspoon of the ashes can be stirred in water or put into a capsule and taken with water every hour, with dose frequency diminishing as symptoms subside. Because of its absorbent properties, charcoal is specific to prevent the absorption of many poisons that may have been inadvertently ingested. For this type of condition, a larger initial dose should be taken, and then smaller teaspoonful doses hourly for at least 8 hours in succession.

Vervain

Verbena officinalis
COMMON NAME: Blue vervain
FAMILY: Verbenaceae
PART USED: Aerial portions
ENERGY AND FLAVORS: Cold, bitter
SYSTEMS AFFECTED: Liver, spleen, nervous system
BIOCHEMICAL CONSTITUENTS: Iridoids, two glycosides (verbenalin and verbenine), essential oil, tannin, bitter principle and mucilage
PROPERTIES: Nervine, emmenagogue, bitter tonic, emetic in larger doses
DOSE: Standard infusion or 10–30 drops of the tincture
USED FOR: Liver disorders, irregular and painful menses, increased milk, colds, flus and fever
NOTES: Vervain is useful for liver congestion and related disorders such as painful or irregular menses. It is also good for hepatitis, jaundice, cirrhosis, ascites, mastitis. In addition to these more chronic symptoms, it can also be taken as a simple infusion for acute symptoms of colds, flus and fevers. Vervain also helps to increase the flow of mother's milk.

For nervousness caused by liver congestion, anger, shock, etc., combine equal parts vervain, skullcap herb, camomile, valerian, Oregon grape and ginger. Take one cup warm three times a day, sweetened with raw sugar or honey as desired. With the addition of one part chaste berries *(Vitex agnus-castus)*, this becomes an ideal treatment for PMS.

Violet

Viola odorata
COMMON NAME: Sweet violet
FAMILY: Violaceae
PART USED: Aerial portions

ENERGY AND FLAVORS: Sweet, mild but pleasantly bitterish, cool
SYSTEMS AFFECTED: Lungs, stomach, liver, heart
BIOCHEMICAL CONSTITUENTS: Saponins, phenolic glycosides, mucilage
PROPERTIES: Demulcent, expectorant, alterative, antipyretic, antiseptic, vulnerary, antispasmodic
DOSE: Standard infusion
USED FOR: Dry coughs and sore throats, softening hard cancerous masses, as a potherb
NOTES: Violet is used as a syrup for sore throat, dryness of the upper-respiratory tract, chronic coughs and asthma with associated dryness. It is also used to soften hard lumps such as tumors and cancerous neoplasms. It is antihypertensive. The steamed fresh leaves can be used as a potherb.

Vitex

Vitex agnus-castus

COMMON NAMES: Vitex, Chaste tree, Hemp tree, Monk's pepper, Chaste-berries
FAMILY: Verbenaceae
PART USED: Fruit
ENERGY AND FLAVORS: Bitter, acrid, cool
SYSTEMS AFFECTED: Liver, spleen
BIOCHEMICAL CONSTITUENTS: Volatile oil, glycosides, flavonoids, castine (a bitter principle)
PROPERTIES: Tonic, emmenagogue
DOSE: 3–6 grams in defusion of the dried and ground berries three times daily; of the tincture, 10–30 drops
NOTES: As the name suggests, chaste berries were used in ancient times to suppress libido in temple priestesses. Supposedly in Italy today, the flowers are still spread before the ground of novices as they enter the monastery. There seems to be little evidence, however, that vitex has anaphrodisiac properties.

   This important female herb seems to regulate the menstrual cycle of women. Its special application is for relieving the symptoms of premenstrual syndrome (PMS) and female menopause. The unique properties of vitex are due to its pituitary-stimulating properties and its ability to increase luteinizing hormone (progesterone), which stimulates the actual sloughing off of the corpus luteum associated with menstruation.

The female menstrual cycle is a good barometer of the overall emotional and physical health of women. After menstruation, the tendency is toward the increase of estrogen. This continues up to ovulation, when the egg drops down from the ovaries and becomes available for fertilization.

Estrogen and progesterone are the two hormones that create all the psychological and emotional qualities associated with femininity. As herbalist David Hoffmann states, vitex is an "amphoteric remedy" because it tends to have a normalizing effect on estrogen even though it favors the progesterone cycle. He further maintains its benefit in helping the body regain "natural balance after the use of the birth control pill."

The diminishing of estrogen and the increase of progesterone is important after ovulation since this hormone is needed to prepare the womb for either the implantation of the fertilized ovum or menstruation. Extensive scientific validation establishes that vitex enhances the progesterone cycle in women and is consequently beneficial for the treatment of painful menstruation, the emotional swings associated with premenstrual syndrome and problems related to menopause.

What this implies is that vitex is the single herb of choice for helping to maintain emotional balance before and during menstruation. Of course, other factors need to be examined to arrive at a more comprehensive treatment for PMS, including treating the liver with bitter herbs such as turmeric or Oregon grape root and the use of the Chinese female tonic herb called tang quai (*Angelica sinensis*), which, among many functions, also regulates hormones, tonifies blood and aids blood circulation.

Walnut
Juglans nigra
FAMILY: Juglandaceae
PARTS USED: Fruit, leaves and bark
ENERGY AND FLAVORS: Fruit has a sweet, warm energy; the leaves, bark and outer hull are bitter and cool
SYSTEMS AFFECTED: Fruit goes to the lungs, kidneys and brain; the leaves, outer hull and bark affect the skin and colon
BIOCHEMICAL CONSTITUENTS: Fruit is rich in oils, juglone, vitamins A, B, C and E, linolenic, linoleic, isolinolenic and oleic acids; juglone is

believed to have an antifungal principle; hulls and leaves contain tannins and juglandin

PROPERTIES: Fruit is roborant, useful for weight gain, and as such can be used freely as is or in soups; the hulls, bark and leaves are antifungal, antiparasitical, antidysenteric; the bark is a mild laxative and alterative

DOSE: Standard infusion, 10–20 drops of the tincture of the hulls; of the fruits, as desired

NOTES: The fruit of the walnut is helpful in promoting strength and weight gain. The extract of the hulls is good for skin diseases, eczema, herpes, psoriasis, skin parasites when taken internally and/or externally. An infusion of the leaves can be taken for skin diseases. The bark is useful for constipation.

For the treatment of amoebic (giardia) or bacterial dysentery, combine equal parts powders of black walnut hulls, goldenseal root, mugwort or wormwood herb, chaparral, and one-half part licorice root. Take two "00" size capsules of this preparation four times daily for seven days while eating a strict diet of brown rice and black or Japanese azuki beans. One clove of garlic can be taken two or three times daily as well. In the evening, take two to four tablets of triphala root powder as needed to maintain bowel regularity.

Wild cherry bark

Prunus serotina

COMMON NAMES: Chokecherry, *P. virginiana*

FAMILY: Rosaceae

PART USED: Bark

ENERGY AND FLAVORS: Acrid, astringent, warm

SYSTEMS AFFECTED: Lungs, spleen-pancreas

BIOCHEMICAL CONSTITUENTS: Hydrocyanic glycoside, isoamygdalin, organic acids, tannin

PROPERTIES: Antitussive, sedative, astringent, carminative

DOSE: Standard infusion

USED FOR: Coughs, asthma, GI tract problems

NOTES: Wild cherry bark calms the respiratory nerves, allays cough and asthma. It is also excellent for digestive weakness including ulcers, gastritis, colitis, diarrhea and dysentery.

The inner bark is best collected, dried and aged in the fall. This is one herb that is best extracted in cool water by macerating an ounce of the bark to a pint of water overnight and then warming slightly. Sustained high heat does diminish its cough-relieving properties.

A good syrup useful for most kinds of coughs, including spasmodic and whooping coughs, is made by combining wild cherry bark, elecampane root, cramp bark and one-quarter part lobelia herb and ginger root with a base of honey. Take as often as needed.

Wild yam

Dioscorea paniculata

COMMON NAMES: Colicroot, Rheumatism root

FAMILY: Dioscoreaceae

PART USED: Root

ENERGY AND FLAVORS: Sweet, bitter, warm

SYSTEMS AFFECTED: Liver, gallbladder, kidneys, spleen-pancreas

BIOCHEMICAL CONSTITUENTS: Steroidal saponins, mainly diosgenin; these are hormone precursors, especially of progesterone and other cortical steroids

PROPERTIES: Antispasmodic, antiinflammatory, cholagogue, diaphoretic, expectorant

DOSE: Standard decoction or 3–9 grams; of the tincture, 10–30 drops

NOTES: Wild yam is used for biliary colic, pains of gallstones, menstrual cramps, arthritic and rheumatic pains, abdominal and intestinal cramps. It is also good for chronic problems associated with gas or flatulence.

For chronic liver problems and chronic gas, combine two parts wild yam root, one part Oregon grape or barberry root and one-half part each of fennel seeds and ginger. Take as a tea or powder after meals.

For gallstones, combine equal parts wild yam root, fringe tree bark, Oregon grape or barberry root, turmeric root and marshmallow root. Take as a tea, simmering one ounce of the combination in a pint of boiling water. It can also be taken as a powder, taking two to four "00" size gelatin tablets every hour or two, tapering off as symptoms subside. If after twelve hours symptoms have not subsided, consider seeking professional help.

Willow

Salix alba

COMMON NAMES: White willow, other species are also useful

FAMILY: Salicaceae

PART USED: Bark

ENERGY AND FLAVORS: Bitter, cold

SYSTEMS AFFECTED: Liver, kidneys and heart

BIOCHEMICAL CONSTITUENTS: Salicin (salicoside) and salicortine and tannin

PROPERTIES: Analgesic, alterative, febrifuge, astringent, antiperiodic and vermifuge

DOSE: One to three teaspoons of the bark soaked in cold water for two to five hours; take one-third cup three times daily. The herb could also be powdered and taken in two "00" size gelatin capsules three times daily. Because of the strong bitter flavor, which can create stomach disturbance, it is good to combine about one-eighth to one-quarter part licorice root along with a small amount of cinnamon bark to counteract some of these possible undesirable side effects.

NOTES: Willow bark is the herbal analogue for aspirin and is an easy substitute with fewer side effects. Therefore, it is good for the symptomatic relief of fevers, headaches and sciatic, arthritic, rheumatic and neuralgic aches and pains. For broader action, combine powdered willow bark, rosemary herb, poplar bark, wintergreen, wood betony and licorice in equal parts. Take two "00" size gelatin capsules every two hours or as needed.

Witch hazel

Hamamelis virginiana

FAMILY: Hamamelidaceae

PART USED: Mainly the bark, but secondarily the leaves and twigs

ENERGY AND FLAVORS: Bitter, astringent, neutral

SYSTEMS AFFECTED: Heart-circulation, stomach and intestines

BIOCHEMICAL CONSTITUENTS: 8–10% tannins, essential oil, various flavonoids, choline and a saponin

PROPERTIES: Astringent, hemostatic, antiinflammatory

DOSE: The bark, which is milder, is usually used internally. It, along with the twigs and leaves, which are higher in tannins, is used externally for douche, varicose veins, enlaged pores, cuts and abrasions.

USED FOR: Healing cuts and abrasions, varicose veins, hemorrhoids

NOTES: Witch hazel is used for diarrhea, dysentery, hemorrhages, excessive mucous discharge, vaginal and penile discharge, menorrhagia, prolapsed uterus or intestines. It is also used as a general tonic after abortions or miscarriages to restore the normal size of the womb. It can be used as a douche for vaginal discharge. The alcoholic extract is similarly applied externally, especially in combination with bayberry bark to relieve varicose veins, for which it is a near specific. Make a strong decoction, combining equal parts witch hazel, bayberry bark, cayenne pepper and prickly ash bark. Moisten a flannel and apply as a warm fomentation over the varicose veins twice daily, each time leaving the warm, moist towel on for at least thirty minutes. In addition, take two "00" size capsules of the above combination three times daily.

For hemorrhoids, make a suppository with finely powdered witch hazel bark, yarrow, comfrey root and oak bark mixed with cocoa butter. Insert one or two one-inch segments into the rectum each night. Wear a protective undergarment in case there is any leakage.

Wood betony
Stachys betonica
COMMON NAME: Betonica officinalis
FAMILY: Labiatae
PART USED: Herb
ENERGY AND FLAVORS: Bitter, cool
SYSTEMS AFFECTED: Nervous system, liver, heart
BIOCHEMICAL CONSTITUENTS: Alkaloids, tannins, choline, betaine, etc.
PROPERTIES: Sedative, nervine, bitter tonic, astringent
DOSE: Standard infusion or 10–30 drops of the tincture
USED FOR: Anxiety-induced headaches, nervousness, various minor aches and pains
NOTES: Wood betony is good for chronic headaches, nervousness, neuralgia and anxiety. Combine with equal parts feverfew, rosemary and skullcap for migraine or nervous headache.

Wormwood (*see also* MUGWORT)
Artemisia absinthium
COMMON NAME: Absinthe
FAMILY: Compositae
PART USED: Aerial portion
ENERGY AND FLAVORS: Bitter, cold
SYSTEMS AFFECTED: Liver, gallbladder
BIOCHEMICAL CONSTITUENTS: Absinthol, which is common to all worm-

woods including southermost and mugwort, essential oils, including pinene, cineol, borneol, phenol, cumin, aldehyde, thujone (which is a mild hallucinogenic but because of the bitter taste it would be difficult to ingest enough to satisfy anyone's interest along these lines), artemisia ketone

PROPERTIES: Anthelmintic, cholagogue, stomachic, antiinflammatory

DOSE: Generally not more than a teaspoon to tablespoonful at a time of the infusion; of the powder, take two "00" size capsules

USED FOR: Fevers, liver problems, inflammatory conditions of the GI tract, worms and parasites

NOTES: Wormwood is traditionally used to counteract fevers, relieve various aches and pains (like willow bark, which is another bitter), hot stomach pains, gastritis, jaundice and hepatitis. It also kills and drives away various internal worms and parasites.

There are many closely related species of wormwood found around the world that have powerful therapeutic properties. One related species (*Artemisia annua*) contains a sesquiterpene lactone with a peroxide group attached, which is referred to as artemisinin. The amount of artemisinin varies according to the growing season and decreases the longer it is stored. Microscopic analysis has determined that this compound works by destroying various and specific membranes of parasites, causing them to starve to death eventually. Clinical studies have demonstrated a 100% cure rate in 485 cases of tertian malaria and a 92.7% cure rate in 105 cases of subtertian cerebral malaria. For these reasons the U.S. Army is presently investigating *Artemisia annua* as a treatment for drug-resistant malaria. It is further endorsed as a natural substitute for chloroquine, to prevent malaria for those traveling abroad.

As for one further use for wormwood, Dioscorides, the early Roman herbalist, described the tea as an effective pesticide to spray on various garden plants to rid them of pests and parasites.

For the prevention and treatment of fevers and intestinal parasites, take a recommended dose two or three times daily.

For intestinal parasites combine equal parts of the powders of wormwood, garlic, goldenseal, black walnut hulls and half parts each of licorice root and ginger. Take two "00" size capsules four times daily for a week, ideally fasting on an exclusive diet of brown rice, and either black beans or Japanese azuki beans or the Indian kicharee (rice and mung beans recipe, described page 55).

Yarrow

Achillea millefolium

COMMON NAMES: Soldier's woundwort, Milfoil, Nosebleed

FAMILY: Compositae

PART USED: Herb

ENERGY AND FLAVORS: Warm bitter, spicy

SYSTEMS AFFECTED: Lungs, liver

BIOCHEMICAL CONSTITUENTS: Essential oil, cineol and proazulene, achilleine

PROPERTIES: Diaphoretic, antiinflammatory, antipyretic, carminative, hemostatic, astringent, antispasmodic, stomachic

DOSE: Standard infusion

USED FOR: Colds, flus and fevers, painful or suppressed menses, bleeding, hemorrhoids

NOTES: Yarrow is used for a wide variety of common acute complaints. These include the treatment of the common cold, flu, fevers, hypertension, painful menstruation and bleeding. It is also applied externally with other herbs such as witch hazel, bayberry and oak bark as a suppository for the treatment of hemorrhoids (see WITCH HAZEL).

Long associated as an herb for the battlefield (and thus being named after the warrior Achilles), yarrow is considered a specific antihemorrhagic wound remedy. In fact, crushed or powdered yarrow can be applied topically or taken internally for any condition of acute bleeding, especially from cuts and abrasions (as opposed to arnica, which is better for sprains and strains).

Having blood-regulating properties, yarrow is a specific for urogenital problems, especially those associated with women. It may be considered for such conditions as amenorrhea, menorrhagia, and vaginal leucorrhea, all caused by poor pelvic circulation and weakness.

For the first stages of colds, flus and fevers combine equal parts elder flowers, yarrow, lemon balm and mint. Steep one ounce of the combination covered in a pint of boiling water until cool enough to drink. Take one or two cups and retire to bed with several covers, lying perfectly still until full sweating occurs. Do not sweat to exhaustion. Conclude with a short, cool-water sponge bath from head to foot, returning to bed immediately.

Yellow dock

Rumex crispus

COMMON NAMES: Broad-leaved or curly dock

FAMILY: Polygonaceae

PART USED: Root

ENERGY AND FLAVORS: Bitter, sweetish, cool

SYSTEMS AFFECTED: Liver, colon

BIOCHEMICAL CONSTITUENTS: Anthraquinone glycosides, rumicin, chrysarobin, tannins and oxalates

PROPERTIES: Cholagogue, alterative, mild laxative, blood tonic

DOSE: Standard decoction; of the tincture, 10–30 drops

USED FOR: Anemia, skin diseases, liver congestion

NOTES: Yellow dock is used for chronic skin diseases including psoriasis, herpes, various eruptions, eczema and acne. It is also used for symptoms of iron deficiency in the blood. Finally it can be used for most inflammatory liver and gallbladder disorders as well as various gastrointestinal diseases. This plant has similar tonic properties to the Chinese ho shou wu (Polygonum multiflorum), except that it might have a little more active laxative properties. However, in smaller doses, it will only serve to regulate bowel movement.

For skin diseases such as eczema, acne and psoriasis, combine yellow dock and burdock roots with burdock seeds, stillingia, red clover and sarsaparilla root. Make into a strong decoction, simmering one ounce of the combination 20–30 minutes. Take three cups daily.

For anemia combine 6 grams yellow dock root, 4 grams each of ho shou wu and tang quai root and 15 grams Chinese astragalus root. Take in decoction twice daily.

Yerba mansa

Anemopsis californica

PARTS USED: Roots, leaves

ENERGY AND FLAVORS: Cool, spicy

SYSTEMS AFFECTED: Lungs, large intestines, bladder; has a particular effect on the mucous membranes and nasal passages, lungs, bronchioles, colon, and urinary passages

BIOCHEMICAL CONSTITUENTS: Methyleugenol, esdragole, thymol methylether, linalool, p-cymene, asarinin, various aromatics

PROPERTIES: This herb, a native of the Pacific West of North America, is an antiinflammatory, similar in properties to goldenseal in that it exerts its effects on the mucous membranes. It is used for either acute or chronic nasal or pharyngeal catarrh (mucus), mouth and throat inflammation, diarrhea or dysenteric catarrh of the intestines, stomach ulcers, gonorrhea, and catarrhal conditions of the urinary tract. It generally relieves irritation and promotes relaxation of the areas affected. One should consider it especially for inflammatory conditions associated with mucous congestion.

DOSE: One can make a tea of the fresh or dried root. In general, it is best to use an alcoholic tincture, since the aromatic oils will tend to dissipate rather quickly when stored. Of the tincture, use 30–60 drops every 2 hours, tapering off as symptoms subside.

Caution: It seems to be especially plentiful in areas where there has been environmental pollution from agribusiness. Therefore, one should avoid using the herb harvested from these areas, such as the Central and Imperial Valleys of California.

USED FOR: Chronic nasal and pharyngeal catarrh, sore throat, diarrhea and dysentery, ulcers, urinary conditions

Yerba santa

Eriodictyon californicum and other species

COMMON NAMES: Holy herb, Mountain balm

FAMILY: Hydrophyllaceae

PART USED: Leaves

ENERGY AND FLAVORS: Spicy, bitter

SYSTEMS AFFECTED: Lungs, spleen

BIOCHEMICAL CONSTITUENTS: Eriodictyol, homoeriodictyol, chrysocriol, zanthoeridol and eridonel along with formic and other plant acids, volatile oil, phytosterol, resin and glucose

PROPERTIES: Expectorant, carminative, sialagogue, alterative

DOSE: Standard infusion; of the tincture, 10–30 drops

USED FOR: Upper-respiratory problems

NOTES: Yerba santa is used for upper-respiratory congestion either as an infusion or as a syrup. It will also promote salivation and thus aid thirst, dryness and digestion. Externally it has been effectively used as an antiinflammatory when combined with grindelia as a treatment for poison oak or ivy dermatitis.

A typical combination for the treatment of upper-respiratory congestion, coughs and colds, is to combine equal parts yerba santa, ma huang (*Ephedra sinica*), mullein leaf, wild cherry bark, elecampane root and one-half part each of licorice and ginger root. Simmer one ounce of the combination in a pint of boiling water and take three cups daily.

Yohimbe

Pausinystalia johimbe

FAMILY: Rubiaceae

PARTS USED: Bark

ENERGY AND FLAVORS: Warm, bitter

SYSTEMS AFFECTED: Kidneys, adrenals

BIOCHEMICAL CONSTITUENTS: Yohimbine (a testosterone precursor) in the form of an alkaloid salt and yohimbine hydrochloride

PROPERTIES: Aphrodisiac, probably stimulates the production of testosterone.

A native of Africa, where it has been used in tribal marriage rituals, yohimbine is probably the strongest purely herbal aphrodisiac effective for both men and women. Yohimbine from the herb is one of the only recognized medical drug aphrodisiacs. It dilates the blood vessels of the skin and mucous membranes, which causes the blood to rise closer to the surface of the sex organs. Because yohimbe increases pelvic circulation and stimulates erections, one should be careful to not aggravate prior irritation of the kidneys, colon, or prostate. It is very stimulating but at the same time, it lowers blood pressure. One wonders why, therefore, there are traditional precautions against its use for individuals with preexisting high blood pressure.

DOSE: Never exceed the recommended dose of 1 or 2 capsules daily with food. One can take it as an aphrodisiac, 1–2 hours before making love.

USED FOR: An aphrodisiac, stimulating erection, impotence, frigity

Yucca

Yucca species

COMMON NAME: Spanish bayonet

FAMILY: Liliaceae

PART USED: Root

ENERGY AND FLAVORS: Sweet, bland, cool

SYSTEMS AFFECTED: Liver, stomach

BIOCHEMICAL CONSTITUENTS: High in steroid saponins

PROPERTIES: Antiinflammatory, antirheumatic, laxative, alterative

DOSE: 10–30 drops of the tincture three times daily; or one-half ounce decocted in two cups of water, one-half cup taken three or four times daily

USED FOR: Arthritic and rheumatic pains

NOTES: Yucca has a long history of use both as a food and medicine by the Southwest desert Natives. Its principal and most outstanding use is for the relief and treatment of arthritic and rheumatic pains. One-fourth ounce of the dried root is boiled in a pint of water for fifteen minutes and taken in three or four doses throughout the day.

Yucca can occasionally be purgative and cause some intestinal cramping. For this reason it is good to combine it with other complementary antirheumatic herbs such as ginger and prickly ash bark. There is some question whether long-term daily use will slow the absorption of fat-soluble vitamins.

· 1 0 ·

CHINESE HERBS

C hina is perhaps unique in the world in its long commitment to preventative medicine through the use of herbal tonics. The tonic herbs have several uses, including direct treatment of acute ailments, building strength in the recovery process, balancing the body's energy and preventing disease from occurring. These herbs are combined to make tonic soups providing nourishment and gentle stimulation to the organs. The Chinese herbs are becoming more readily available in the West, and many of the ones described here can be purchased in herb stores around the United States.

To make the herbal soup, combine six to seven grams (about one-quarter ounce) of each of the desired herbs in a large nonmetallic pot. Use a quart of water per ounce of herbs and simmer for an hour. Drink one cup of tea, once per day, reheating the soup each day until it is all used. Always include some licorice in the formula.

Most of the Chinese herbs mentioned in this book are considered to be tonics of either the Yin-body, Yang-energy, Yin-blood or tonics for specific organs. Usually these herbs are used in a powerful Chinese herb soup. They are never cooked in a water soluble metal container as this will dilute their properties. For the more difficult diseases involving deficiency, they should be regularly used over a long period of time to help "build up the deficiency," the primary therapeutic principle of Chinese medicine. This is in contrast to Western herbalists who, coming from a tradition of excess meat eating and the use of rich foods, advocate a more eliminative approach to health.

Since the herbs discussed here are among the most frequently used in Chinese medicine, I would like to suggest some approaches for the novice in beginning to integrate them into his health regime.

First we should classify the herbs according to their tonic capacities. Yang or energy tonics include the following: aconite, astragalus, don sen, ginseng, eleuthero, ephedra, fu ling, licorice, ho shou wu, pai shu, and salvia (dang shen). Yin or blood tonics include: dong quai, ho shou wu, lycii, rehmannia, peony, and tienchi.

There are also some herbs that are Yin-cooling, thus helping to detoxify the blood and remove inflammation and heat from the internal organs and body in general. These include: bupleurum, honeysuckle, chrysanthemum, and rehmannia (raw).

Herbs that are stimulating and warming to metabolic functions include: cinnamon, ginger, aconite, and citrus peel (especially tangerine). These have more extreme warming or stimulating action and also help digestion. Other herbs that help to build warmth include pai shu, dong quai, Korean ginseng, prepared rehmannia, don sen, eleuthero, astragalus and tienchi.

Following the principles of Yin and Yang, one might determine what energy is most deficient in and use a combination of those herbs that tend to augment the areas of Yin or Yang deficiency. However, it is important to remember that Yin and Yang are interconnected, and while one who is deficient in "chi" or energy might want to take a combination of ginseng, don sen, and astragalus, he should also add a small amount of herbs that would nourish the Yin such as peony root, ho shou wu, or especially jujube date, which is commonly used for this purpose. In addition, it is customary to add assisting herbs that help to "move the Chi," acting as catalysts for the body's utilization of the power of the herbs being taken.

A basic combination used as weekly soup stock in many traditional Chinese families is as follows:

Astragalus—5 grams
Don sen—8 grams
Fu Ling—5 grams

Ginger—5 grams
Jujube date—5 grams
Licorice—2 grams (to harmonize)

The proportions are my own and are subject to individual variation. One could substitute ginseng root for don sen, add 1.5 grams of aconite to increase the metabolic stimulant action, longan berries and/or lycii in addition to or along with jujube date. So there are many possibilities for adjusting this basic combination to suit one's particular needs.

Those who suffer from anemia, poor circulation and menstrual irregularities should use combinations using dong quai as the major herb. The basic combination for stimulating and tonifying the Yin-blood is dong quai and ginger. Just as most Chinese households keep a quantity of ginseng or don sen and astragalus on hand to tonify Yang-energy, they also keep available a quantity of dong quai and fresh ginger root to tonify Yin-blood.

Again this basic combination can be creatively adjusted to accentuate the intention of the formula with other herbs. A basic combination that is frequently over and beyond the simple dong quai and ginger mentioned above is:

Dong Quai—6 grams (to tonify the blood)
Ligusticum—4 grams (to tonify and move the blood)
Peony—4 grams (antispasmodic, helps move the blood)
Rehmannia—4 grams (tonifies the blood, helps the kidneys)

To this basic formula ginger, dried citrus peel, cinnamon or aconite can be added in small amounts to help catalyze and move the energy of the herbs.

The above formulas are especially good for deficiencies and are best taken in the form of Chinese herb soup. This is done by simply cooking the above ingredients in one or two quarts of water for one hour. Strain if you don't want to encounter pieces of Chinese herbs in your soup broth. Add two to four ounces of lean pork, beef, or a whole chicken to the broth and continue cooking. Add some whole grains, vegetables and salt to taste. One or two bowls of this soup mixture should be taken daily for chronic deficiencies. For maintenance, serve this delicious soup to the family on a weekly basis.

Following is a combination of herbs that utilizes elements from both the Yang and Yin tonics:

Ginseng—2 grams
Astragalus—2 grams
Dong Quai—2 grams
Fu Ling—2 grams
Aconite—1.5 grams (one slice of the root)
Rehmannia—2 grams
Ho Shou Wu—2 grams
Lycii—2 grams
Longan berries (Dragon's Eyes)—2 grams
Pai Shu—2 grams
Jujube date—2 grams
Ginger (fresh)—2 or 3 slices
Licorice—1 or 2 grams
Chrysanthemum—1 gram (as a cooling detoxifying herb)

This mixture is made in the same way as the preceding and has general energy and blood building characteristics.

One can also emphasize the herbs that will help tonify specific organs as follows:

Liver: dong quai, bupleurum, peony, lycii, ho shou wu
Kidneys-adrenals: rehmannia, fu ling, ho shou wu
Spleen-pancreas: ginseng, don sen, pai shu, fu ling, jujube, longan, astragalus
Lungs: astragalus, platycodon, eleuthero
Heart: lycii, rehmannia, longan berries, ginseng

Long Life Tea

Yellow chrysanthemum flower tea is commonly drunk in the heat of summer in China. Heat is a term used for toxins, whereas warmth denotes a more normal metabolism. Chrysanthemum flower tea is used as a blood purifier to get rid of excess heat and to calm and relax the body and mind. It is often combined with honeysuckle flowers to enhance the cooling properties, then a small amount of cinnamon, licorice and ginseng is added to balance the cooling and warming properties.

The prescription of Chinese herb teas is based upon an analysis of the individual's symptoms and constitution. Thus several different formulas can be given for the same basic pathology, depending on the unique manifestation of the symptoms and on the constitution of the patient. To demonstrate this, three basic but extremely important Chinese herb formulas follow that are generally prescribed for fever, cold, flu syndrome.

The first, Cinnamon Herb Tea, emphasizes warming herbs that tend to tonify Yin-cold conditions:

Cinnamon Herb Tea
(Kuei Chih Tang)

1. Cinnamon—4 grams (warms; tonifies Yang-circulation)
2. Ginger—4 grams (warms the stomach; tonifies Yang-digestion)
3. Peony alba—4 grams (helps circulate blood and energy; antispasmodic)
4. Jujube—4 grams (warms the spleen-pancreas)
5. Licorice—4 grams (harmonizes the herbs in the formula)

This tea is used for people of Yin confirmation suffering from chills in the abdominal region and with "flushing up" (headache, shoulder stiffness, and sweating). It is given to patients with low blood pressure and weakened digestion. It can be used for the early stages of colds, flus and stomachache with chills. With the addition of six grams of peony alba, this basic formula becomes more effective for abdominal pains associated with diarrhea, distension and chills. The use of this formula by extreme Yin people should be followed after twenty minutes with a warm bowl of brown rice.

The second formula for treating the common cold, fevers, flu, and respiratory diseases is more suitable for Yang-excess syndrome. It relies heavily on elimination through the diaphoretic (sweating) action of ephedra, and is called Mao Huang Tang.

Ephedra Herb Tea
(Mao Huang Tang)

1. Ephedra—5 grams (diaphoretic-stimulant)
2. Apricot Kernel—5 grams (nourishes the lungs)
3. Cinnamon—4 grams (warming)
4. Licorice—1.5 grams (harmonizing)

This basic formula is used for people with a more Yang constitution suffering from common cold, asthma, congestion, and arthritic and lower back pains. It is a warming formula designed to remove coldness from the lungs, which is characterized by clear mucus secretion. However, because the ephedra is an adrenal stimulant, it is inadvisable to prescribe this combination to someone who is in a very weakened state.

The third formula is specifically for individuals whose constitution is between Yin and Yang, but who suffer from symptoms of cold, flu, stiffness, chills, perspiration and fever. It is a combination of both cinnamon and ephedra teas headed by pueraria root (Kudzu), which is a cooling herb with diaphoretic-antispasmodic properties of special benefit to the lungs and gastrointestinal tract.

Pueraria Tea
(Ko Ken Tang)

1. Pueraria—6 grams (diaphoretic-antispasmodic)
2. Peony alba—4 grams (antispasmodic, helps circulation)
3. Ginger—4 grams (warms the center)
4. Licorice—1.5 grams (harmonizes)
5. Jujube date—4 grams (tonifies the spleen-pancreas)
6. Cinnamon—4 grams (warms; helps circulation)

One can see from the above examples the principle of using Chinese herbs according to symptoms and constitution. There are hundreds of tried and tested herbal formulas which are studied and prescribed according to individual requirements by Chinese herbalists. The Western methods of herbal prescribing are not as well developed in this scientific way as the Chinese. However, many of these same principles are followed in the Western formulas and prescriptions given in this book.

I feel that by studying the Oriental systems of herbology we can apply these ancient principles to the prescription of Western herbs, foods and medicines. In this way we will be evolving a system of healing that I call "Planetary Herbology," which will use the best from all cultures.

This is only a brief introduction to the use of Chinese herbs. I hope it will give the lay person the confidence to purchase and use these centuries-old health aids on a regular basis. In Appendix 2, "Sources for Herbs and Herb Products," I have listed possible sources for some of the herbs mentioned in this text.

Aconite (FU TZU)
Aconitum carmichaeli
FAMILY: Ranunculaceae

PARTS USED: The prepared root

ENERGY AND TASTE: Warm; acrid taste, toxic

SYSTEMS AFFECTED: Nervous system, circulation, spleen, urinary system, heart and small intestine

PROPERTIES: Antispasmodic, Analgesic, Stimulant, Diuretic, Diaphoretic, Tonic

DOSE: 0.5–1 gram

NOTES: Aconite is considered the most Yang of all Oriental herbs. Because of its powerful Yang properties, it should be avoided, or used with caution, by those with a Yang condition. It can be toxic if used to excess. Much of the toxic properties of aconite have been neutralized by the Chinese in their processing and preparing the herb for medicine. It is used for Yin, weak people, and will stimulate sexual potency and relieve flatulence, excess moisture, coldness, numbness, pain, arthritis, sciatica and other severely painful conditions.

This herb is always used in combination with other herbs such as ginseng or licorice, or to balance Yin, eliminative herbs. In any case, it is never used in a dosage of more than two grams or so and is not prescribed for individuals who are hypertensives (have high blood pressure).

Externally, aconite is made into a liniment applied locally for the relief of neuralgia and rheumatism.

Apricot seed (KU XING REN)

Prunus armeniaca

FAMILY: Rosaceae

PART USED: Kernel

ENERGY AND TASTE: Mild energy with sweet taste

SYSTEMS AFFECTED: Lungs, large intestines

PROPERTIES: Expectorant, Demulcent, Lung nutritive

DOSE: 3–5 grams

NOTES: The apricot kernel, while highly regarded as an anti-cancer source of laetrile, seems to be used only as a nutritive tonic for the lungs in traditional Chinese medicine. It is not recognized for any of its purported anti-carcinogenic characteristics.

My theory is that herbs seem to have a powerful eliminative property when first taken by someone whose diet and lifestyle are characterized by excess leading to toxicity and cancer. In this regard, many herbs could be of even greater benefit to help cure cancer. However, it is best to treat such a disease with a strict balanced diet as given in this book as the first prerequisite for treatment and then using other blood purifying herb combinations as suggested in the formulas chapter.

Astragalus (HUANG CHI)
Astragalus membranaceus
COMMON NAME: Bok kay
FAMILY: Leguminosae
PART USED: Root
ENERGY AND TASTE: Warm; pleasant taste, tonic
SYSTEMS AFFECTED: Spleen, kidneys, lungs and blood
PROPERTIES: Stimulant, Diuretic, Tonic
DOSE: 4–18 grams
NOTES: Astragalus is used to increase the energy and build resistance to weakness and disease. It has warming properties and is tonic to the spleen, kidneys, lungs and blood.

Astragalus is combined with other herbs to promote their effects. It is a valuable diuretic.

Astragalus balances the energy of all the internal organs. It helps neutralize fevers and improves digestion.

It is one of the most valuable tonics, being used especially for those under thirty-five years of age. It is a specific for all wasting and exhausting diseases because it strengthens the body's resistance.

Bupleurum (CH'AI HU)
Bupleurum chinese
FAMILY: Umbelliferae
PART USED: Root
ENERGY AND TASTE: Slightly cold energy, bitter taste
SYSTEMS AFFECTED: Liver, gallbladder, pericardium
PROPERTIES: Antipyretic, Alterative, Analgesic for pains in the head or chest
DOSE: 2–5 grams
NOTES: Bupleurum is regarded as one of the finest herbs for detoxifying the liver. It ranges from Northern China and Asia to Europe, where it is called "Thorough Wax." It is prescribed as an antipyretic, analgesic, antinauseant, and to counteract anxiety, dizziness, and to strengthen

the eyes and limbs. It seems to be especially good for toning up the leg muscles.

Chrysanthemum (CHU HUA)

Chrysanthemum morrifolium
FAMILY: Compositae
PART USED: Flowers
ENERGY AND TASTE: Cold; bitter but pleasant taste
SYSTEMS AFFECTED: Blood, nerves, digestion and liver, clears heat
PROPERTIES: Alterative, Antipyretic, Carminative
DOSE: 4–10 grams
NOTES: Yellow chrysanthemum flowers are valuable to counteract inflammation and pneumonia and in the treatment of fevers, headaches and dizziness. It helps purify the blood, calm the liver and brighten the eyes. Chrysanthemum is used to reduce inflammation, abscesses and boils. It is a cooling herb very popular in China for treating many Yang ailments.

Chrysanthemum is a carminative and is made into a healthful summer beverage in China.

Citrus peel (CHEN PI)

Citrus reticulata
COMMON NAME: Orange, tangerine peel
FAMILY: Rutaceae
PART USED: Peel
ENERGY AND TASTE: Warm energy, bitter and acrid taste
SYSTEMS AFFECTED: Stomach, spleen-pancreas, lungs
PROPERTIES: Stimulant, Digestant, Stomachic, Expectorant, Antitussive, Antiemetic
DOSE: 5 grams
NOTES: This herb counteracts the formation of mucus. The inner part of the orange is actually cold, and therefore mucus forming, while the peel is warming and helps eliminate it. It is added to herbal formulas to improve digestion and as a stimulant to promote the circulation of energy. It counteracts diarrhea, vomiting, colds, indigestion and abdominal swelling. The quality of this herb seems to improve with drying and age.

Cnidium (CHUANXIONG)

Ligusticum chuanxiong
COMMON NAME: "Chinese Lovage"

FAMILY: Umbelliferae
PART USED: Root
ENERGY AND TASTE: Warm energy, acrid taste
SYSTEMS AFFECTED: Bladder and reproductive organs
PROPERTIES: Emmenagogue, Antispasmodic, Stimulant
DOSE: 3–5 grams
NOTES: This herb is often used in connection with or as a substitute
for dong quai. Probably the Western herb lovage has very similar
properties. It is used to help regulate the menstrual cycle and bowels,
for abdominal pains, headache at the top of the head and to treat
various skin diseases such as boils and itch.

Deer antler (LU RONG)

Cervus nippon
PART USED: Cross section of the antler
ENERGY AND TASTE: Warm energy with sweet, pungent and salty taste
SYSTEMS AFFECTED: Hormonal system
PROPERTIES: Tonic, Stimulant
DOSE: 3–5 grams
NOTES: The antler of the Sika red deer of Northern China is one of the
most potent Yang tonics. It is as prized as expensive ginseng, and its
price reflects the high regard the Chinese have for its tonic properties.

Generally, it is taken by itself as an alcoholic extract made by steeping one ounce in a half gallon of high proof alcohol (I use cognac).
This brew is taken in teaspoonful doses two or three times a day,
mainly through the cold winter months by people over the age of
forty. It is a powerful aphrodisiac for both men and women.

Dong quai

Angelica sinensis
FAMILY: Umbelliferae
PART USED: Root
ENERGY AND TASTE: Warm energy, bitter and acrid taste
SYSTEMS AFFECTED: Uterus, blood and muscles
PROPERTIES: Uterine tonic, Antispasmodic, Alterative
DOSE: 4–7 grams
NOTES: Dong quai is used for the treatment of almost every female gyne-
cological ailment. It is particularly useful for the treatment of men-
strual cramps, irregularity, delayed flow and weakness during the

menstrual period. It is also used to relieve the symptoms of menopause.

Dong quai is a useful antispasmodic for treating insomnia, hypertension and cramps. It is nourishing to the blood and useful in treating anemia. Dong quai is a valuable blood purifier. It is warming to
the circulation and is used to moisten the intestines to treat constipation.

Dong quai, also known as tang kwei, should not be used during
pregnancy, or with excessive menstrual flow.

The Western herb angelica, *Angelica archangelica,* can be substituted in some cases. However, its action is harsher and it is a stimulant that reduces cramping through its warming quality, while dong
quai accomplishes this through its antispasmodic components. Both
are useful blood purifiers.

Don sen *(TANG SHEN)*

Codonopsis pilosula
FAMILY: Campanulaceae
PART USED: Root
ENERGY AND TASTE: Slight warm energy, bittersweet taste
SYSTEMS AFFECTED: Spleen, pancreas, heart and stomach, assists Yang,
   increases energy
PROPERTIES: Spleen tonic, Stomach tonic
DOSE: 7–14 grams
NOTES: Don sen is used to strengthen the vital energy (*chi*) and is considered to be close in its properties to ginseng. It has the advantage
   of being cheaper, as well as useful at any time of year in both cold
   and warm climates, and it can be taken on a daily basis by both men
   and women. Its action is milder and safer than ginseng and it can be
   used for a longer treatment. It is recommended in combination with
   astragalus for increasing energy and building resistance to disease.

Don sen strengthens the functions of the spleen and pancreas. It is
thus used in treating infection and inflammation and for diabetes. It
is given in all diseases associated with weakness, debility and anemia.

Don sen strengthens the stomach and is used to treat hyperacidity
and weak digestion.

Eleuthero

Eleutherococcus senticosus
FAMILY: Araliaceae

PART USED: Roots and leaves
ENERGY AND TASTE: Warm energy, biting taste
SYSTEMS AFFECTED: Heart, circulation, nerves and lungs
PROPERTIES: Cardiac tonic, Antispasmodic
NOTES: Eleuthero is a relative of ginseng that is used for its general tonic properties and for its calming effects. It is used in conditions for which ginseng would be considered too stimulating.

Eleuthero is considered by the Chinese to be the best medicine for treating insomnia. It is also extensively used for bronchitis and chronic lung ailments.

In the treatment and prevention of heart disease, eleuthero is used to lower blood pressure and reduce cholesterol levels. It has been used to treat arthritis, low blood oxygen, impotence and stress. It is a mild herb and must be used in large doses, about eight to thirty grams per day, depending upon the severity of the ailment. The leaves are stronger and are taken two to eight grams per day.

Ephedra (MA HUANG)

Ephedra sinica
FAMILY: Ephedraceae
PART USED: Stems and branches
ENERGY AND TASTE: Warm energy, acrid taste
SYSTEMS AFFECTED: Adrenals, lungs and heart
DOSE: 3–10 grams
PROPERTIES: Stimulant, Diaphoretic, expectorant, astringent
NOTES: Ephedra is useful for asthma, bronchitis, coughs and other congestive conditions. It should be used only for those with a Yang constitution and are not deficient, as it is a strong stimulant that would debilitate the adrenals of one who is already exhausted and low in energy. It is good for colds and flus and for those fevers that are without sweating. Ephedra increases blood pressure, and therefore should not be used by people with hypertension.

There is also an American ephedra (desert tea), which is used similarly but is much milder.

Fu ling

Poria cocos
FAMILY: Polyporaceae
PART USED: Whole fungus

ENERGY AND TASTE: Neutral; pleasant taste

SYSTEMS AFFECTED: Kidneys

PROPERTIES: Diuretic, Nervine, expectorant

NOTES: This fungus is considered one of the finest diuretics. It is used to rid the body of excess moisture and the attendant emotional imbalances of insecurity, apprehension, fear and instability. It is used to treat kidney weakness, lung congestion and insomnia. It helps to expel and transform mucus.

   It is nutritive and tonifying, helping the spleen, pancreas, stomach and nerves. Thus it is prescribed in all wasting diseases. It is also used for the treatment of hyperactivity in children.

   Fu ling comes in both red and white colors. The red fu ling, called muk sheng, is considered best for nervous, restless conditions.

Gelatin

PART USED: Traditionally derived from cooking the hides of black donkeys

ENERGY AND TASTE: Mild energy; sweet, fetid taste

SYSTEMS AFFECTED: Lungs, liver, kidneys

PROPERTIES: Tonic for the blood, Coagulant

DOSE: 5–10 grams

NOTES: This is one of the most potent Yin-nourishing substances used in Chinese medicine. It is given to anyone suffering from Yin deficiency. It seems to be particularly useful for women as a blood tonic. It comes in hardened black pieces which are dissolved in warm water or wine. It is excellent combined with dong qua and a small amount of ginger as a women's hormonal tonic to be taken on a regular weekly basis for health maintenance, or in small amounts (one or two tablespoons) every morning. For the latter formula I recommend cooking it in rice wine (sake).

Ginseng (JEN SHENG, REN SHENG)

Panax ginseng

FAMILY: Araliaceae

PART USED: Root

SYSTEMS AFFECTED: Heart and circulation; general effects on the whole body

PROPERTIES: Alterative, Cardiac tonic, Hepatic tonic, Stimulant

DOSE: 5–10 grams

NOTES: Ginseng is considered the king of all tonics. It provides a stimulation to the entire body energy to overcome stress and fatigue and to recover from weakness and deficiencies.

Ginseng has a very beneficial effect on the heart and circulation and is used to normalize blood pressure, reduce blood cholesterol and prevent atherosclerosis. It nourishes the blood and is thus used to treat anemia. By reducing blood sugar levels, it is useful in managing diabetes.

Ginseng is not used with any diseases where there is inflammation, burning sensations, high fever and other Yang conditions (see the "Diagnosis and Treatment" chapter). Ginseng is used for women with deficiency diseases, lowered resistance and lack of hormonal balance, but is not used with Yang conditions, such as excessive menstrual flow.

There are many grades of ginseng available. *Panax ginseng* comes from China and Korea, and is either dried (white), steamed and dried (which changes the color naturally to red) or extracted. I suggest using the red ginseng, the best being shiu chu roots from China.

Honeysuckle *(JAPANESE YIN HUA)*

Lonicera japonica
FAMILY: Caprifoliaceae
PART USED: Flowers
ENERGY AND TASTE: Cooling; bitter taste
SYSTEMS AFFECTED: Blood and liver (clears heat)
PROPERTIES: Alterative, Antipyretic
DOSE: 10–17 grams
NOTES: Honeysuckle figures prominently in all Chinese detoxifying formulas. It is mostly used for all acute infectious and inflammatory conditions. It is very valuable for inflammatory skin diseases such as poison oak and various other rashes. It can be used alone or together with chrysanthemum flowers for treatment of acute flus, fevers and other similar conditions. It is not considered to be a medicine for chronic diseases and so is not intended for extended usage.

The infusion, prepared by steeping an ounce of the flowers in a pint of water, may also be applied externally for skin infections.

Ho shou wu (also known as Fo-Ti in the United States)

Polygonum multiflorum
FAMILY: Polygonaceae

PART USED: Root
ENERGY AND TASTE: Warm energy, bitter and acrid taste
SYSTEMS AFFECTED: Kidneys, liver, blood, pancreas and spleen
PROPERTIES: Hepatic tonic, Alterative, Diuretic
DOSE: 7–15 grams
NOTES: Ho shou wu is a rejuvenating tonic that will restore energy, increase fertility and maintain strength and vigor for those who are advanced in years.

I recommend its use as a strengthener of the kidneys, liver and blood. It plays an important role in the treatment of all deficiency diseases. Ho shou wu is excellent for use in treating both hypoglycemia and diabetes.

The Chinese claim that it will keep the hair black, and benefit the muscles, tendons, ligaments and bones. Ho shou wu accomplishes this by preventing premature aging. An alcoholic preparation called "shou wu chic" is sold in Chinese herb stores and contains shou wu and other tonic herbs useful for tonifying the liver and kidney.

Jujube date (DA T'SAO)
Ziziphus jujuba
PART USED: Whole date
ENERGY AND TASTE: Neutral energy, sour taste
SYSTEMS AFFECTED: Spleen-pancreas, nerves, stomach
PROPERTIES: Nutritive, Digestive, Nervine, Tonic
DOSE: 5–10 grams
NOTES: The Chinese jujube date is commonly used in a wide variety of herbal formulas. It is found in dried form in most Oriental markets. The people use it to enhance the taste and health benefits of their soups and stews. It gives energy to the body and is used to relieve nervous exhaustion, insomnia, apprehension, forgetfulness, dizziness and clamminess. It is usually given in prescription with a variety of other suitable Chinese herbs. The tree from which this fruit comes seems to be able to grow in the warmer climates of America.

Licorice (GAN T'SAO)
Glycyrrhiza glabra
FAMILY: Leguminosae
PART USED: Root
ENERGY AND TASTE: Neutral; pleasant taste

SYSTEMS AFFECTED: Lungs, stomach, intestines, spleen and liver; general
effects on the whole body
PROPERTIES: Expectorant, Alterative, Demulcent, Laxative
DOSE: 3–10 grams
NOTES: Licorice contains substances similar to the adrenal cortical hormones. For this reason, it is very beneficial in treating adrenal insuf-
ficiency and other glandular problems. However, large and frequent
doses will exacerbate hypertension.

Licorice can safely be added to tonics and detoxifying herbal formulas to alleviate the harsh stimulating aspects of bitter herbs without interfering with the beneficial aspects associated with their use.
It is considered one of the most important herbs of Chinese medicine
and is frequently prescribed as part of Chinese herbal formulas.

It is a proven remedy for all kinds of stomach and intestinal ulcers.
It also has a stimulating action and helps counteract stress.

By itself, licorice is a good remedy for flu, colds, debility and all
lung problems. It is a very good expectorant for treating coughs and
bronchial congestion. For colds and flu, combine licorice with stimulating herbs, such as black pepper, sage, juniper, cayenne or ginger.
Licorice root can be smoked for relief of sore throat and hoarseness.

Licorice is beneficial to the liver and for this it is often mixed with
equal parts of peony root. It is a safe sweetener for diabetics. It is a
good mild laxative that can be given to children and persons who are
debilitated.

As a detoxifier of the blood, it can be combined favorably with
echinacea, dandelion, red clover, burdock, sassafras or sarsaparilla.

Herbal pills can be made by decocting licorice with other herbs,
straining and then slowly simmering down the liquid until a thick
paste is formed. It is then rolled into little pills and dried at low heat
or in the sun.

Licorice should not be given to people who tend to retain water in
their bodily tissues.

Longan berries (LONG YEN ROU)

Euphoria longana
COMMON NAME: "Dragon's Eyes"
FAMILY: Sapindaceae
PARTS USED: Berries
ENERGY AND TASTE: Neutral energy, pleasant, sweet taste

SYSTEMS AFFECTED: Heart, spleen-pancreas
PROPERTIES: Nutritive tonic
DOSE: 10–15 grams
NOTES: This berry is a powerful tonic that is used in medicine, foods
and confections. It strengthens the reproductive organs of women
and counteracts anemia, forgetfulness and hyperactive mental activity. Cooked with millet and aduki beans and served with sweet
squash it is an effective remedy for hypoglycemia and conditions associated with sweet cravings.

Lycii (GAY GEE)
Lycium chinensis
FAMILY: Solanaceae
PART USED: Berries
ENERGY AND TASTE: Neutral; pleasant taste
SYSTEMS AFFECTED: Blood, liver, kidneys and lungs
PROPERTIES: Nutrient tonic (Yin), Antipyretic, Alterative
DOSE: 6–10 grams
NOTES: Lycii berries are a cooling tonic used to reduce fevers and thirst,
and to treat bronchial inflammations. They aid in the removal of tox-
ins from the blood by nourishing the liver and strengthening the
kidneys. Lycii is often prescribed in the treatment of diabetes.

It is an ideal herb for meat eaters, as it is nourishing to the liver
and kidneys like ginseng, but is a cooling, Yin tonic to balance the
Yang effects of the meat.

Lycii is never used for acute fevers and colds because it is said to
drive the fever deeper. It is best used for chronic, deficient, low-grade
fevers with perspiration.

Lycii is good for those who suffer from cloudy vision. It clears the
eyes.

Pai shu
Atractylodes macrocephala
FAMILY: Compositae
PART USED: Root
ENERGY AND TASTE: Warm energy; acrid but pleasant taste
SYSTEMS AFFECTED: Kidneys, spleen, pancreas and stomach
PROPERTIES: Diuretic
DOSE: 5–10 grams

NOTES: Pai shu increases the energy of the body by eliminating excess moisture through a process that first eliminates excess sodium and other electrolytes. This process is effected without directly interfering with the kidney filtration process and thus as a diuretic, pai shu does not exhaust the kidneys as some other diuretics do. It is of very low toxicity and a major ingredient of the famous "Mu" tea blend. It is a tonic for the spleen and pancreas.

Pai shu is given for diarrhea, indigestion, edema, chest tightness, abdominal distension and vomiting.

It is often combined with other Chinese tonic herbs, such as those described in this chapter, to enhance their tonic properties.

Peony (SHAO-YAO)

Paeonia lactiflora
FAMILY: Ranunculaceae
PART USED: Root
ENERGY AND TASTE: Slightly cold; bitter and acrid taste
SYSTEMS AFFECTED: Liver, blood, uterus and skin
PROPERTIES: Alterative, Antispasmodic, Hepatic tonic
DOSE: 5–10 grams
NOTES: Peony root is a liver tonic and is almost always used together with licorice root for treating all diseases stemming from an imbalanced liver function. It is also a good blood purifier, useful in treating skin eruptions and infections.

Peony is very useful in treating all female complaints, especially menstrual irregularity and abdominal pains associated with the menstrual cycle. It is nourishing to the blood and is used to treat anemia.

Platycodon (JIE GENG)

Platycodon grandiflorum
FAMILY: Campanulaceae
PART USED: Root
ENERGY AND TASTE: Slightly warm energy; bitter, acrid taste
SYSTEMS AFFECTED: Lungs
PROPERTIES: Expectorant, Lung tonic
DOSE: 2–5 grams
NOTES: This is a tonic expectorant useful for treating asthma, cough, sore throat, lung and bronchial congestion. It is useful as a strong

expectorant and helps to counteract pneumonia and clear infected mucus from the lungs.

Pueraria (KO KEN)
Pueraria lobata
COMMON NAME: Kuzu root
FAMILY: Leguminosae
PART USED: Root
ENERGY AND TASTE: Mild energy with sweet taste
SYSTEMS AFFECTED: Lungs, stomach
PROPERTIES: Antipyretic, Refrigerant, Diaphoretic, Spasmolytic, Demulcent
DOSE: 4–11 grams
NOTES: Kuzu root or Kudzu Vine, as it is sometimes called, is commonly used as a treatment for cold, flu and gastrointestinal problems. For colds and flu it is excellent to take mixed with a small amount of licorice, cinnamon, ginger and tamari-soya sauce. It also neutralizes acidity in the body and thus relieves minor aches and pains.

It is a mild acting substance high in starch. The starch extracted from the root is dried into chunks and used as a sauce-thickening substitute for arrowroot. It grows wild in the Southern states, where it is considered the scourge of the South. Its fast growing, hardy vines seem to creep over everything and are most difficult to eradicate. I wonder why there has been no industry exploring the many beneficial uses of this valuable healing herb?

Rehmannia (SOK DAY-SANG DAY)
Rehmannia glutinosa
FAMILY: Scrophulariaceae
PART USED: Root
ENERGY AND TASTE: Cool; bitter but pleasant taste
SYSTEMS AFFECTED: Blood, kidneys, bones and tendons
PROPERTIES: Cardiac tonic, Diuretic, Alterative, Uterine tonic, hemostatic
NOTES: Rehmannia is an important herb encountered frequently in Chinese herb formulas. It is used to purify and nourish the blood, strengthen the kidneys and heal the bones and tendons.

There are two forms commonly sold. One is the unprocessed root ("sang day"), which is considered the best for treating the kidneys and eliminating excess acids from the body. The other is a processed form ("sok day"), which is preferred for treating the blood. It is useful in treating anemia and heart weakness.

Rehmannia is useful in helping build the body during recovery from illness, and it helps relieve fatigue. It is given to women to treat menstrual irregularities and infertility, as a tonic during pregnancy and to stop postpartum hemorrhage.

Salvia (DANG SHEN)
Salvia miltiorrhiza
FAMILY: Labiatae
PART USED: Root
ENERGY AND TASTE: Slightly cold energy, bitter taste
SYSTEMS AFFECTED: Heart, liver
PROPERTIES: Emmenagogue, Alterative, Blood stimulant
DOSE: 5–10 grams
NOTES: This is one of the most important Chinese herbs for removing blood stagnation and regulating the menses. It is also useful as an alterative, thus making dang shen a complete blood tonic.

It is used for a variety of diseases, including both excessive and obstructed menstruation in women, abdominal distension, boils, erysipelas, itch, and spasmodic rheumatism.

In China this herb is used both in tea form and as a liquid extract directly injected into acupuncture points and affected areas with a hypodermic needle.

While this is a type of sage-root related to the many species of sage growing through the world, this particular variety has reddish colored roots unlike any found growing in America.

Scutellaria (HUANG CHI)
Scutellaria baicalensis
COMMON NAME: Skullcap
FAMILY: Labiatae
PART USED: Root
ENERGY AND TASTE: Cold energy, bitter taste
SYSTEMS AFFECTED: Heart, lungs, liver, gallbladder, large intestines
PROPERTIES: Diuretic, Laxative, Antipyretic, Hemostatic, Astringent
NOTES: This is another species of plant of which there are many varieties found in different parts of the world. In Western herbology, the skullcap is considered a very important herb for the nerves, and its leaves

are used in medicine. In Chinese herbology, "scute" root is primarily used as a cooling, antipyretic herb that sedates by removing the congestion of heat toxin from the heart, lungs, and liver. It is given for jaundice, suppurating infections, carbuncle, sores, pneumonia, and insecure motion of the fetus.

Sileris
Ledebouriella divaricata
COMMON NAME: "Fang-feng"
FAMILY: Umbelliferae
PART USED: Root
ENERGY AND TASTE: Warm energy, acrid taste
SYSTEMS AFFECTED: Liver
PROPERTIES: Antispasmodic
NOTES: This herb is used as an antispasmodic to relieve flu, headache, chills, rheumatoid numbness, pain of the joints and tetanus.

It is combined in a wondefully effective formula called "Jade Screen Powder" to build up the immune resistance to colds and flu for Yin-weak constitutions. This formula, consisting of 12 to 15 grams astragalus, 10 to 12 grams of atractylis and 6 to 9 grams sileris, can be taken on a daily basis as a tonic for the immune system.

Tienchi
Panax notoginseng
FAMILY: Araliaceae
PART USED: Root
ENERGY AND TASTE: Warm energy, sweet and slightly bitter taste
SYSTEMS AFFECTED: Blood, heart and liver
PROPERTIES: Hemostatic, Cardiac tonic
DOSE: 5–10 grams
NOTES: Tienchi is one of the best treatments for hemorrhage. It may be applied directly to a wound or taken internally to stop bleeding (dose, three to nine grams). When cooked for about an hour in a tonic soup, it makes an excellent tonic for the heart, normalizing blood pressure and heart rate and improving circulation.

Tienchi is used to help maintain normal body weight, to prevent fatigue and to withstand stress.

A patented medicine from China called "Yunan Baiyao," using tienchi as its main ingredient, is considered the best herbal medicine to use for wounds, gunshot, bleeding, cuts and chronic stomachache. It is commonly available in Chinese Herbal Pharmacies.

Wild Ginger *(XI XIN)*
Asarum heterotropoides
FAMILY: Aristolochiaceae
PART USED: Root
ENERGY AND TASTE: Warm energy, acrid taste
SYSTEMS AFFECTED: Heart, lung, liver and kidney meridians
PROPERTIES: Emmenagogue, Stimulant, Antispasmodic, Diaphoretic
NOTES: This herb is used for any obstruction in the flow of energy in the meridians. It is also used for obstructed flow of the menses and congestion in the lungs, nose and head. Its warm, pungent action serves to relieve spasms and congestion in general. There is a milder-acting American variety of wild ginger which is effective for similar conditions. The Chinese variety should only be used in small quantity as it can possibly be mildly toxic if taken in doses larger than 3 to 5 grams.

· 11 ·

OBTAINING AND STORING HERBS

In order for herbal remedies to be effective in the recommended doses, the herbs used must contain their full complement of active constituents. The potency of herbs depends on many factors:

1. the species
2. the growing location and climatic conditions
3. the time of harvest
4. the method of drying and preserving
5. the storage conditions
6. the form of the herb
7. the duration of storage

Whether you harvest your own herbs or purchase herbs from a store, it will be of value to be familiar with all the factors that affect the potency of the herbs you use in healing.

Species

In some cases, more than one species of plant will be sold under the same generic name. For example, "echinacea" is used to refer to both *Echinacea angustifolia* (Kansas snakeroot) and *Echinacea purpurea* (Missouri snakeroot). *Echinacea angustifolia* is probably more potent and is most commonly mentioned as the plant used in traditional Native American medicine. Both have similar properties. However, *Echinacea purpurea* is more readily available and about one third the price of *Echinacea augustifolia*. Thus most herb stores will provide products made from *Echinacea purpurea*.

Similarly, "ephedra" may be used to describe *Ephedra sinica* (ma huang or Chinese ephedra) or to refer to an American species of ephedra (desert tea or Mormon tea). But only the Chinese species contains large amounts of the active principle "ephedrin." In this case the availability and price in stores are similar, so that one or the other is likely to be carried.

In the case of ginseng, the term is properly used to describe both the Oriental ginseng, *Panax ginseng,* and the American variety, *Panax quinquefolium.* Both have similar properties, but the Chinese regard Oriental ginseng as warming and thus it is used as a winter tonic, while American ginseng is considered cooling and is used more as a summer tonic. An entirely different species, *Eleutherococcus senticosus,* which is a cousin of *Panax ginseng* with some similar properties, is often sold as "Siberian ginseng." Yet another plant, *Panax notoginseng,* is sold as "Tienchi ginseng."

There are two commonly used species of angelica, the Chinese variety, *Angelica sinensis* (dong quai), and the American and European species, *Angelica archangelica.* The Chinese variety is primarily used for its effects as a uterine tonic and antispasmodic, while the American species is used primarily for its warming, stimulant properties and in the treatment of lung diseases. The warming quality of the American species will help calm muscle spasms, and thus can partially match the antispasmodic properties of the Chinese species. However, the two are not equivalent in their effects and the Chinese species is superior as a treatment for all ailments of the female reproductive system.

Whenever there is any question as to the species of plant to use, it is best to investigate the matter more fully by consulting several sources of herbal information (see the Bibliography at the end of this book for some suggestions).

Growing Location and Climatic Conditions

For any given species of plant, different growing conditions will affect the content of active principles. This will include the nutrient quality of the soil and the particular weather conditions during the plant's growth. In general, too little is known about how these factors influence the medicinal properties of the plant to allow much control in choosing the best quality.

For one who is following the principles of Simpling (see the chapter on "Theory of Using Herbs"), the local area is ideal. However, one should avoid picking herbs along heavily trafficked roads, since the exhausts from the vehicles will leave a residue on and in the plants.

When purchasing herbs from a store, one should realize that though many of the medicinal plants are available in the United States, the ones that are available commercially are often imported. This is because herb growing is a labor intensive enterprise and labor costs are too high in the United States compared to other countries, especially those of Eastern Europe, South and Central America. The major exception to this is the wildcrafting of herbs in the Appalachian region. Here, the poorer people can gather wild herbs in the surrounding forest area for a little extra income. The efforts of many individuals are revealed as a substantial quantity of herbs is brought to a central collecting area. These are then shipped around the country.

Herbs that survive a harsher climate are often believed to better help one through the harsher ailments.

Time of Harvest

Herbs must be picked when they contain the highest amount of medicinal essences. This varies greatly throughout the year. The following are some general rules.

Leaves are picked just before the plant is about to begin flowering. At this time, the energy of the plant is focused in the upper portions. These and other plant parts should be picked after the morning dew has dried but before the hot sun has evaporated away the essential oils.

Flowers are picked just before they first reach full bloom. They will lose much of their value if picked later.

Berries and fruits are picked at the peak ripeness, as they are about to fall naturally from the plant.

When the aboveground portion of the plant is used, this usually refers to the combination of stems and leaves and is picked just before the plant begins to flower.

Barks and twigs of shrubs and trees are collected in the spring when the sap rises, when the leaves first appear.

Roots and rhizomes are collected in the fall, when the sap returns to the ground as the leaves just begin to change color and the berries or seeds are mature. In some cases, such as sassafras, these are harvested in the early spring before the sap rises.

Method of Drying and Preserving

Plant tops are gently washed, allowed to dry, then picked and hung in a well ventilated, dry, shaded area. Unless the whole plant is going to be used, the plant is hung upside down so that the sap will run from the stems into the leaves as it dries. They may be tied in small bunches, or they may be spread on a screen. If a screen is used, the plants should be turned each day to assure uniform drying.

Roots and barks are carefully scrubbed and then chopped before drying. The pieces should not be more than an inch thick after drying. Spread the pieces on a screen and turn daily. Those roots lacking volatile oils may be dried in direct sunlight, while the others should be dried in a warm shaded area.

A dryer that passes warm (about 100°F.) dry air upward through a series of screens can be used if air drying is not possible.

Drying will usually take three to four days. Most plants will lose half to three-quarters of their weight upon drying. They will generally retain about 10% of their weight as moisture.

Herbal properties may also be retained by other methods of preservation. Fresh herbs are used directly for making vinegar extracts (liniments), essential oils and salves (see "Methods of Application" chapter).

Storage Conditions

Herbal properties are destoryed by heat, by bright light, by exposure to air, by the activity of plant enzymes and by bacteria and fungi. Enzyme activity and growth of microorganisms are promoted by heat and moisture. Volatile substances are readily lost to the air, and oxygen will destroy the properties of oils and other important substances in the herb.

Herbs should be kept in a cool, dry place with minimum exposure to air and sunlight. However, it is a mistake to hide herbs away in a dark closet or in dark jars if that will inhibit your use of them. It is much better to have them easily seen or readily accessible—they will not sit unused for long. Containers should be tightly capped. Clear plastic bags are almost useless, as they allow air to circulate and volatile substances are rapidly lost. Do not place herbs on a windowsill where they will have exposure to direct sunlight. Keep them at a safe distance from the kitchen stove and other sources of intense heat.

Form of the Herb

When purchasing herbs, three forms are usually available: whole, cut/sifted and powdered. While herbs keep best, since air and microorganisms cannot get at the interior of the herb, but it is also more difficult to extract the essences. Whole herbs may be used for making tinctures, liniments and decoctions. Some herbs, such as small leaves and flowers, are usually available only in whole form or as powders. Herbs are cut and then sifted to remove powders for use in making teas. They are easy to strain when in this form and may also be used for most herbal applications, except for gelatin capsules and boluses. Powders do not keep as well because there is so much surface area exposed to air, moisture and light. Powdered herbs are specifically used for gelatin capsules, pills and boluses. It is often difficult to powder herbs finely enough for capsules, even with an electric coffee grinder, so it is advisable to purchase them already ground up. Powders may be used for most other applications, but they are more difficult to strain and must be separated through a cloth. An advantage to using powders is that they extract very quickly. Thus a tincture can be made in three days using powdered herbs but will require about fourteen days using whole herbs.

Duration of Storage

If herbs begin to lose their smell, taste and/or color they should be set aside for use in herbal baths for the body or for foot and hand baths. For this purpose, the older herbs can be mixed together indiscriminately. In general, one should restock one's herb collection every year or two. If herbs are purchased at a store, they have probably already been stored for one or two years since being harvested. These will then have a shelf life in the home of not more than one year. After that, they will have diminished potency. Herbs with aromatic oils will lose potency first, while heavy roots and barks and some seeds will maintain potency for considerably longer.

It is generally not necessary to keep a hundred herbs in stock. Rather, one should have a collection of about two dozen culinary herbs and spices regularly used in cooking, and about three dozen medicinal herbs, including those used most often and those that are more difficult to obtain. Then if other herbs are needed for treating a specific condition, one can purchase them at that time.

When making herb teas, it is often convenient to make a large batch, one quart to one gallon, and store it in a tightly closed bottle in the refrigerator. These teas will last for no more than about three days. When reheating, do not boil the tea. Tinctures and vinegar extracts, because of their antibacterial properties, will last for three years if stored in a cool place.

Oils, when stored with a minimum contact to air and kept in a cool place, will last for up to seven years. A small amount of Vitamin E added to the oil will greatly aid in preservation.

Salves and lotions may be preserved for several years by adding a small amount of tincture of benzoin. This is an important addition, since these may be applied to broken skin and thus must be kept relatively free of bacteria.

Poultices, boluses and fomentations should be made as needed and not stored at all.

· 1 2 ·

MAKING AN HERBAL
FORMULA

W hen using potent herbs, herbalists generally prefer using a mixture of several herbs according to a basic formula rather than
using a single herb. This is because the single herb may have an effect
that is too direct or too strong, or because a set of effects is desired that
no single herb provides. One can think of the herbs as different colors.
By mixing them together one can produce a tremendous variation in
shades that aren't found in nature. The effects of the combination of
herbs are different from the mere sum of the individual herbs going into
the formulation.

An appropriately combined herbal formula is essential in the treatment of chronic ailments where many organ systems have been affected.
The design of a tonic formula for a chronic ailment is a subtle art that
must be developed with considerable experience. However, one may
learn the way of herbs through the treatment of the acute ailments and
thus gain experience to tackle the more difficult work with chronic
problems.

For acute ailments, a general formula outline is:

1. use a large proportion (about 70%–80% by weight) of one to
   three herbs that possess the primary property required to treat the

ailment (expectorant for coughs, antibiotic and blood purifying properties for infections, warming properties for colds, etc);·

2. add a small amount of stimulant herb to promote the action of the primary medicine;

3. add a small amount of antispasmodic herb to reduce tensions in the body;

4. add a small amount of carminative or demulcent herb to provide gentle action and protection to the system.

The primary medicine makes up the major bulk of the herb formula and determines the basic action of the formula on the body. It is important that the secondary medicines—the stimulants, antispasmodics and demulcent/carminatives—not dilute the primary medicines. This is why about 70–80% of the herb formula is usually primary medicines.

Any herb may be a primary medicine, and the choice of the herbs to use will depend on the major symptoms of the body. Herbs always have a number of properties. By combining two or three herbs that share the property of greatest importance in treating the ailment, one will also get the other properties of these herbs. If the primary herbs are properly chosen, these additional properties will complement its action, providing other important effects that will assist in healing the body.

Of the secondary medicines, it is often the case that several essential properties can be found in a single herb, thus the formula may be simplified and the primary medicine will not be greatly diluted. Ginger, licorice, fennel seed, anise seed and cumin seed are examples of herbs that provide all three properties required of the secondary medicines. In some cases, however, specific herbs for each of the secondary properties will be desired. For example, if a strong demulcent is needed, an herb which is high in mucilage would be added.

The stimulant herbs have been discussed in the section on "Stimulation" in the "Herbal Therapies" chapter. A stimulant herb can be added to provide about 10% of the formula. Ginger root and cayenne pepper are two very commonly used herbs for this purpose.

Antispasmodics are important for two reasons. First, they relieve spasms directly associated with the ailment or as a result of tension/ nervousness in reaction to the disease symptoms. Second, they help prevent a reaction to strong effects of the primary medicine. Sometimes the bitter flavor of some herbs will upset one for a while, or the herbs will cause a slight nausea in the stomach. The antispasmodic relieves these reactions. Commonly used antispasmodics are lobelia, valerian and skullcap. Licorice is very useful for overcoming the strong bitter taste of some herbs. Antispasmodics make up about 10% of the formula.

Demulcent and carminative herbs soothe the system and counteract any irritating principles in the primary medicines. It is essential to use demulcents when giving diuretics, since if kidney stones are present, the diuretic may help release the stones, which would damage the tissues in the absence of a soothing demulcent. It is also necessary to use demulcents when using the more irritating diuretics (such as horsetail or juniper berries) and laxatives (such as cascara sagrada). Carminatives are particularly useful to relax the stomach and intestines so that the herbal properties may be better assimilated. Demulcent herbs also help assimilation by softening the internal tissues, making them more absorbent. Demulcent/carminative herbs usually make up about 10% of the formula.

The treatment of chronic diseases requires a different approach. Because of the weakness developed during prolonged illness, one can't push the body too strongly in one direction. The herbs used must have a mild action and they must simultaneously strengthen all the affected systems. Since all herbs have a cleansing and eliminating effect, special care must be taken to use herbs whose eliminative power is mild.

I prepare a "signature formula" for the treatment of a chronic ailment, comprising a variety of herbs whose effects are matched to the particular condition of the person. All systems are affected to some degree. Because of the assortment of herbs with differing actions, I often add a small amount of licorice to balance the formula, harmonize the action of the herbs and avoid side effects. This practice has been successfully applied in China for many centuries. In fact, the Chinese refer to licorice as the "peacemaker."

A properly composed formula for the treatment of a chronic ailment should result in only gradual changes in the body's condition. If stronger symptoms of the disease arise after taking an herb tonic, the formula should be changed. As the chronic condition improves, the body becomes stronger and may eventually have the power to manifest the ailment as an acute disease (this process is called the "healing crisis"). At this time, it is possible to use stronger herbs with a more direct effect.

To maintain a mild character in a tonic herb formula, it is best to use complementary herbs. Hence if one uses a pungent or spicy herb, the irritating effects can be balanced by the use of a demulcent herb. When a diuretic or laxative is used, its effects can be toned down by adding an astringent. If anything in the formula is strong, it should be buffered by an appropriate complementary herb.

Just as one would use a mild action to treat chronic ailments because the energy is weak, one must generally avoid diluting the herbal formulas for acute diseases with many mild tonic herbs. In the acute disease, the individual is relatively strong and can best be helped to throw off the sickness by stimulating the natural defenses directly. A tonic may later be used to recover the full vitality of the body, which has been drained in the process of healing.

Choosing the Herbs

Choosing herbs with the proper complement of effects is a relatively simple matter once the major properties of the important herbs are noted. Hence when a demulcent herb is to be used, marshmallow root is one of the best in a diuretic formula because it is also a diuretic; licorice is a demulcent preferred for tonics because it harmonizes the many herbs in that formula; slippery elm is used when extra nutrition is needed because of its high content of vitamins, minerals and carbohydrates. In choosing an antispasmodic, lobelia is used in treating acute ailments because of its strong direct action; valerian is used in more Yang tonics to treat superficial chronic ailments; skullcap is preferred to treat deeper and more debilitating chronic ailments affecting the nerves. Of the carminatives, cumin, fennel and anise seeds are very useful since they also have stimulant and antispasmodic properties, but they are without tonic value and are therefore used only in medicines for acute ailments.

A Note on Following the Recipes

The recipes that follow are designed for use with the herbal powders or the cut form of the herb. Proportions are given in parts by weight. When using a powder, let the powder settle to the bottom of the liquid extract and carefully pour off the clear extract for use. Alternatively, the liquid may be strained through a cheesecloth or paper filter. If the cut form is used, the extract is simply strained through a tea strainer. The advantage of powders is that they extract more fully and quickly than the cut form. They have the disadvantage of losing potency more quickly during storage and being more difficult to strain.

When whole herbs or seeds are used, they should first be crushed or bruised using a mortar and pestle. In making formulas that are to be capsuled, if the powder cannot be purchased, the herbs may be ground in an electric coffee and spice grinder. Pills can be made with a coarser powder. Alternatively, the formula may be used to make a tincture, in which one teaspoon (sixty drops) is taken in place of two gelatin capsules. (Note that dosages have assumed a body weight of about 150 pounds; people who weight less will require a proportionately smaller dose.)

In some cases, the herb components of the formula have been divided into primary and secondary categories to demonstrate the use of this method of formulation. However, it is often the case that the primary and secondary properties are contained in the same herb and in these cases no division has been made. Some of the herbs contributing to the secondary properties (stimulant, antispasmodic, demulcent/carminative) have been indicated.

These formulas have been developed and used by me in my clinic. They are safe and easy to use and will prove to benefit the health. For simple diseases, a single formula might be sufficient. For more complicated problems, more of the internal organs are involved and it may be necessary to use a combination of the formulas simultaneously to restore normal function of the internal organs.

This approach, called "Rasayana" in Ayurvedic medicine, constitutes an herbal body purification program which may be undertaken for anywhere from one week to 3 months depending on the individual. For best results, one should also follow the balanced diet as given in Chapter 7.

Herb recipes are given in parts by weight, so that the total amount of the formula to be made can be adjusted to your needs and the availability of the ingredients. As a simple guide, use one-half ounce of herb for a one part measurement. When taking the herbs for acute ailments, it is best to divide the daily dosage into smaller doses taken frequently throughout the day if it is convenient to do so. This way, the herbal properties will be continuously available for the body to use as needed. If there is any bowel sluggishness or constipation, one must work to remove this condition as it can become the cause of more serious diseases later. Following are some effective formulas that can be used for regulating the bowels.

Dr. Christopher's Lower Bowel Tonic

This is a very useful formula for treating all bowel problems. It will help to regulate bowel movements and restore tone to weakened bowels. This formula is also used in the treatment of hemorrhoids. Take two capsules, two or three times per day.

PRIMARY: Cascara sagrada—2 parts
                Barberry root—1 part
                Rhubarb root—1 part
                Goldenseal—1 part
                Raspberry leaves—1 part
SECONDARY: Lobelia—1 part (antispasmodic)
                Ginger root—1 part
                (stimulant/carminative)

Combine the powdered herbs and fill gelatin capsules, or add one part slippery elm and make small pills.

The Wonders of Triphala

A traditional Ayurvedic formula from India that is a common household remedy for acute and chronic constipation consists of three fruits that, when combined, serve as both a mild laxative and a tonic to clean out and sharpen the entire digestive system.

Triphala consists of chebulic myrobalan, which regulates the nervous system; emblic myrobalan, which is the highest known source of vitamin C and is antiinflammatory; and belleric myrobalan, which is anticholesterol and clears mucus from the channels of the body.

Each of these contribute to this gentle, non-habit-forming laxative, blood and liver detoxifier and tonic. Thus, unlike other laxative formulas, triphala is safe even for vegetarians, who are often more sensitive to cleansing and eliminative therapies, as it will cleanse and sharpen the digestive tract, improving assimilation and elimination, yet create no laxative dependency.

This remarkable formula, a mainstay of the vegetarian Hindu culture, is also used as an aid in weight reduction and as an eyewash for relieving eyestrain and sharpening vision. It is no wonder that an Indian saying states, "If you have no mother and have triphala, everything will be all right!"

For some, constipation is caused by bowel dryness. While triphala is useful for this condition, it is better to use psyllium-seed husks or a demulcent laxative to help retain moisture in the intestines. Again a principle of Planetary herbalism is to combine synergistic herbs, which in this case serve as demulcent laxatives to create a broader range of effect. I use psyllium-seed husks, flax seeds and the tonic nutritive chiao seeds, together with triphala, to create a sure and effective combination that again has some tonic as well as eliminative properties.

Antispasmodic Formula (Acute Medicine)

This is an all-purpose first aid remedy for a variety of emergencies, including shock, cramps, hysteria and poisonous bites and stings. It is also a good gargle to clear the voice, cut mucus and treat pyorrhea and sores in the mouth. Applied externally, it is used to treat pains and muscular spasms. Use fifteen drops in a half glass of hot water every hour or as needed for internal applications.

PRIMARY: Lobelia—1 part
Skullcap—1 part
Valerian—1 part
Myrrh gum—1 part
Black cohosh—1 part
SECONDARY: Licorice—½ part
(demulcent/harmonizer)
Ginger root—½ part (stimulant)
Cayenne—½ part

Steep the herbs in boiled water, one pint for six ounces of herbs, for one-half hour. Strain and add one pint apple cider vinegar.

Nerve Tonic (For Chronic Ailments)

Use this nerve tonic to treat chronic nervousness, muscular spasm or emotional instability. Take two teaspoons, three times a day.

Black cohosh—1 part
Hops—1 part

Lady's slipper root—1 part
Skullcap—1 part
Lobelia—1 part
Valerian—1 part
Camomile—1 part
Wood betony—1 part
Hawthorn berry—1 part (demulcent)
Ginger root—1 part (stimulant)

Mix the herbs thoroughly and use four ounces of herbs per pint of alcohol to make a tincture. Shake daily and allow to extract for two weeks. Then strain.

A formula which I use, called Stress Free, combines some effective Chinese herb along with organic calcium. Calcium is an important mineral to strengthen and quiet the nervous system.

Sleep Formula

To achieve a sound sleep, drink this tea throughout the day, one-quarter cup three times, after meals, and one-quarter cup before going to bed.

PRIMARY AND	Hops—1 part
SECONDARY	Valerian—1 part
QUALITIES	Passion flower—1 part
COMBINED	Spearmint—1 part

Use one ounce of herbs steeped in a pint of boiled water for twenty minutes.

Female Corrective Tonic (For Women Who Have Meat in the Diet)

This tonic is used over an extended period of time to strengthen the genitourinary tract. Take two capsules or one teaspoon of tincture morning and night. After six weeks of use, go without using the formula for one week. This and other female tonic herbs should be taken for at least three months to show their effects.

Blessed thistle—1 part
Cramp bark—1 part

False unicorn root—1 part
Squawvine—1 part
Uva ursi—1 part
Goldenseal—3 parts
Ginger root—1 part (stimulant)
Angelica or dong quai—1 part (antispasmodic)

Mix the powdered herbs and place in "00" capsules, or make a tincture using four ounces of herbs per pint of alcohol. Use with a half cup of raspberry leaf tea.

Female Corrective Tonic (For Vegetarians or Women Who Eat a Low Protein, High Carbohydrate Diet)

Of great benefit in correcting all menstrual irregularities.

Dong quai—1 part
Lovage—1 part
Peony—1 part
Rehmannia—1 part
Ginger root—½ part (stimulant)

Combine pieces of the herbs in water (four and one-half ounces of herbs per quart) and cook slowly for forty-five minutes. Use as soup. The herbs may be cooked a second time.

Women's Treasure is a similar formula that combines both Chinese and Western herbs for regulating the menstrual cycle and balancing female hormones. For symptoms associated with premenstrual syndrome, one may need to combine the liver tonic along with the anti-stress formula as well as the female tonic.

Menstrual Cramps Formula

PRIMARY:　　Cramp bark—1 part
　　　　　　Angelica or dong quai—1 part
　　　　　　Squawvine—1 part
SECONDARY:　Ginger root—½ part (stimulant)
　　　　　　Lobelia—½ part (antispasmodic)

Mix powdered herbs and fill "00" capsules. Take two or three as needed.

Composition Powder

This is a mixture of stimulant herbs that may be used for stimulant therapy (see the chapter on "Herbal Therapies") or to enhance the effects of other herbs. In the early stages of an acute disease, composition powder should be taken hourly.

PRIMARY: Ginger root—2 parts
                  Bayberry bark—1 part
                  White pine—1 part
                  Cloves—⅛ part
                  Cayenne—⅛ part
SECONDARY: Licorice—¼ part (demulcent/harmonizer)

Steep one teaspoon of the combined powders in a cup of boiled water for fifteen minutes, covered. Drink the liquid poured off from the sediment.

One variation of composition powder in which I add some licorice root to smooth out the effect is aptly called Herbal Uprising and can be used for all the same indications as the traditional composition powder previously described.

Liver Tonic

This tonic helps rebuild the liver. It is useful in the recovery from hepatitis, liver sclerosis and toxicity from a bad diet.

Oregon grape root—1 part
Wild yam root—1 part
Dandelion root, raw—1 part
Licorice—¼ part (demulcent)

Simmer the herbs in distilled water (three ounces of herbs in one quart of water) for forty-five minutes. Refrigerate. Take two tablespoons, three or four times a day between meals. Do not add sweetening. If desired the licorice content may be slightly increased.

Bladder/Kidneys Tonic

This is a good tonic for the entire genitourinary tract and will serve as a good all-purpose diuretic. If you are ever in doubt as to what systems of the body are imbalanced, according to some practitioners of Chinese medicine it is generally best to treat the water element (bladder and kidneys). Take one-half cup of the tea four times a day, after meals and before going to bed.

Buchu—1 part
Uva ursi—1 part
Parsley root—1 part
Cleavers—1 part
Juniper berries—1 part
Marshmallow root—1 part (demulcent)
Ginger root—¼ part (stimulant)

Combine the herbs and simmer one ounce of herbs in one pint of distilled water for twenty minutes.

Nerve Stimulant Formula

This is a powerful vitalizer for the entire nervous system; it is a general stimulant, and aids in digestion and elimination. Take three to four tablespoons, three or four times a day.

Prickly ash bark—4 parts
Irish moss—1 part (demulcent)
Bayberry bark—1 part

Combine three ounces of herbs per quart of distilled water and let stand for two hours with occasional stirring. Then bring to a boil for thirty minutes and strain while hot. Add one cup of black molasses and one cup of glycerine to the strained liquid. Boil slowly for five minutes, stirring constantly. When it is cool, bottle and cap tightly.

Kidney and Gallstone Formula

I have had several occasions when this formula was instrumental in dissolving and expelling kidney- and gallstones and relieving the severity of the symptoms. The balanced diet (Chapter 7) must be followed strictly with daily or occasional applications of ginger fomentation externally over the affected parts.

PRIMARY: Dandelion root—1 part
             Gravel root—3 parts

Parsley root—1 part
Lemon balm—1 part
Marshmallow root—2 parts
SECONDARY: Ginger root—½ part (stimulant)
Licorice—½ part
(demulcent/harmonizer)

Simmer the roots in water (two quarts water for every two ounces of herbs) for about an hour, reducing the volume by half through evaporation. Add the lemon balm and let steep for twenty minutes without additional heating. Strain and take one-half cup every two hours.

Interestingly enough, tumeric root is an effective liver and gallstone eliminator. Stone Free formula adds this valuable herb to the above with good effect.

Internal and External Infections and Inflammations

Use this combination to treat acute infections, inflammation, colds, flu, and skin boils.

PRIMARY: Chaparral—3 parts
Echinacea—3 parts
SECONDARY: Marshmallow root—1 part
(demulcent)
Cayenne pepper—¼ part
(stimulant)

Fill "00" gelatin capsules with the combined herb powders and take two capsules every two hours.

Heartburn Formula

In this formula, the herbs each contain primary and secondary characteristics.

Marshmallow root—2 parts
(demulcent)
Hawthorn berries—6 parts
Peppermint—3 parts (stimulant)
Wild yam root—6 parts

Fennel seed—3 parts
Ginger root—3 parts

Simmer marshmallow root, hawthorn berries and wild yam root (one quart of water for every three ounces of herbs) for twenty minutes. Remove from heat and add the peppermint, fennel seed and ginger root. Let steep ten minutes. Strain and drink one-half cup to one cup after meals or more often as needed.

Heart Tonic

Useful for treating high or low blood pressure or arrhythmia. Take one teaspoon of the tincture with one tablespoon of wheat germ oil, three times daily.

Hawthorn berries—6 parts
Motherwort—3 parts
Ginseng—3 parts
Don sen—3 parts
Ginger root—2 parts
(stimulant/carminative)
Comfrey root—2 parts (demulcent)

Combine four ounces of the herbs with a pint of alcohol (vodka, gin, or brandy). Cap tightly and shake once or twice daily for fourteen days. Pour off the extract and strain out the herbs.

Life Pulse is a similar heart tonic formula and combines a number of valuable Chinese herbs including Chinese red sage root and Tienchi ginseng, which promote circulation, relieve arteriosclerosis and regulate the heart. It also contains polygala, which works not only on the physical heart but the emotional heart as well. Polygala has mind- and heart-calming actions that make it an invaluable addition to a heart tonic formula.

Children's Nervine

For hyperactive children and all nervous problems. Give three to seven drops of the tincture as needed.

Camomile—2 parts
Lemon balm—2 parts
Catnip—2 parts

Valerian—2 parts
Lady's slipper—1 part
Hawthorn berries—1 part

Add four ounces of the herbs to a pint of brandy and extract for two weeks, shaking daily.

Calm Child formula has a similar but more profound action than this children's nervine formula. It is available as a glycerite extract and contains a balanced combination of essential oils of anise and cinnamon, which improve the flavor tremendously.

Prostate Tonic

This formula will dissolve kidney stones and clean out sediments and infection in the prostate.

Gravel root—1 part
Uva ursi—1 part
Parsley root—1 part
Goldenseal root—1 part
Cayenne—1 part (stimulant)
Juniper berries—1 part
Marshmallow root—1 part
(demulcent)
Licorice—½ part (demulcent)

Mix together the powdered herbs and fill "00" gelatin capsules. Take two capsules, morning and night.

Witasu is a similar formula intended for the male prostate.

Glandular Balance Formula

This formula provides natural hormone-like substances useful for change of life, adolescence, maturity, sterility, frigidity, forgetfulness, anemia, general weakness, and tiredness.

Licorice—1 part (demulcent)
Black cohosh—1 part
Sarsaparilla—1 part
Dong quai—2 parts
Ginseng—2 parts

Kelp—1 part
Goldenseal—½ part
Ginger root—1 part (stimulant)
Lobelia—½ part (antispasmodic)

Mix the herb powders and fill "00" capsules. Take two capsules, three times a day.

Lifebreath Tonic Decongestant for the Lungs

Thyme—4 parts
Mullein herb—3 parts
Elecampine—3 parts
Wild cherry bark—3 parts
Lobelia herb—2 parts
Ginger—2 parts
Licorice—2 parts

Simmer one ounce of the herbs in a pint of water for twenty minutes and take one cup three times daily, or more or less as needed.

Breeze Free is a stronger decongestant formula because it adds Chinese ma huang to many of the above herbs.

East-West Stomach Bitters

An effective old-fashioned remedy for weak digestion. Combine powders of the following:

Gentian root—4 parts
Calamus—4 parts
Dandelion—2 parts
Centaury—2 parts
Anise seed—2 parts
Mugwort—1 part
Licorice root—1 part

Add one ounce of the powdered formula to a pint of rice wine (sake), vodka, gin, or good quality red wine. Allow to soak for two weeks.

Dose: 1 teaspoon of the tincture before meals.

"Dit Da" Liniment

For sprains, strains, injuries, and arthritic pain.

Prickly ash bark—3 parts
Myrrh gum—3 parts
Goldenseal—3 parts
Hyssop—3 parts
Calendula flowers—3 parts
Cinnamon—3 parts
Tienchi ginseng—3 parts
Cayenne pepper—3 parts

Soak three and one half ounces of powdered herbs in a quart of gin or vodka to make a tincture. Allow to stand in a closed jar for at least two weeks, shaking daily, before use. This liniment is most useful for injuries and blows followed by poor circulation and blood stagnation (black and blue marks). It is a special formula commonly used for injuries and accidents in oriental martial arts.

Eyewash

For red, tired or strained eyes, wash eyes twice a day.

Goldenseal—1 part
Eyebright—1 part
Bayberry bark—1 part
Red raspberry leaves—1 part

Mix herbs and make a tea, using one teaspoon of herbs in one-half pint of water. Allow to cool and keep refrigerated. Make fresh each week.

Healing Salve

This salve is very useful in the treatment of all skin rashes, swellings, wounds, eruptions, and burns.

Calendula flowers—1 part
Plantain leaves—½ part
Mugwort or wormwood—½ part
Comfrey leaves—½ part

Gently sauté the herbs in lard or clarified butter (one pound of lard for every four ounces of herbs) over low heat until leaves are crisp. Strain and store in a wide-mouthed jar. The ointment can also be made with oil and beeswax (see the chapter on "Methods of Application").

Chickweed Salve

For the treatment of itching and rashes.

Fresh chickweed—12 ounces
Vegetable shortening or oil—16 ounces
Beeswax—2 ounces

Melt the shortening and beeswax in a pan, then combine ingredients and place in the oven in a stone jar for about three hours; strain through a fine wire strainer while hot.

Comfrey Paste

This formula, provided by Dr. Christopher, can be used topically to heal burns, fractures, sprains and cuts. For third degree burns, wash the affected area thoroughly and apply with a bandage. Do not disturb for three days, thus allowing formation of new skin tissue to take place. The honey will keep the burn from getting infected.

Comfrey leaves or root—3 parts
Lobelia—1 part
Wheat germ oil—½ part
Honey—½ part

Combine herb powders with other ingredients and store in a wide-mouthed jar.

Poultice

This is used for drawing infections and in treating painful and swollen joints.

Plantain—3 parts
Comfrey—3 parts
Marshmallow root—1 part

Lobelia—1 part
Cayenne—⅛ part

Blend the herb powders together and add enough honey/wheat germ oil mixture (equal parts) to form a paste. Spread on gauze and apply over the affected area. Cover and leave on all day and night.

Bolus

This is used to draw out toxins and reduce cysts and tumors in the vagina or rectum. (See the chapter on "Methods of Application".)

Squawvine—1 part
Slippery elm—1 part
Yellow dock—1 part
Comfrey—1 part
Marshmallow root—1 part
Chickweed—1 part
Goldenseal root—1 part
Mullein leaves—1 part

Mix the powdered herbs together and add a tablespoon of the herbs to a small amount of melted cocoa butter to form a pie-dough consistency. Roll the mass to form the bolus. Refrigerate to solidify the cocoa butter and then allow to reach room temperature before applying.

River of Life Blood Purifier

Useful to help purify the blood in the treatment of drug toxicity, acne, boils, infections, inflammations, eczema, psoriasis, cancer. This valuable tonic is also used for treating acute ailments such as sore throats, colds, flu, infections, urethritis, abscessed teeth. Take two to four capsules twice daily.

Echinacea—2 parts
Chaparral—2 parts
Yellow dock—1 part
Garlic—1 part
Sarsaparilla—1 part
Sassafras—1 part
Ginseng—1 part

Golden seal—1 part
Ginger—1 part
Licorice—1 part
Poke root—1 part

Note: Because of current regulations, sassafras and poke root may be commercially unavailable at this time. However, the formula can be used without these valuable blood purifiers.

Combine the powdered herbs and fill gelatin capsules, or make a tincture using four ounces of herb to a pint of alcohol, taking one-half to one teaspoon doses.

Trikatu Anti-Mucus and Digestive Powder

An ancient formula made up of three herbal stimulants in equal amounts: powders of black pepper, pippli pepper, and ginger. If the pippli is unobtainable one can substitute anise seed. This is mixed with honey to form a thick paste. One half to one teaspoon is taken before meals. Its benefits are to warm the digestion and prevent the formation of mucus. It acts as a natural antihistamine and can be added to other herbal formulas whenever this action is needed.

Tree Flower Oil

An herbal first-aid kit in itself. If I had only one herbal product to carry with me all the time it would be this one. It can be used both externally and internally for all acute ailments such as the first sign of colds, flu, headache, pain, bruises, sprains, indigestion and low spirits. Since it is very concentrated only a drop or two at a time should be used. It consists of a blend of the following herbal oils; cinnamon, thyme, camphor, cajeput, eucalyptus, marjoram and olive oils.

· 13 ·

TREATMENTS FOR
SPECIFIC AILMENTS

The suggestions in the following pages are typical types of treatments for specific ailments. On the basis of the information in preceding chapters, you can design alternative treatments to fit the particular nature of the ailment and to utilize those herbs and foods immediately available. Proportions are given in parts by weight.

In case you wish to make a formula but are lacking one or two ingredients, try to use a substitute with similar properties. If an ingredient were simply left out, the other ingredients would then be present in unusually high proportion and the effects might be somewhat different. When instructions are given to make a tea, it is also possible to make a tincture (see the chapter on "Methods of Application"), and when the instructions are given to fill gelatin capsules it is possible to use pills—or again one may simply use a tincture. The most consistent rule is to use common sense in determining the best method to apply the therapy. Remember to adjust the dose of internal medicines to the body weight of the person being treated (see the section on "Herbs for Children" in the "Cautionary Notes on Herb Use" chapter).

Continue to use the therapy for several days and follow the appropriate instructions on diet. Do not expect to get immediate changes in the condition after drinking a single cup of tea, although in several cases this will occur.

Abscesses

Internal:
Prepare capsules of:

> Echinacea powder—3 parts
> Chaparral powder—3 parts
> Marshmallow root—1 part
> Cayenne pepper—¼ part

Take two capsules every two hours. After the infection subsides, reduce frequency of dose to every four hours.

External:
Make a poultice of:

> Plantain leaves—2–3 leaves, crushed
> Comfrey leaves—1–2 leaves, crushed
> Cayenne pepper—a pinch
> Marshmallow root powder—a pinch

> Apply directly to affected area.

Note: This combined treatment is very effective for any type of infection, provided a balanced diet is strictly adhered to. It may be helpful to accompany this treatment with an herbal laxative or lower bowel tonic.

Acne and Skin Problems

Internal:
Use a good blood purifier, such as:

> Echinacea—2 parts
> Red clover—1 part
> Kelp—1 part
> Burdock—1 part
> Dandelion root—1 part
> Licorice—½ part

Fill gelatin capsules with the powdcxer and take two capsules every two hours until the condition is greatly improved.

Or make a tea of:

Sassafras—1 part
Sarsaparilla—1 part
Dandelion—1 part
Burdock—1 part
Licorice—½ part

Simmer one ounce of herbs in a pint of water for thirty minutes. Take one cup, three times daily.

External:

Use aromatic steam from:

Elder flowers—2 parts
Eucalyptus leaves—1 part

Use one ounce of herbs in a pint of boiled water in a bowl. Cover the head with a cloth and lean over the bowl to get the full benefit of the aromatic steam for five minutes.

Note: Skin eruptions are often caused by dietary imbalanced, either by consuming too much meat, white sugar, denatured flours, eggs and stimulants (including spices) or by lack of wholesome foods such as whole grains, fresh vegetables, fruits and balanced protein. Skin ailments will often follow or accompany ailments of the lung or colon.

Arthritis and Rheumatism

Internal:

Use a good blood purifier, such as:

Oregon grape root—6 parts
Prince's pine or parsley root—6 parts
Sassafras—3 parts
Prickly ash bark—3 parts
Black cohosh—3 parts
Guaiacum—3 parts
Ginger root—2 parts

Make a tea using one ounce of herbs to a pint of water, simmered for thirty minutes. Add a small amount of senna if necessary to regulate the bowls. Take one-half cup of the hot tea every two hours to induce perspiration. Between doses, take a nerve tonic tincture or powder with warm water. A simple combination of equal parts skullcap, valerian and lady's slipper will prove useful. Take two capsules or one teaspoon of the tincture.

External:
Apply warming herbs to promote circulation. Make a poultice, fomentation or liniment using:

Ginger root—2 parts
Cayenne—1 part
Lobelia—½ part

Note: The intake of animal foods, alcohol, sugar and denatured foods should be reduced as these promote the deposit of uric acids in the joints. Avoid dampness and coldness of the joints, and use rubefacients or circulation-promoting herbs externally.

Back Pain

Internal:
Use a diuretic tea, such as:

Juniper berries—1 part
Uva ursi—1 part
Parsley root—1 part
Marshmallow root—1 part

Simmer two ounces of the herbs in two pints of water for fifteen minutes in a tightly covered pan. Strain and take one-half cup, three to four times daily.
Or use a diuretic, antispasmodic combination, such as:

Prince's pine—6 parts
Valerian—1 part
Lobelia—1 part
Ginger root—1 part
Marshmallow root—1 part

Simmer two ounces of the herbs in two pints of water for thirty minutes and take one cup three times a day or more often until relief is obtained.

In cases where there is inflammation, try:

Echinacea—4 parts
Lady's slipper—1 part

Make a tincture and take five to ten drops every two hours.

External:
Apply as a fomentation *equal* parts of:

Comfrey root
Horsetail
Gravel root
Marshmallow root
Lobelia
Ginger root

Simmer once ounce of the herbs in a pint of water for thirty minutes. Dip red flannel or a piece of thick cotton cloth into the solution and apply or wear to bed as warm as possible each night, using a plastic sheet to protect the bed from dampness.

Note: When there is back pain it is often symptomatic of deeper organic defects. Most back pain originates from kidney and bladder weakness. Various toxins otherwise eliminated through the kidney and bladder urine are deposited in surrounding tissue areas, especially the spinal joints of the lumbar region. If the back pain is accompanied by inflammation, it is often the case that nerves will become irritated, resulting in shooting pains called sciatica.

Burns

Internal:
Make a tea of:

Comfrey leaf—2 parts
Red clover blossoms—1 part
Nettles—1 part
Skullcap—1 part
Marshmallow—1 part

Use one ounce of herbs per pint of water. Drink one-half cup every two hours, along with two capsules of equal parts echinacea and comfrey root powders.

External:
Apply immediately the gell pressed from aloe vera leaves. Make a poultice of calendula mixed with comfrey mucilage (see "Comfrey" in the "Western Herbs" chapter) and a pinch of lobelia. For pain, add a pinch of echinacea or kava kava powder.

Cancer

Cancer is a metabolic disease affecting the blood and lympatic systems. The major causes are the consumption of processed and denatured foods containing synthetic drugs, chemicals, coloring and preservatives. Other contributing factors include environmental toxins, stress and for some, an inherited predisposition. This latter factor need not be a significant issue so long as one is eating a healthy balanced diet free of unnatural toxic byproducts which the body is unable to fully metabolize and use or eliminate.

When these toxic byproducts reach a dangerously high level in the blood and lymph, the body's only recourse is to concentrate them in the form of tumors and cancers in specific areas depending upon the individual's predisposition and weaknesses.

Statistically, it has been shown that patients who receive no radical chemical treatments such as radiation and chemotherapy have a longer rate of survival without degrading the side effects that these medicines cause. Yet, perhaps the biggest enemy of the cancer patient is the fear that allows him to surrender all personal responsibility to the orthodox medical establishment. I believe there is a right use for everything that exists, and even the methods of Western medicine can be appropriate when judiciously applied along with wholesome diet, herbs, and natural physiotherapies. The major problem in the use of strong Western therapeutic measures is the tendency to debilitate the deep life force, without which the body is unable to heal itself.

Recently a renowned neurosurgeon, Dr. Anthony Satilaro, cured himself of cancer by following the macrobiotic diet as outlined in this book. He is one of countless cancer patients who have been able to cure themselves even after radiation and chemotherapy by changing their attitudes toward disease and their diets according to the principles outlined in this book.

The first step in healing, therefore, is to eliminate overly rich animal protein in the form of meat, dairy products and eggs from the diet and to substitute vegetable sources of protein balanced with 50% whole grains. For people who have had a history of consuming heavy protein and rich processed foods, a short period of 2 to 3 weeks on raw vegetables and juices would help detoxify the meat protein to a safer level. Then they should eat only lightly cooked foods using 50% whole grains, 10% beans, 25% steamed vegetables, 5% sea vegetables and 10% fruit, either baked or in season.

In addition the following herbal formula can serve as a decisive aid in helping the body to naturally detoxify itself. It is a formula which I have created to promote balanced elimination and detoxification and combines the most powerful blood purifiers in the herbal kingdom, echinacea and chaparral. It also has rare Chinese herbs which help to support the life force and are traditionally recognized as having anti-carcinogenic properties.

Pure-Blood Formula
Echinacea—25%
Chaparral—25%
Red Clover blossoms—6%
Cascara Sagrada—3%
Kelp—3%
Astragalus—10%
Grifola—6%
Ginseng (American)—10%
Poria cocos (fu ling)—4%
Licorice—4%
Cayenne—4%

Approximately two "00" size capsules of a powder of the above formula should be taken three or four times daily.

Two important South American herbs that have been effective for some in the treatment of cancer are pau d'arco, which is contained in the Complete Pau d'Arco formula, and suma. For further information see their sections in the chapter "Western Herbs."

Coldness and Cramps

Internal:
Make a winter tonic using:

  Cramp bark—2 parts
  Angelica root—2 parts
  Squawvine—2 parts
  Raspberry leaves—2 parts
  Camomile—1 part
  Ginger root—1 part
  Lobelia—1 part

Add about six ounces of this combination to a quart of good quality dry wine. Heat gently in a covered container, but do not boil. Let stand for a day, then strain and bottle for use. Take one tablespoon three times daily, twenty minutes before meals.

External:
Apply a fomentation of ginger root.

Note: Avoid eating cold and watery foods. This formula is usefulf or the treatment of coldness, negative emotional states, deficiency, irregular menstruation and menstrual cramps. It will also be useful for all muscular cramps.

Colds, Flus, Fevers and Upper Respiratory Diseases

Internal:
If the ailment is due to overeating, use of alcohol, exposure to weat, damp, cold or excessive activity, use sweating therapy. For this a tea is made with *equal* parts of:

  Elder flowers
  Peppermint

Catnip, yarrow or lemon balm tea may be used instead. Take one or more cups of the infusion and follow immediately with a hot bath. Then go to bed with several covers to provoke perspiration. Use regular doses (every four hours) of one teaspoon garlic oil and two capsules of composition powder (see the chapter on "Making an Herbal Formula"). In case of fever make a tea of sweet basil with a pinch of black pepper. If the disease is caused by blocked food in the stomach, a lobelia emetic might be beneficial (see the "Herbal Therapies" chapter) to clear the stomach through vomiting.

If the ailment is accompanied by weakness, emaciation, paleness, low fever, clear or white discharge or is occurring in a person who has a deficient diet, low in protein, use a tea of *equal* parts:

Dandelion root
Burdock root
Angelica root
Chicory root
Elecampane

Take one-half cup of the decoction every two hours. After the acute stage has passed, take one or two capsules of ginseng root a day to help overcome the deficient condition and build the body's defenses.

External:
Apply a rubbing oil of eucalyptus oil or a commercial combination such as Tiger Balm. For coughs, see the section on "Coughs and Sore Throats" in this chapter.

Note: Before treating a cold, flu or fever, determine whether the disease is due primarily to excess (Yang condition) or deficiency (Yin condition) as described in the chapter on "Diagnosis and Treatment." Those with a Yang condition should use a warm liquid diet and sweating therapy, while those with the Yin condition should avoid cold foods and should rely on teas, broths, mucousy grains, steamed vegetables, seaweeds and chicken soup. A Chinese tonic soup is of great benefit for treating the deficient condition. See the section on "Tonification" in the "Herbal Therapies" chapter and the chapters on "Chinese Herbs" and "Western Herbs."

Constipation and Diarrhea

Internal:
For a good remedy for either diarrhea or constipation take:

Rhubarb root—6 parts
Slippery elm—1 part
Cinnamon—1 part

Add enough water to make a mucilage from the combined powders and form little pea-sized pills. Dry with low heat, and then dip them in a little melted beeswax. Take two to seven pills, three times a day. The beeswax covering allows the pill to enter the small intestines before releasing its properties. One of the best formulas for all bowel complaints is Dr. Christopher's lower bowel tonic (see the chapter on "Making an Herbal Formula"). Use two capsules three times daily—the amount may be increased if results are not adequate. For constipation, one may also use a bulk laxative made by mixing:

Psyllium seed
Flax seed
Chia seed

Use in any combination, soaking two to three tablespoons overnight in a cup of tea made from equal amounts of licorice and raisins. Take three tablespoons at a time, each hour.

For diarrhea and dysentery, make a tea of blackberry root bark (see the "Western Herbs" chapter) and take one-half cup every two hours until the condition is relieved.

Note: Diarrhea is another form of constipation where the underlying cause is failure to assimilate food properly. The use of whole grains, bran and a balance of a few fruits and vegetables will help eliminate this problem, provided harmful denatured foods are removed from the diet. For children or persons who are weakened, a mild laxative is a tea of licorice and raisins or a tablespoon of sesame or olive oil taken in the evening.

Coughs and Sore Throats

Internal:
Make a cough syrup using *equal* parts:

Elecampane
Wild cherry bark
Licorice
Comfrey root
Coltsfoot
Lobelia

Cook down the decoction until a syrupy consistency is achieved (see the section on "Syrups" in the "Methods of Application" chapter). Take a tablespoon every hour or as needed.

Fill gelatin capsules with the powders of *equal* parts:

Slippery elm
Bayberry bark
Comfrey root
Mullein

Take two capsules every two hours along with one teaspoon of garlic oil and five to ten drops tincture of echinacea. An enema using white oak bark tea is also helpful.

Note: Coughs and sore throats are often benefited by a short fast or a diet using warm vegetable broth and soupy grains.

Cramps and Spasms

Internal:
For a tea that is warming and antispasmodic, use:

Ginger root—1 part
Cramp bark—2 parts

Take as needed. Or use the tincture of lobelia, five to fifteen drops, the antispasmodic formula (see the chapter on "Making an Herbal Formula") or a tea of equal parts camomile and ginger.

External:
Use a ginger compress or heating oils such as camphor, wintergreen or Tiger Balm.

Note: Cramps are often caused by cold, thus one should keep warm and take warm foods and drinks. Usually it is better to abstain from solid food for a while. Calcium is an important mineral nutrient in the prevention of cramps.

Fevers with Sweating

Internal:
For fevers accompanied by excessive sweating, make a tea using:

Cinnamon—2 parts
Peony root—2 parts
Ginger root—2 parts
Licorice—1 part

Simmer one ounce of the herbs in a quart of water along with four dates for twenty minutes. Take three or four cups a day, and one-half hour after taking the tea, eat a small bowl of watery brown rice.

External:
Make a tofu plaster by squeezing out the water from tofu and then mashing it together with 20% pastry flour and 5% grated fresh ginger root. Apply directly to the skin.

Headaches

Internal:
Make a tea of *equal* parts:

Skullcap
Valerian
Rosemary
Camomile
Peppermint

Take one-half cup of the decoction (prepared in a tightly covered pot) every hour.

External:
Apply a stimulating oil such as ginger, peppermint, wintergreen, Tiger Balm or Essential Balm (the latter two being commercial preparations from China) to the forehead and temples.

Note: Headaches are usually caused by bowel and stomach disorders, or may be due to tension, stress, weak kidneys or sluggish liver function. The bowels and digestion should be regulated, perhaps with the use of a laxative such as a lower bowel tonic.

Hemorrhoids

Internal:
Prepare a tea with:

Dandelion root—2 parts
Chicory root—1 part
Cascara sagrada—1 part
Oregon grape root—1 part
Licorice—½ part

Using one ounce of herbs to one pint of water, make a decoction. Take one-half cup of the tea, two or three times a day.

External:
Combine:

Witch hazel leaves—2 parts
Bayberry bark—1 part
Goldenseal—1 part

Make a strong tea using one ounce of herbs per pint of water. Add a pint of glycerine, and insert a small amount directly into the rectum with a dropper three times daily. Or make boluses and apply frequently (see the "Methods of Application" chapter). Also, see "Stoneroot" (in the chapter on "Western Herbs").

Note: Hemorrhoids are often caused by sluggish liver function or liver obstruction. Hence the use of liver tonics is recommended. Another major cause of hemorrhoids is constipation. This is best corrected by balancing the diet and insuring that sufficient fiber is taken. The hemorrhoids are shrunk by the application of astringent herbs. Goldenseal is also applied, as it is beneficial for the inflamed mucous membrane surface of the rectum.

Herpes

Venereal disease is on the rise as a condition of the general breakdown of the ethical and moral standards of our times. There are dangerous and accumulative side effects to taking massive doses or antibiotics, and so far there is no effective orthodox treatment for herpes virus. I have found the following herbal approach extremely effective when strictly combined with the therapeutic diet (Chapter 7).

Herb-Plex
Echinacea—25%
Chaparral—25%

Sarsaparilla—12%
Oregon grape root—12%
Poria cocos—10%
Licorice root—8%
Ginger—8%

Take two "00" capsules of the powder three or four times daily for at least 3 months along with the therapeutic macrobiotic diet.

Hoarseness of Voice

Internal:
Use equal parts of powdered:

Licorice
Calamus

Mix with a little honey and take one teaspoon, three to four times daily.
Warm the body with a tea made from:

Sage—4 parts
Fresh ginger—4 parts
Black pepper—a pinch
Cinnamon—½ part
Cardamom—½ part
Licorice—½ part

Simmer two ounces of the mixture in a quart of water in a glass or enamel pot for twenty minutes. Add a little milk and continue to heat for ten minutes. Flavor with honey if desired. Add garlic, ginger and black pepper to cooked foods.

Note: One should avoid cold foods, fried foods and sour-tasting foods (such as yogurt and citrus). Gargling with salt water is beneficial, using one teaspoon salt to a glass of warm water.

Indigestion

Internal:
Make an extract in any white wine using:

Dandelion root—1 part
Calamus root—1 part
Gentian—1 part
Angelica—1 part
Valerian—1 part
Ginger root—½ part

Use two ounces of herbs to one pint of wine and let extract for two weeks. Take one teaspoon before and after meals.

Infections and Blood Poisoning

Internal:
Combine the powders of:

Goldenseal—1 part
Chaparral—2 parts
Echinacea—3 parts

Fill "00" capsules with the mixture. Take four every four hours. As the symptoms subside, the dosage should be reduced to three times a day for one week.

External:
Make a poultice of:

Plantain—2 parts
Lobelia—1 part
Marshmallow—1 part
Cayenne—⅛ part

Insomnia

Internal:
Make an infusion using *equal* parts:

Camomile
Valerian
Skullcap
Catnip
Wood betony
Spearmint

Use one ounce of herbs per pint of water. Let steep ten minutes and drink before going to bed.

For incredible dreams and for nights when you can't allow sufficient time for sleep, make an infusion of:

Kava kava—4 parts
Alfalfa—1 part
Spearmint—1 part
Raspberry leaves—1 part
Lemon balm—1 part

Vary the strength according to your needs, and sweeten with honey. The kava kava will produce a numbing effect on the tongue.

External:
Stuff a small pillow with hops and mugwort, and sleep on or next to it. Before bed, take a bath using herbs that are antispasmodic, nervine and/ or sedative.

Note: Reduce the intake of strong stimulants, especially coffee and black tea, and normalize the daily schedule of meals and activities.

Kidney and Bladder Infections

Internal:
Make a tea of *equal* parts:

Plantain
Parsley root
Marshmallow root

Take one-half cup every two hours. Also alternatively take two capsules of echinacea or two capsules of chaparral along with the tea.

External:
Apply a hot ginger fomentation over the lower abdomen.

Note: The treatment should include a fast of one to three days, taking only warm vegetable broth and the herbs mentioned above.

Kidney Stones

Internal:
Make a decoction of:

Gravel root—2 parts
Parsley root—2 parts
Marshmallow root—2 parts
Lobelia—½ part
Ginger root—½ part

Simmer two ounces of herbs per quart of water for about an hour until the liquid is reduced by half. Add an equal volume of vegetable glycerine to preserve. Take one-half cup, three times daily. Alternatively, one may make a tincture of the above herbs and take fifteen drops, three times daily.

Kidney Weakness

Internal:
A valuable Chinese formula is:

Ginseng—3 parts
Rehmannia (unprocessed)—3 parts
Fu ling—2 parts
Licorice—1 part
Ginger root—1 part

Make a decoction, using one ounce of the herbs for one pint of water. Take one-half cup, three times daily for three days.
A Western herbal formula is:

Dandelion root—4 parts
Parsley root—4 parts
Marshmallow root—2 parts
Ginger root—1 part

Simmer one ounce of the herbs in a pint of water for thirty minutes. Take one cup, three times daily. (See also "Buchu" and "Uva ursi" in the "Western Herbs" chapter.)

Note: I would say that about 90% of the people in America suffer from weakened kidneys due to our dietary habits. This formula is thus useful for almost everyone.

Leukorrhea (White Vaginal Discharge)

Internal:
Make a decoction of *equal* parts:

Uva ursi
Parsley root
Dandelion root
Burdock root

Use one ounce of herbs per pint of water. Also, alternately take two capsules of equal parts echinacea, goldenseal and myrrh every two hours along with one half cup of the tea.

External:
Once a day use a douche made with white oak bark or bayberry bark tea.

Note: The treatment should begin with a one to three day fast, unless weakness or severe deficiency is present. Follow the fast with a light nourishing diet of whole grains, steamed vegetables and a small amount of beans and seaweeds.

Liver Ailments and Indigestion

Internal:
Mix *equal* parts of the powdered herbs:

Calamus
Wild cherry bark
Gentian
Oregon grape root
Cascara bark
Goldenseal
Dandelion root
Wild yam root
Lobelia
Ginger root
Licorice

Fill "00" capsules. Take two capsules three times a day, with one cup of dandelion root tea, one-half hour before meals to improve digestion or after meals to influence the liver and stimulate the secretion of bile.

Note: This formula is good for cirrhosis of the liver, scrofula, indigestion, gas and constipation.

Menstrual Cramps and Irregularity

Internal:
Combine *equal* parts of:

Dong quai
Peony root
Rehmannia
Licorice

Either make a tea by simmering one ounce of the herbs in a pint of water or use the powders in gelatin capsules. Take one-half cup of the tea or two gelatin capsules three times daily. This is a good tonic for regulating the menstrual cycle and reducing cramping.

For painful menstruation, one can also make a tea of:

Angelica root—1 part
Cramp bark—1 part
Camomile—1 part
Ginger root—¼ part

Steep one ounce of the herbs in a pint of water. Take one-half cup of the tea, two or three times a day regularly.

Another valuable formula is:

Squawvine—4 parts
Cramp bark—2 parts
Wild yam root—1 part
False unicorn root—1 part

Simmer one ounce of the herbs in a pint of water for twenty minutes. Strain and take two to three tablespoons, three times a day.

Note: Avoid exposure to cold (eating cold foods, swimming or bathing in cold water) around the time of the menstrual period. Make sure there is adequate calcium in the diet.

Mucous Congestion (see No. 29 Trikata)

Nausea

Internal:
Mix together the powders of:

Cinnamon—3 parts
Cardamom—1 part
Nutmeg—1 part
Cloves—1 part

Use one-quarter to one-half teaspoon in a cup of boiling water, steeped covered for ten minutes. Strain and drink one cup every four hours or as needed. It can also be added to scalded milk with a little honey.

Nervous Diseases

Internal:
As an all-purpose nerve tonic, blend together *equal* parts:

Lady's slipper
Valerian
Wood betony
Skullcap
Spearmint
Lemon balm

Use the powders to fill gelatin capsules and take two, three times a day, or steep two tablespoons in a cup of boiling water for ten minutes, adding honey to taste. Drink one cup, two or three times per day.

For treating hysteria, withdrawal from alcohol and drugs (delirium tremens—the "D.T.'s") and insomnia, make a tea of *equal* parts:

Lady's slipper
Skullcap

Simmer in a closed pot for twenty minutes, strain and add honey to taste. Take one-quarter cup every hour, tapering off as symptoms subside.

To promote memory and mental clarity, use:

Gota kola—3 parts
Calamus root—1 part

Heat an ounce of the mixture in half pound of clarified butter (ghee) for forty-five minutes. Strain and store for use. Dosage is one teaspoon in a cup of warm milk with a little honey (if desired), taken twice a day.

Note: Nervous debility comes from a combination of lack of balance in diet, recreation, exercise and rest. The herbs will help speed recovery as these important factors are brought into better balance.

Poison Oak and Poison Ivy

Internal:
Use a blood purifying combination, such as:

Chaparral—1 part
Yellow dock—2 parts
Echinacea—2 parts

Combine the powders in gelatin capsules, and take two capsules every two hours.

Calm the itching and reaction to the pain using antispasmodics, such as:

Kava kava—2 parts
Valerian—1 part
Black cohosh—1 part
Lobelia—½ part

Combine the powders in gelatin capsules and take two capsules, three times a day.

Make a detoxifying tea using Chinese chrysanthemum and honeysuckle flowers in roughly equal portions.

External:
Apply a poultice of:

Comfrey root
Marshmallow root
Slippery elm
Aloe vera
Witch hazel

Use roughly equal parts of each. Or use mugwort, plantain and comfrey leaf.

Prostatitis

Internal:
Make a decoction of:

Gravel root—1 part
Uva ursi—1 part
Echinacea—1 part
Parsley root—1 part
Ginger root—¼ part
Lobelia—½ part

Use one ounce of the herbs per pint of water and drink three or four cups of this tea daily until relief is obtained.

Note: This formula will help the blood and kidneys, which in turn will be of benefit in relieving problems of the prostate gland. (See also the prostate tonic described in the chapter on "Making an Herbal Formula.")

Stomach Acidity

Internal:
As a decoction or in gelatin capsules, use:

Dandelion root—1 part
Slippery elm—1 part
Goldenseal—⅛ part
Calamus root—⅛ part

Take one-half cup of the tea or two gelatin capsules of the powder every hour or as needed. Alternatively, combining a pinch of several kitchen spices, to total one teaspoon, in a glass of water will be very effective (see the "Medicines in the Spice Rack" section of the "Kitchen Medicines" chapter).

Note: Stomach acidity is due to imbalanced diet and must be controlled in the long run by becoming more in tune with the digestibility of the foods being eaten.

Ulcers

Internal:
Combine *equal* parts of the powders of:

Slippery elm bark
Licorice

Comfrey root
Marshmallow root

Fill "00" gelatin capsules. Take two capsules, three or four times daily, especially before meals.

Note: The condition is treated by balancing the diet and using less meat and more vegetable protein, as is found in a combination of whole grains and beans. The bowels can be regulated with lower bowel tonic if necessary.

Vaginitis

Internal:
Combine powders of:

Echinacea—1 part
Goldenseal—1 part
Chaparral—1 part
Squawvine—1 part

Fill gelatin capsules. Take two capsules, three times a day, before meals. Also, take a teaspoon of garlic oil with meals.

External:
Make a tea of equal parts:

Goldenseal
Chaparral
Comfrey root
Kava kava

Use an ounce of herb per pint of water, and simmer gently for thirty minutes. Strain, cool and add one tablespoon vinegar per pint. Use as a douche once per day for one to three days.

Note: See also the section on "Leukorrhea" in this chapter.

Weakness

Internal:
Simmer in an open pot:

Alfalfa—8 parts
Comfrey root—2 parts
Burdock root—2 parts
Ginseng—1 part
Dong quai—1 part

Use four ounces of herbs per quart of water. Cook this mixture for about one hour and strain. Return the liquid to the pot and add equal amounts of honey and barley malt syrup, totaling the same as the amount of herbal extract, so that the volume of the whole is doubled. Continue to heat and stir for five minutes to blend the ingredients. Take two tablespoons, three or four times a day, especially before meals.

A valuable Chinese formula is:

Astragalus—6 parts
Ginseng—3 parts
Dong quai—3 parts
Licorice—1 part

Simmer one ounce of herbs per quart of water in a nonmetallic container down to a pint. Take one cup of the tea, two to three times a day for three days.

Note: These formulas can be used as a good tonic for thinness, emaciation and general weakness.

Weight Reducing

The following formula provides the mild detoxification and tonification necessary for treating most chronic overweight problems. The basic consideration is that obesity is a toxic condition involving a breakdown of the normal eliminative functions of the body. The consequent discharge of acids into the digestive tract creates an irresistible craving to eat more. This tendency must be regulated and normalized first by the regular intake of three wholesome, balanced meals a day with occasional special dieting following the contraction diet (Chapter 7).

This formula represents another blending of the finest of both the Western and the Chinese herbal traditions using herbs that help normalize elimination, detoxification and circulation as well as aiding in the breakdown of fat tissue.

Herbal Lite Formula
Kelp—12%
Stephania (Chinese)—8%
Astragalus—8%
Atractylodes—6%
Poria cocos—4%
Ginger—4%
Cascara sagrada—5%
Rhubarb—5%
Fennel seed—5%
Echinacea—10%
Chaparral—8%
Watercress—5%
Mate—5%
Mustard seed—8%
Licorice root—3%
Cleavers—4%

Kelp serves to normalize thyroid metabolism; stephania; atractylodes, cleavers and poria cure edema and help dissolve fat; cascara and rhubarb help normalize elimination; echinacea and chaparral are detoxifiers; mustard seed, cayenne and ginger act as metabolic stimulants; licorice and fennel are harmonizers; and watercress provides essential vitamin and mineral supplementation.

Approximately two "00" capsules of these powdered herbs should be taken three or four times daily. For even greater effectiveness drink the following weight reducing tea, using a half cup each time you take the Pure lite blend. Since triphala complex is a specific, reducing all excesses in the body, and spirulina helps supply important nutrients and substances that seem to satisfy hunger, two formulas that I recommend for this purpose are Rainbow Light's Spirulina Diet formula, or Triphala Diet formula, which is similar to the formula described above but adds triphala complex.

Fasting Tea
Violet leaves
Chicory root (roasted)
Anise seed
Chickweed
Rose petals

Mix equal parts of the herbal combination and steep one ounce in a pint of water. Dose: one cup three times daily.

The single most effective diet I have used for balanced fast weight reduction is the contraction diet (Chapter 7) using only whole grains for one week and strictly limiting the amount of fluids to two or possibly three cups a day. The combination of grains can be varied or combined or mixed with a small amount of aduki beans. A simple sauce can be made by mixing water and a small amount of miso and sesame-tahini butter together with a little grated lemon rind. Or one may use gomasio sesame salt with a low salt ratio. Generally speaking, one should be careful to only use the finest quality sea salt and no more than ¼ teaspoon a day on the average (that much is needed whereas more is possibly harmful).

This type of diet will quickly eliminate the body's excess water. A long daily walk, moderate stretching and exercise is also important. After completing the above program for one week, one should only gradually add steamed vegetables and other foods to the diet.

Excess weight is easily put on by attempting to use large amounts of nuts as a source of protein. The amount of protein compared to calorie content (mostly from fats) in nuts is too low to make them a substantial component of the diet. Weight gains are also a common result of using high-carbohydrate snacks to compensate for low-protein meals. A low-protein diet will lead to poorly regulated blood sugar levels that in turn produce cravings for carbohydrates and little willpower to maintain healthful eating habits. A cup of dandelion tea, taken two or three times a day, will help you compensate for this hypoglycemic condition sustained by a history of poor eating habits.

· 1 4 ·

CAUTIONARY NOTES
ON HERB USE

When properly used, herbs are the safest and surest medicines available. However, one must be well aware of the power of herbs both to heal and, if misused, to cause imbalance. Herbs produce no side effects when used in the amounts required to effect a cure. Negative effects occur only when one fails to observe the cautions that herbalists have recognized after many years of experience.

Essential Oils

All essential oils are very concentrated substances that are irritating in large doses. Externally, one should avoid contact with the eyes, nose, mouth and all mucous membranes. Many of the essential oils are rubefacients intended to cause a mild irritation reaction to stimulate circulation in the area. If applied to the skin in large amounts they may cause a burning irritation.

Internally, essential oils are used only a drop or a few drops at a time, diluted in a cup of tea. In larger amounts they may cause severe toxic reactions. Recently, a fatal poisoning occurred from the ingestion of an ounce of pennyroyal oil. On the other hand, teas made from the herbs that yield these oils, and the use of small amounts of the oil as directed, cause no toxic reactions.

Emetics and Laxatives

Some herbs cause fairly strong reactions, and these are intended as part of the therapy. Thus emetics are meant to cause vomiting and laxatives are meant to cause strong bowel movements (strong laxatives are called cathartics or purgatives). The force of this reaction will depend upon the amount of herb taken. When these responses are expected, there is no problem, but the use of strong laxatives, such as senna leaf and cascara bark, will provide a very uncomfortable condition for anyone ignoring these properties. Many of the strong, bitter-tasting herbs will act as emetics if taken in large enough doses.

It must be remembered that emetics and laxatives, while stimulating the elimination of wastes, will also reduce the body's energy. Thus they should not be used by one who is already weak, nor should they be used repeatedly over an extended period of time.

When used in very small doses, emetic and laxative herbs will not cause noticeable eliminative responses, but they may reveal other properties. The most important example of this is lobelia, which is a strong emetic, most commonly used in small doses to act as an antispasmodic.

Cumulative Effects

Most herbs can be safely used in small quantities over a long period of time, but there are some that provide cumulative effects, which will be harmful if the herb is taken regularly without a break. These include goldenseal, which will affect blood pressure and digestion if taken continuously, and kava kava, which contains a substance that will be stored in the liver, and which taken in regular large doses may cause skin eruptions. Horsetail taken regularly may irritate the kidneys and cause some toxic reactions. These herbs should be used with adequate resting periods after any treatment lasting more than six days.

Excessive Doses

Mild herbs can be taken in large quantities, and this is the practice in the art of Simpling. But more potent herbs will cause toxic reactions in large quantities. These include: poke, lobelia, goldenseal, horsetail, black cohosh, blue cohosh, aconite, mandrake and many of the very bitter-tasting herbs. With some herbs, such as black cohosh, you will be aware of taking more than a therapeutically useful dose by feeling nausea. The dose needs to be decreased. Sometimes, however, a mild nausea will be felt as a reaction to the bitter taste. The addition of a little licorice or ginger will often act to counteract this reaction.

Sensory Effects

Lobelia may cause a feeling of scratchiness at the back of the throat when taken in teas and tinctures. Both kava and cloves will cause a numbing effect on the tongue. Strong astringents, such as bayberry bark and myrrh, will cause a tightening sensation within the mouth when taken in teas and tinctures. Strong laxatives, known as purgatives, may cause intestinal cramping (called griping), and this is usually counteracted by using specific herbs (as mentioned, for example, in the chapter on "Western Herbs"). Cayenne pepper will cause a very warm feeling in the stomach, and may also cause a burning sensation during defecation. Prickly ash bark will cause a strong sensation of heat in the stomach and may produce profuse perspiration.

Tannins

Most herbs contain tannins, substances that bind up proteins and in so doing provide the property of being astringent. There appears to be a correlation between extensive drinking of tannin-rich teas and the occurrence of esophageal and stomach cancer. It is believed that the repeated effect of the tannins on the throat and stomach, especially in combination with other agents in the diet, may result in the formation of cancerous cells. In those countries where black tea (*Camellia sinensis*) is consumed in large quantities, the rate of esophageal cancer tends to be high. However, where the black tea is commonly taken with milk, the elevated cancer rate is not seen. This is because the tannins are rendered insoluble by the milk, the proteins of the milk being bound to the tannin.

One should use astringent teas as needed, but avoid excessive use. When an astringent herb is being used for properties other than astringency, a little milk should be added to neutralize the tannins. There is

292 THE WAY OF HERBS

no reason to fear the occasional use of astringents internally or externally.

Herbs that are particularly high in tannins are the barks, such as bayberry, cascara and blackberry; some of the roots, such as yellow dock, sarsaparilla and comfrey; and a few leaf herbs, such as peppermint, uva ursi and cleavers.

FDA Evaluation of Herbs

The Food and Drug Administration has surveyed some of the available literature on chemical composition and pharmacology of herbs and has suggested that some herbs, commonly used as herbal medicines, are "unsafe." However, it must be realized that these herbs were not judged unsafe on the basis of proper usage, but only based on the presence of a known toxic substance or on the report of severe overdose reaction. Virtually all goods and medicines contain substances that are toxic in large enough doses, so this does not shed much light on the true toxicity of the herb. Among the herbs listed that are also mentioned in this book are calamus, lily of the valley, lobelia and mandrake.

In addition, by extracing ingredients from some herbs and feeding very large doses to laboratory animals, tumors have been induced in these animals. These substances are very weak carcinogenic agents and there is no evidence that the use of the herb itself is at all a health threat. Among the herbs which have been shown to contain a weak carcinogen are sassafras, nutmeg, cloves, basil and tarragon.

Pregnancy

Pregnant women should carefully avoid using herbs that are emmenagogues. Oxytocic agents, which promote delivery, should only be taken during the last month of pregnancy. In general, strong uterine tonics such as dong quai and false unicorn are also not taken during pregnancy, except as directed.

Strong herbs and any king of substance that has a strong effect on the body should be used with great care as they will also affect the developing fetus. Whenever possible, local applications, such as fomentations, liniments and salves, should be used in place of internal medicines.

High Blood Pressure

Persons with a history of very high blood pressure should avoid herbs that stimulate the heart action or constrict the blood vessels. These include goldenseal, ginseng, licorice, lily of the valley and ephedra. Such persons should generally use only small amounts of stimulating substances and should use more of the antispasmodic, nervine and sedative herbs. However, two stimulants, cayenne pepper and garlic, also seem to be useful for reducing blood pressure.

Caution with Handling Herbs

When handling large amounts of poke root, for example when harvesting the roots, gloves must be worn because the roots contain substances that can pass through the skin and are toxic in large amounts. Nettles must also be picked with gloves, as the sting is very painful. Yellow dock applied to the area will be an antidote for nettles sting.

Cascara sagrada must be dried and stored for about one year before it is usable. Before this time it is too toxic. Blue cohosh powder must be handled with care as it is extremely irritating to the mucous membranes. Similarly, one must be careful handling cayenne powder.

Some herbs may cause allergic reactions; a couple of common examples are mugwort and orris root.

Aloe vera should only be taken internally in combination with ginger root, because alone it might cause cramping of the bowels.

Herbs for Children

When giving herbal remedies to children, the dosage should be decreased. As a general rule, the dose should follow the body weight, so that a forty pound child would get no more than half the dose of an eighty pound child. The doses recommended in this book are the adult doses, representing a body weight of about 150 pounds for purposes of calculation. *Therefore women weighing less than 150 pounds, for example, should begin with a lower dosage.* When treating very young children, only the very mild herbs should be used, such as lemon balm and catnip.

Gathering Wild Herbs

Though it is a rare occurrence, it is possible to mistakenly identify herbs found in the wild, substituting a toxic plant for a healing herb. Always be sure of the identification of the plant species before gathering and using quantities of an herb. Recently, an elderly couple picked a plant they thought to be comfrey. They made a tea of this herb and were fatally poisoned. They had consumed a toxic dose of foxglove, a potent heart stimulant that is the source of digitalis. It is easy—and wise—to learn to distinguish foxglove and comfrey, but these people had not taken the time to become familiar with even the obvious botanical characteristics.

Pesticides and Chemicals

Most of the herbs from the Appalachian region of the United States are collected from the forests, so these are completely natural products. However, the majority of other herbs are grown in large fields in foreign countries. The growers often use pesticides in producing these herb crops, so there may be some minor residues associated with these herbs.

When herbs are imported from certain tropical countries, they are fumigated with chemicals that destroy insects and their eggs when they arrive at United States ports. This is done in order to prevent exotic insects from entering the country.

A few herb manufacturers in the United States sterilize the herbs to destroy bacteria and fungi. It is not uncommon for dried herbs to contain thirty million bacteria per ounce! These are harmless bacteria, though they will contribute to the deterioration of the herb in the presence of excess moisture. The standard for drugs in the United States is to have not more than about one million bacteria per ounce. Those manufacturers attempting to match this standard will sterilize practically every herb. This is done by applying ethylene oxide gas. There are some minor residues thus left in these herbs.

Through consumer awareness of these practices, it may be possible to effect a shift away from the use of chemicals with a return to more natural methods of control, as has been done with organic produce.

Diagnosis and Treatment

This book provides basic principles for the diagnosis and treatment of a wide variety of ailments. These techniques are of particular value in treating minor acute ailments, curing long-term chronic ailments for which modern medicine is usually ineffective and as an adjunct to other therapies.

Every culture in the world has as an integral part of its social structure a group of healers who have a special knowledge of health, disease and the treatments of common ailments. Whenever one's own knowledge and experience of personal health and well-being are inadequate for treating these ailments, it is important to consult a trained healer. The herbal remedies in this book can be self-applied, but whenever there is an uncertainty about the nature of the ailment or the efficacy of the cure, a trained professional should be consulted.

Today there are many practicing herbalists and many doctors open to the idea of using natural methods of healing, including herbs. Seek out these individuals in your area and go to them for consultation when this seems appropriate.

Very special care must be taken if strong herbal remedies are used in conjunction with modern pharmaceuticals, as there might be adverse effects of the combinations. In such cases a doctor familiar with the pharmaceuticals must be consulted.

· 1 5 ·

A BOTANICAL
APPROACH TO CANCER
TREATMENT

With an estimated one in five Americans having cancer in their lifetime, the multibillion-dollar war on cancer seems to be a faltering campaign. This means that the treatment of cancer with such alternative methods as herbs and diet is practically ignored. Critics of alternative treatment modalities for cancer complain about such things as the lack of credible research and double-blind studies. The problem is that there is little emphasis on prevention because it involves a series of radical considerations of our lifestyle, food chain, water supply, and environmental issues overall. In our economic system, if there is no profit motive, a serious focus on prevention would wreak havoc on the economic status quo, and further, there is no incentive for a highly vested pharmaceutical company to conduct research on herbs or such other low-tech cancer treatments as herbal medicine. For these reasons, I feel that it is important to share some of my personal findings and experience in the botanical treatment of cancer of all kinds.

This is not the place to exhaustively define cancer. However, a basic understanding may help us to visualize how a cure is possible with wholesome diet, herbs, and lifestyle changes. Fundamentally, cancer is a weakening of the immune system that causes the mutation of cells that eventually colonize, destroy, and displace healthy tissues, eventually leading to death. The immune system involves many complex functions that originate with digestion. Food and its proper assimilation, therefore, are fundamental to strengthening the immune system.

Even with all of this, most cell mutations are weaker than healthy cells and simply die. The proliferation of those that survive is limited by normal feedback controls that prevent their growth. As a result, they live out their normal life span and die. Those cells that may eventually become potentially cancerous produce abnormal protein, which triggers the B-lymphocytes to form an army of antibodies to destroy the mutated cancer cells.

Oncogenes or precancerous cells can be inherited; however, until the requisite number of mutations occurs in life, cancer will not develop. Viruses can also produce oncogenes. Since they proliferate by invading and taking over surrounding healthy cells, they are protected by a coat of protein. The science of virology substantiates that there are mechanisms in a healthy organism that can and do inhibit the invasion of viruses. Again, this depends on a healthy immune system. There are physiological mechanisms that can destroy viruses, and there are herbs, such as bloodroot, hydrastis, burdock, and dandelion, for instance, that have anticancer properties and are effective in overcoming viruses and harmful bacteria.

CANCER INTERVENTION

Apoptosis versus Necrosis

Necrosis involves the cell death of areas of tissue or bone. As a medical procedure, it employs the methods of chemo- and radiotherapy to destroy cancer cells. Unfortunately, this is not purely a selective method, so healthy cells are also destroyed. Necrosis is also associated with such diseases as gangrene and the spread of advanced stages of certain types of cancer, such as that of the breast. Necrosis has long been understood to be a cause of cell death. Only since the 1990s have researchers understood a second cause of cell death, namely, apoptosis. In apoptosis, cells are programmed at birth to die at old age or when various extenuating conditions no longer benefit the host.

The difference is that whereas necrosis in cancer is associated with inflammation and damage to adjacent cells, apoptosis affects scattered individual cells and is a more organized method of removing old, damaged, or otherwise undesirable cells. Apoptosis therefore represents a more selective delimitation of cancer cells.

Angiogenesis

Angiogenesis or *neoangiogenesis* refers to development of vascular tissues. The process occurs in benign tumors in healthy adults during the healing of wounds, ovulation, menstruation, and pregnancy. By inducing their own blood supply, tumor cells are greatly assisted by oxygen and nutrients to grow and proliferate.

Compared to normal tissue, angiogenesis in a tumor is limited and imperfect and characteristically associated with chaotic vessel growth. Vessels tend to be thin walled and break easily. Eventually, this leads to an occlusion of blood flow and hypoxia-induced central necrosis with the formation of open tumorous sores. Because of increased interstitial pressure, the uptake of chemotherapy drugs and herbs as well as the ability of the immune cells to function is greatly impeded. Be that as it may, capillary density in a tumor is a predictive metatastic measure for women with breast cancer. During the angiogenic phase, tumor growth is exponentially metastatic.

Angiogenesis is, at different stages, both desirable—in terms of facilitating the effective delivery of chemotherapy and various anticarcinogenic substances derived from herbs—and undesirable—when it evolves to the stage of enhancing the proliferation of tumor cells and the devolution into necrotic stasis and sores.

Since angiogenesis is precipitated by congestion of tumor cells and blood, the therapeutic strategy from this perspective is to break up congestion through the use of emmenagogue or blood-moving herbs. Another method is the suppression of reactionary mast cells that secrete histamine and serotonin characteristic during the first stages of inflammation that cause local edema and inflammation and the proliferation of phagocytes.

The Holistic Treatment of Cancer

No cancer treatment should be focused on treating only the manifestations of the disease—the tumor. Instead, the focus of treatment should be the balanced promotion of the health of the whole body, mind, and spirit. This may mean making significant lifestyle changes, but these will ensure success in overcoming the immediate manifestation of the disease as well as its dread recurrence.

To recover from cancer, it is not enough to commit to changing one's diet or to simply taking some herbs. These in themselves for many can be a formidable undertaking. Creating a healing environment and allowing time to process emotional and spiritual issues that may adversely effect healing are also necessary. Healing from any disease with any modality always involves a certain act of faith; for this reason, daily meditation and/or prayer is of inestimable benefit to maintain as positive an outlook as possible. Further, because the treatment of cancer can be such a daunting task, it is very important to develop a reliable support system—at least one other individual—to assist, encourage, and help you each day on your road to recovery.

Diet for Cancer Patients

Diet—what to eat and what to avoid eating—is of primary importance in the treatment of cancer. Most of us renew our covenant with life three times a day or each time we eat. For the cancer patient and indeed anyone with degenerative disease, the Hippocratic principle "Let your medicine be your food and your food your medicine" should determine the choices we make. In general, I would suggest that the cancer patient follow the dietary suggestions set forth in another section of this book. However, it may be useful to point out certain foods and classes of foods that have particular beneficial and detrimental impact on cancer patients.

We all have come to realize that certain vitamins—vitamins A, C, D, and K; folic acid, beta-carotene, selenium, and the B-complex group—are all beneficial in inhibiting carcinogenesis. In addition, fiber from whole grains and citrus pectin have the beneficial effects of inhibiting and preventing cancer of the large intestine and prostate.

A major factor involved in the process of carcinogenesis and all degenerative conditions is a high level of cancer-causing, oxygen-scavenging free radicals, which are unstable particles that damage the outer protective membrances of cells and are incrementally self-replicating. Free radicals, which result from an internal process of oxidation, also serve a beneficial function, when in balance, helping to kill invading pathogens and thereby preventing inflammation. According to an article in the *New York Times*, on April 28, 1988, "free oxygen radicals, the main type formed in living organisms, have been implicated in more than 60 disorders, including heart disease, cancer, Alzheimer's disease, cataracts, and rheumatoid arthritis."

Vitamins A, C, and E are powerful free radical scavengers. These are found in most fruits, vegetables, and whole grains. One of the most powerful, pycnogenol, is present in large amounts in pine bark and grape seeds. It certainly would not hurt to eat a bunch of organic grapes and chew the seeds when these are seasonally available. In addition, I would recommend that cancer patients take a daily high dose of pycnogenol from 25 milligrams of pine bark (OPC 85) and 25 of grape seed (OPC 85 +).

Phytochemicals found in a variety of herbs offset cancer in many ways. First, they stimulate the vital process of detoxification in the body that eliminates carcinogenic factors; second, they powerfully stimulate and strengthen the body's immune system to help it to inactivate, fight, and destroy cancer cells; and third, many herbs have free radical scavenging properties. It is important to realize that just because one substance is researched and then marketed for having particular properties and effects does not mean that those same effects are not present to an even greater degree in other substances. There are literally thousands of herbs that are known to have therapeutic value. Less than 1% of them have been researched.

Foods High in Beta-Carotene

Foods carrying a great deal of beta-carotene include yellow-orange vegetables, such as carrots, yams, squash, pumpkin, paprika, cayenne pepper, turnips. Carotenoids other than beta-carotene include canthaxanthin, phytoene, lutein, xanathophylls, and lycopenes, many of which, according to herbalist Donny Yance of the American Herbalists' Guild (AHG), may offer greater anticarcinogenic effects than does beta-carotene. He further states that carotenoids have antioxidant properties, protecting phagocytes, lipids, and cells against oxidation, strengthening the immune system, increasing the production of certain interleukins, and—with their special effect on the skin—protect against cancer-causing sun damage.

Cruciferous Vegetables

Vegetables in the cabbage family (cruciferae) contain high amounts of anti-cancer constituents called indoles and isothiocyanates. They are also high in vitamins A, C, E, beta-carotene, anti-carcinogenic minerals and fiber. Because when eaten raw, these vegetables contain a high amount of thyroid lowering agents, they should always be cooked. Some vegetables in this category include cabbage, collards, kale, broccoli, brussels sprouts, cauliflower, mustard greens, turnips and radishes.

Dark Green Leafy Vegetables

Dark green leafy vegetables are high in chlorophyll and other anticarcinogenic compounds and should be eaten daily, in both raw and cooked forms. Again, this is a place to include uncultivated herbs, such as dandelion, chicory, chickweed, malva, watercress, nettles, and mustard greens. In addition, romaine lettuce, arugula, and spinach are valuable.

One of the most powerful wild greens, purslane, hardly included in North American cuisine, is a prized delicacy in many other areas, including Central America and France. Purslane is high in omega-3 fatty acids; antioxidants; vitamins E, C, and K; beta-carotene; glutathione; and psoralens. Psoralens have powerful antioxidant properties, which—besides fighting cancer—are particularly beneficial for normalizing skin pigmentation.

Greens with a bitter flavor, such as dandelion and chicory, more powerfully stimulate detoxification, especially from the liver. They are also potassium-rich foods. They can be served steamed or lightly sautéed with a little olive or sesame oil.

Garlic and Vegetables in the Onion Family

In preparing dark green leafy vegetables, one can add chopped garlic, which is high in anticarcinogenic sulfur compounds, including allicin. Other foods that contain similar compounds to a lesser extent include onions, leeks, chives, and shallots.

Mushrooms

Traditional peoples around the world hve always valued the health benefits of edible mushrooms. Mushrooms are high in minerals, especially potassium, which is important in the regulation of intracellular fluid and the absorption of nutrients into the cell. All mushrooms have potent health-giving, anticarcinogenic properties, but the one that is the most practical to use regularly is the shiitake mushroom (*Lentinual edodes*). These can be economically purchased dry, by the pound in Chinese grocery stores and pharmacies as black mushrooms. They can then be soaked and reconstituted in water before using. Shiitake mushrooms are high in vitamins B_1, B_2, and B_{12}; niacin; and pantothenic acid. B vitamins are necessary for cell energy and hormone production.

They also contain high amounts of protein, enzymes, and eight essential amino acids and have been found to be useful for cancer, heart disease, acquired immunodeficiency syndrome (AIDS), flu, tumors, viruses, high blood pressure, obesity, and aging. Lentinant, a polysaccharide found in the root and cell wall of shiitake, has a triple-helix structure, a shape considered important to the healing properties of shiitake. Lentinant stimulates the production of T-lymphocytes and macrophages that ingest foreign invaders. It also helps the production of interleukin-1 and interleukin-2*, known to inhibit the growth of cancer and viruses.

In Japan, lentinan, the polysaccharide found in shiitake, is an approved drug used together with chemotherapy to treat cancer patients. Research has substantiated that it increases the life span of cancer patients and may also prevent the recurrence of cancer after surgery.

Best of all, the oral ingestion of shiitake by animals and humans has shown that shiitake has strong antitumor activity, stimulating the body's innate immune system to fight abnormal cells. It helps the body produce more interferon† to defend itself from viruses and other harmful matter. Shiitake is also very beneficial for the cardiovascular system, in the treatment of human immunodeficiency virus (HIV), and in the treatment of viral/bacterial infections.

Asparagus

Surprisingly, asparagus has a cleansing effect in the lymphatic system and the kidneys. It is high in potassium and other anticancer vitamins

---

*Interleukin-1 is a substance from monocytes and macrophages, which are important in initiating the immune response for various acute inflammations and infections. Interleukin-2 is a lymphokine that stimulates the growth of T-lymphocytes. When this combines with the immune system's T-lymphocytes, they produce together lumphokine-activated killer (LAK) cells that lyse, or dissolve, cancer cells.

†Interferon is a protein that is formed when cells are damaged by viral or other foreign invaders. Interferons are part of the immune system and have antitumor activity.

and minerals but also contains certain protein compounds that, according to herbalist Donny Yance, act as "cell growth normalizers in cancer cell division." He further states that "asparagus therapy has been used to treat various forms of cancer, and reversal of the disease has been reported in a number of cases." He says that when used as a form of cancer therapy, asparagus is always cooked and puréed in a blender. It can then be stored in the refrigerator. The dose is 4 tablespoons two or three times daily alone or mixed in hot or cold water.

Fruits

Apples, grapes (with the seeds), apricots, peaches, and berries all have powerful anticancer properties. They also tend to have a stronger cooling or antiinflammatory effect, so they are best eaten in the season and climate in which they naturally occur. Citrus peel contains D-limonene, which has powerful anticancer properties. It has been used in trials in England as a monotherapy for individuals with pancreatic and large-intestine cancer. Always use organic unsprayed citrus fruits, especially if you are going to use the peel. Orange, tangerine, or lemon rinds make a zesty condiment when grated into soups, salads, and sauces. They are also very beneficial for digestion and assimilation, and a variety of citrus peels are used in teas.

Grains

Whole grains provide the most important biochemical balance for health. The most balanced grain is brown rice,* which should constitute a large part of the diet. Other grains are also very beneficial and include millet, quinoa, whole wheat, corn, oats, and barley, all containing various anticarcinogenic compounds and properties.

Barley contains coixenlide, amino acids, saccharides, and alkaloids. In traditional Chinese medicine (TCM), barley is used to drain dampness, meaning it has mild diuretic properties. Dampness is one of the symptomatic issues of arthritic conditions and cancer. Coix, a type of

---

*The pH of blood is 7.4, which is slightly alkaline. The body must maintain this balance; any slight variation higher or lower can result in severe sickness and death. Brown rice has a pH similar to that of blood—around 7.4 to 7.5—which is why it is considered the most balanced food.

barley, is used for a variety of cancers, but especially cancer of the breast, larynx, uterus, and stomach.

Brown rice also has anticancer and diuretic properties. If digestion is weak, TCM advocates the use of long-cooked white rice for easier digestion and assimilation.

Congee: Chinese Rice Porridge

One of the most assimilable foods is congee or rice porridge. Traditionally, it is used by Chinese people as a basic breakfast because it is easily digested. In general, congee is made with white rice because it is considered easier to digest than brown rice and is particularly beneficial for convalescence and for the treatment of such chronic diseases as cancer. The basic recipe is 1 part by volume of white rice in 7–10 parts of water, cooked slowly for 6–8 hours (a slow cooker can be used).

For protein supplementation, one can add a good-quality soy or whey powder. There are infinite variations on this basic congee recipe that should be selected according to individual requirements. One can substitute or mix different grains, such as barley for arthritis and cancer. Congee is also an ideal medium in which to combine various vegetables or tonic herbs according to one's condition as follows:

Immune tonic: astragalus root, 9 grams
Low energy: codonopsis or Chinese ginseng combined with poria cocos mushrooms (or shiitake), approximately 9 grams each
Liver and blood deficiency: lycii berries (high in beta-carotene) and *Polygonum multiflorum,* 9 grams each
Dryness, Yin, or wasting conditions: ophiopogon root and Chinese asparagus root, approximately 9 grams each
For general weakness, immunodeficiency, emaciation, spontaneous perspiration, and loss of appetite: astragalus root, 60 grams; Chinese ginseng, 12 grams; white rice, 90 grams; shredded lean beef, 4 ounces; whole brown sugar (Sucanat) added to taste after cooking

Congee offers a wonderful opportunity to add grated orange or tangerine peel as desired, both for flavor and for their anticarcinogenic properties. Orange or tangerine peel in tea or with congee is good to help overcome the nausea caused by chemotherapy.

It is not possible to offer all the possible variations for making congee. As one can see, congee is the perfect medium for a variety of health-giving, easily digested and assimilated food and herb combinations.

Beans and Various Legumes

Isoflavones are flavonoid compounds commonly found in various legumes, including soybeans. One of the most important currently is genistein because of its close molecular resemblance to human estrogen. For this reason, it is very important to include beans, especially soybeans, in an anticancer diet. Fermented soybean products, such as miso, tempeh, and shoyu tamari, go through complex chemical processes that are of particular benefit in the prevention and treatment of cancer.

Protein Foods

Cancer is fundamentally involved with malutilization of protein. Oncologists generally agree that the actual cause of death in cancer patients is cachexia, a condition of severe weight loss and wasting associated with protein malabsorption. In fact, cancer cells are able to grow by making the amino acids of protein available for their growth at the expense of the body as a whole. Meat, especially red meat, being the most readily assimilable protein, becomes a banquet for cancer cells. Plant sources of vegetable protein, such as legumes and beans that contain cancer-fighting compounds, should be a prominent part of an anticancer diet.

Legumes and beans supply high-quality protein necessary to rebuild the tissues and maintain a healthy immune system. They are also an important source of insoluble fiber that slows the release of glucose into the bloodstream, keeping blood sugar levels in balance. It has been found that sugar speeds up metabolism and causes tumors to grow at a much faster rate. Fiber is also fermented in the colon mostly by beneficial bacteria that produce short-chain fatty acids (SCFAs) that help prevent colon cancer. Legumes also serve as protease inhibitors, which are protein-splitting enzymes found to be important to block cancer growth. Finally, legumes are an important source of such valuable phytochemicals as saponins, which tonify the immune system and inhibit the deoxyribonucleic acid (DNA) synthesis of cancer cells.

Another important source of protein is from fish, especially salmon, which is high in omega 3 fatty acids. Poultry with the skin removed is a less dense protein than is red meat and can also be occasionally used.

The following recipe for the treatment of cancer was given to me by one of my esteemed former teachers. It is a basic stew; if not all the ingredients are available, it still has great benefit.

Dr. Miriam Lee's Bean Soup Treatment for Cancer

> 10 tablespoons brown rice
> 1 tablespoon pinto beans
> 1 tablespoon azuki beans
> 1 tablespoon pine nuts
> 1 tablespoon mung beans
> 1 tablespoon split peas
> 1 tablespoon soya beans
> 1 tablespoon black beans
> 1 tablespoon corn or cornmeal
> 1 tablespoon barley
> 1 tablespoon millet
> 1 tablespoon buckwheat
> 1 tablespoon oats
> 1 tablespoon peanuts (nip removed)

Add 12 grams of each of the following Chinese herbs: qian shi (euryale seeds; also called foxnuts); mai men dong (ophiopogon root), bai guo (ginkgo seed) with the skin removed (this is the most difficult to obtain and can be omitted), bai he (tiger lily bulb), lian zi (lotus seed), shan yao (Dioscorea batatas), fu ling (poria cocos).

Preparation: Simmer the entire contents in 18 cups of water. As soon as it comes to boil, reduce heat and simmer the soup for another 2 hours. (Do not use too high a flame, as doing so will destroy the nutrients.) Consume the soup over a period of 3 days. Keep the unused portion in the freezer. Continue this food therapy for many months. All these herbs are available from Chinese pharmacies (see sources in the appendix).

Soybean Extract: Special Nutrition for Cancer Patients

One of the most valuable anticancer food agents I have found is a special fermented soybean extract that was first developed in a cancer hospital in China. It is made by concentrating approximately 25 to 27 pounds of organic soybeans down to 8 ounces of liquid. This is then fermented for several days to form and release thousands of bioactive phytochemicals that have antiinflammatory, antibacterial, antiviral, antiosteoporotic, antimutagenic, anticarcinogenic, and other properties. The phytochemicals generated from the concentrated fermented soybean extract are able to prevent cancer by capturing free radicals and prevent them from damaging DNA. In animal studies, they have been found to be effective in the prevention and treatment of most cancers, including breast, colorectal, and prostate. They assist in detoxifying the liver, lowering the number of histamines in the blood to help clear various allergic reactions (including bronchitis and nasal congestion), and also to help relieve pain, lower cholesterol, heal stomach ulcers, and stop menstrual cramps.

Research* has shown that soybean products contain five cancer-preventive or -reversing chemical agents:

1. Protease inhibitors, which hold off activation of the specific oncogenes that cause cancer

2. Phytate, which binds iron in the intestines to prevent it from generating free radicals that result in cancer

3. Phytosterols, which neutralize the breakdown of cholesterol and reduce the development of colon tumors and skin cancer

4. Saponins, which stop cellular mutations that could inevitably lead to cancer

5. Isoflavones, which are plant estrogens with strong inhibiting effects in hormone-related malignancies, such as prostate, ovarian, cervical, and breast cancers.

The isoflavones are a group of phytochemicals that include genistein. Genistein is an estrogen precursor that binds to receptor sites and either blocks estrogen uptake if there is too much or supplies it if there is too little. This is thought to be why Asian women have a noticeable lack of gynecological problems associated with menopause, fibroids and more than a 45% lower incidence of breast cancer. The assortment of other isoflavones found in soy are effective against a wide variety of cancers, including lung, brain, breast, colon, prostate, skin and even blood dyscrasias, including leukemia and Hodgkin's disease.

---

*St. Clair, A. R., W. H. Billings, P. C. Kennedy. The effects of the Bowman-Birk protease inhibitor on C-MYC expression and cell proliferation in unirradiated and irradiated mouse color. *Cancer Letters* 52: 145–152, 1990.

Juices. Cancer patients should have one or two 8-ounce glasses of fresh organic vegetable juice each day. A good combination is carrots, beets, celery, garlic, and, if available, fresh burdock root. For an occasional flavor variation, add an apple.

Green Drink. I also recommend the use of chlorella, which is a highly nutritive one-cell blue-green algae that is a powerful immune system stimulant that also has demonstrated anti-tumor effects. Research has shown that chlorella is able to repair DNA and increase serum albumin levels.

Beverages. Green tea contains catechin polyphenols that have been shown to have potent anticarcinogenic properties. Other beverages that can be used are red clover tea, the anticancer tea described on page 313, and roasted root and grain beverages, many of which contain a roasted extract of dandelion root, which is a potent liver detoxifier with anticancer properties.

HERBAL TREATMENT

The basic strategy in the treatment of cancer involves improving the health and natural immunity of the patient overall and secondly dissolving the tumor by killing the more vulnerable cancer cells. Herbs and herbal preparations have the ability to treat cancer both through necrosis and apoptosis.

Internal Herbal Treatment

FORMULA 14 (BLOOD PURIFIER AND ALTERATIVE)

Echinacea root
Goldenseal
Chaparral
Honeysuckle flowers
Forsythia blossoms
Sarsaparilla root
Yellow dock root
American ginseng
Ginger root
Red clover

Cinnamon twigs
Licorice

The blood-purifying effects of formula 14 are good for inflammatory conditions, skin eruptions, fevers, toxicity of blood and lymph, boils, sores, and arthritic conditions. It can be used for both bacterial and viral infections. It is also a good antibiotic herbal formula useful for many acute inflammatory symptoms, including flu and sore throat. The majority of the herbs in this formula have known anticarcinogenic compounds, which make it useful for the treatment of cancer. The tablets should be taken at least two or three times daily.

CHAPARRAL

Chaparral contains the powerful antioxidant nordihydroquaiaretic acid (NDGA), which has known anticarcinogenic properties.

GOLDEN SEAL

Goldenseal (*Hydrastis canadensis*) is another important North American blood purifying antiinflammatory herb. Its major constituents, berberine, hydrastine, and hydrastinine, are effective against gram-positive and gram-negative bacteria, yeast, fungus, and protozoas. Berberine, a major compound in goldenseal, has been found to inhibit cellular respiration especially of cancer cells, which are more sensitive to berberine than are normal cells.*

HONEYSUCKLE FLOWERS

Honeysuckle flowers contain flavones, luteolin, inositol, and saponins and are used for the treatment of cancer generally but especially that of the lungs.

FORSYTHIA BLOSSOMS

Forsythia blossoms contain oleanolic acid, flavonoid glycoside, and saponin and have anticarcinogenic properties similar to those of honeysuckle flowers.

---

*Minyi Chang. *Anticancer Medicinal Herbs* (Hunan Science and Technology Publishing House, 1992).

SARSAPARILLA ROOT

Sarsaparilla root is rich in phytochemicals, including various saponins that have immune-potentiating and cancer-inhibiting properties.

YELLOW DOCK ROOT

Yellow dock root is effective for cancer and has been used in TCM for acute leukemia.

AMERICAN GINSENG

American ginseng contains ginsenosides and polysaccharides that inhibit Ehrlich's ascites carcinoma and various other types of cancers, including sarcoma-180 and adenocarcima-755.

LICORICE

Licorice and its various constituents, including glycyrrhizin, have been found to be prophylactic against cancer.

ECHINACEA

Echinacea is perhaps the most famous Western herb for the treatment of inflammatory diseases. While it may have little direct activity against cancer, its ability to stimulate the immune system makes it a useful addition to the formula. Echinacea has shown anticarcinogenic properties.

FORMULA 15 (PAU D'ARCO–MUSHROOM COMPLEX)

Pau d'arco bark
Pau d'arco extract
Burdock root
Echinacea root
Echinacea root extract
Red clover blossoms
Poria
Reishi mushroom in soy culture
American ginseng
Kelp

Cool-natured and dispersing, formula 15 is a mild diuretic, helping to resolve tumors, cysts, and lymphatic congestion. It can be used for all degenerative diseases associated with the appearance of abnormal growths. For patients undergoing chemo- or radiotherapy, it can be taken with formula 75, Reishi Mushroom Complex (see page 319), to offset some of the negative side effects and to optimize the effects of the Western treatments for these conditions. This formula can also be combined with formula 14 (see page 308).

Dosage: 2–4 tablets three times daily with warm water or a tea made from a combination of equal parts of red clover blossoms, burdock root, and chaparral.

PAU D'ARCO

Pau d'arco (*Tabebuia heptaphylla;* also called lapacho, taheebo, and ipe roxo) is cooling, bitter, alterative, antibiotic, antifungal, antitumor, antiviral, antineoplastic, digestive, diuretic, fungicidal, antidiabetic, anodyne, analgesic, astringent, parasiticide, and hypotensive. Its constituents are lapachol, a quinone and a recognized antitumor agent found in the wood and barely in the bark. According to H. Wagner, head of the Institute of Pharmaceutical Biology at the University of Munich in Germany, much of the basis for pau d'arco's reputation is its immune-stimulating properties. Quinones (also present in *Cascara sagrada* and rhubarb root) are present throughout nature. They are involved with the transference of hydrogen and of electrons.

Lapachol, found in the inner bark, activates human immune cells (lymphocytes and granulocytes) in low concentrations. Lymphocytes include cells that mediate immunological reactions, such as T-cells. Granulocytes are white blood cells found in the blood that devour foreign cells and bacteria. Lapachol is barely soluble in water.

The best-quality pau d'arco comes from Argentina. It has significant antifungal properties and has been shown in several studies to be effective at treating cancer. Pau d'arco is a first-rate alterative and blood purifier and can be used for a wide variety of conditions, including all skin diseases, for the treatment of the flu, herpes, and hepatitis; and for environmental allergies, asthma, and leukemia and pernicious anemia.

BURDOCK ROOT

Burdock root (*Fructus et radix arctii;* Chinese *niu pang*) is classified as an acrid, bitter antipyretic resolving masses and lumps and removing the stagnation of *qi* in the viscera. The root is classified in Chinese medicine as cold, bitter, and of a slightly biting flavor. It is used to clear fever, detoxify, and dispel wind (spasms and the proliferation of pathogenic influences). The dried root, seed, and whole plant are used. It contains arctiin, fatty oil, sterol, vitamin A–like substances, and vitamin B in the fruit; volatile oil and vitamin B in the leaf; and 5% inulin, mucilage, a tannic substance, and proteins in the root. For cancerous edema, 60 grams is fried and pulverized for oral administration, with 6 grams taken three times daily. Doses of the root often combined with the seed range from 9 to 30 grams daily.

RED CLOVER BLOSSOMS

Red clover blossoms (*Trifolium pratense*) are classified as bitter, cold, antiinflammatory, diuretic, antipyretic, and able to improve acuity of vision because of a high beta-carotene content. They contain isoflavones, which possesses estrogen-like actions (genistein): the level of activity of 100 grams of the dried plant corresponds to 0.55–0.56 micrograms of estradiol. The plant's anticancer properties are enhanced by the presence of active carotene (richest in the blossoms) and vitamin E.

PORIA COCOS

Poria cocos has a neutral energy and bland flavor. It contains beta-pachyman (93% of the weight of poria), choline, adenine, and other constituents. It has been found to inhibit mice sarcoma-180 at an effective rate of 96.88%.* It increases phagocytosis and promotes the formation of immunoglobulin.

REISHI MUSHROOM

The reishi mushroom (*Ganoderma lucidum*) has a sweet and warm energy, is both sedative and tonic, is a supreme deep immune system tonic, and nourishes the spirit, essence, and vital energy. It has strong anticarcinogenic properties and is rich in a number of complex phytochemicals, including ergosterol, fumaric acid, aminoglucose, and mannitol; coumarins; alkaloids; lactone; and various enzymes. It is effective

---

*Minyi, Chang. *Anticancer Medicinal Herbs* (Hunan Science and Technology Publishing House, 1992).

for all cancers and immune system deficiencies. As such, it is specific for individuals recovering from chemotherapy.

KELP

Kelp (*Laminaria* species) is salty and cold in nature and has trace amounts of iodine, which activates thyroid function. It is generally used in Chinese medicine to soften any hard lumps or tumors. It is rich in polysaccharides, which have known anticancer properties. It also is able to inhibit the growth hormone of tumors.

With these formulas 14 and 15, I combine other herbs and formulas for detoxification and elimination:

Formula 12 for detoxifying the blood through the liver (see page 314)

Formula 23 (Triphala) for gentle purification of the liver, blood, and gastrointestinal tract (see page 317)

Formula 2 to assist the process of detoxification through the urinary tract (see page 316)

Formula 75 (Reishi Mushroom Complex), taken as a digestive and immune tonic before meals (see page 319)

RED CLOVER, BURDOCK, CHAPARRAL, AND PAU D'ARCO TEA FOR CANCER

Simmer 1 handful of these herbs each morning in 3 cups of boiling water. Have 1 three times daily with the other herbal formulas. Warm each cup before use.

In addition, two formulas that may be considered include Stress Free (formula 8) and the Ayurvedic *guggul raj* formula, which is used in traditional Indian Ayurvedic medicine for circulatory disorders, lowering blood cholesterol and creating the correct ratio of low-density lipoprotein (LDL) to high-density lipoprotein (HDL) cholesterol. *Guggul raj* is also regarded as an effective Ayurvedic treatment for various types of cancer. Stress Free (formula 8, page 320) may be useful to feed the nervous system and counteract nervous stress, which is understandably associated with cancer and can affect one's recovery.

Herbs and the Liver

The liver is the most important organ of detoxification in the body. It has numerous functions, including filtering out stored internal toxins caused by stress and external toxins caused by ingested substances and environmental pollutants. All the herbs in the formula below have anti-cancer properties. Milk thistle seeds are particularly valuable to help nourish and rebuild the liver. A good nutritional supplement I recommend can be made by lightly dry-roasting whole milk thistle seeds (available from http://supplies.planetherbs.com/mall/) and then grinding them with a little rock salt or roasted sea salt. These can be eaten by the spoonful several times a day or sprinkled on food as a condiment.

FORMULA 12 FOR THE LIVER (LIVER DETOXIFYING FORMULA)

> Bupleurum
> Milk thistle seed extract (83.5% silymarin)
> Cyperus
> Dandelion root
> Oregon grape root
> Wild yam root
> Dong quai
> Dong quai extract
> Lycii berries
> Fennel seed
> Ginger
> Green citrus peel

Formula 12 is used to help regulate liver metabolism. It both dredges deep-seated toxins stored in cells throughout the body and detoxifies the liver while supporting the liver Yin (blood). It is useful for hepatitis, chest pains, colitis due to liver irregularities, constipation, cirrhosis, gynecological disorders, and general blood detoxification. Unlike many other cholagogues, it also helps tonify live blood, so it is especially good for deficient conditions of the blood and Yin. It contains a number of anticancer herbs, including the following.

DANDELION

Dandelion (Herba taraxaci; Chinese, pu gong ying) clears heat and is sweet, bitter, mild, and cold with no toxicity. The whole herb is used.

It is especially effective for curing female breast abscess. It goes to the liver and spleen. It contains taraxasterol, choline, inulin, and pectin.

Interestingly Dr. Chang Minyi M.D. states that "the drug (herb) has been processed into an extract or pills and is widely used for treating various sorts of cancer." This statement seems very unsubstantiated in my experience.

The hot-water extract inhibits sarcoma-180 in mice with an effective rate of 43.5%, whereas the alcohol extract has no effect. The hot-water extract contains a polyose substance that is anticarcinogenic and promotes immunity. According to *Elucidation of the Materia Medica*, "the drug cures female breast cancer because breast abscess is distributed to the liver channel, which dominates all the body activities during menstruation." This seems to suggest that because dandelion activates liver function, it helps the liver neutralize estrogen, which can activate certain cancer cells.

BUPLEURUM

Bupleurum (*Bupleurum falcatum*) contains saikosaponins that have antiinflammatory properties similar to those of prednisoloe.* It is a primary ingredient in a number of herbal formulas whose action involves liver detoxification. It has the ability to inhibit cancer growth by inducing apoptosis (slow death of cancer cells) and inhibiting angiogenesis (blocking the vascularization of tumors). It is used for breast, liver, and colon cancer and it has been found to increase the effectiveness of the chemotherapeutic agent 5-fluorouracil (5-FU).

OREGON GRAPE

Oregon grape root (*Berberis acquifolia*), like goldenseal, is high in berberine, which has antineoplastic properties and tends to block oxygen uptake specifically to cancer cells.

Herbs and the Urinary Tract

The kidneys serve as a filter of soluble wastes from the blood. Urea, one of the waste by-products of urine, is formed from ammonia, which in turn is the result of protein degradation. These are discharged along

---

*Boik, John. *Cancer and Natural Medicine: A Textbook of Basic Science and Clinical Research*, p. 186 (North Princeton, MN: Oregon Medical Press, 1995).

with other cellular wastes from the liver to combine with other wastes and nutrients in the blood. When the blood passes through the small tubules of the kidneys, the waste by-products that are smaller than proteins pass into the tubules for excretion. Other important nutrients, such as amino acids, certain vitamins, calcium magnesium, and sodium, are reabsorbed. Urine contains water, urea, urates, nitrates, sulfates, and phosphates. The dietary need for potassium is obviated by the fact that there is a certain loss of potassium by secretion with urates in the urine.

Herbs have a number of effects on the urinary tract. They can stimulate the excretion of urine and thus have a more flushing effect. They also possess potent antiseptic and antimicrobial properties, which help prevent and cure urinary tract infections. Many urinary diuretic herbs have antilithic, or stone-dissolving, properties. Still another important effect is to soothe the lining of the bladder and greatly relieve pain and irritation.

Finally, such mushrooms as poria cocos have potent anticarcinogenic properties. Because of their high potassium and mineral content, they help regulate cellular nutrition and inter- and extracellular fluid balance.

FORMULA 2 (URINARY SYSTEM DETOXIFYING FORMULA)

Cleavers
Dandelion root
Poria
Marshmallow root
Parsley root
uva ursi
ginger root

Formula 2 is dispersing and diuretic, regulates fluid metabolism, and overcomes thirst, swelling, cystitis, and kidney weakness. It has a cool to neutral energy and is effective for most damp heat (inflammatory) urinary tract disorders. Interestingly, the formula has also proved corrective for frequent urination in both women and men with benign prostate enlargement that causes incomplete and dribbling urination. This formula can be used as a safe and effective diuretic as well as for urinary disorders and infections.

Herbs Maintaining Balanced Elimination and Detoxification

FORMULA 23 (TRIPHALA)

Terminalia emblica
T. belerica
T. chebulae

Triphala (*tri,* three; *phala,* fruits) is a combination of the fruits of the chebulic, beleric, and emblic myrobalan trees. These are popularly known in India as *harada, behada,* and *amla,* respectively. Triphala is widely regarded as a purgative and laxative, but in fact it is considered a *rasayana* and rejuvenator. Its special value, therefore, is both as a regulator of elimination as well as rejuvenator of the whole body.

Harada and *behada* have a warm energy, while *amla* is cool. Triphala, being a combination of all three, is therefore balanced, making it useful as an internal cleansing, detoxifying formula for everyone, including more sensitive individuals and vegetarians.

Daily use of triphala will promote normal appetite, good digestion, the increase of red blood cells and hemoglobin, and removal of undesirable fat. Triphala will also eliminate what is called deficient heat in Chinese medicine. This is a feeling of heat and burning on the chest, legs, palms, and/or soles of the feet, all representing a B-vitamin deficiency in Western medicine. Triphala, taken regularly, will promote absorption and utilization of the B vitamins and will completely relieve the symptoms of deficient heat. Triphala is very beneficial for creating a favorable chemical environment for the proliferation of beneficial intestinal bacteria and an unfavorable environment for nonbeneficial intestinal bacteria.

Of primary importance is the use of triphala as a bowel regulator. It is considered as safe as food and is not habit forming, even when taken on a daily basis. No wonder that in India there is a saying comparing the importance of triphala to that of a mother.

Since triphala is a tonic, cleanser, and blood purifier, there is still one other important use for it—as a strengthener of the eyes, useful for cataracts, conjunctivitis, and glaucoma. Triphala can be used as daily eyewash to strengthen vision, counteract many eye defects, and eliminate redness and soreness.

When using triphala as a blood purifier, reducing and cleansing agent, take 2 tablets three times daily. When using triphala as an occasional tonic laxative, take 2–6 tablets in the evening. When using triphala as an eyewash, steep 1 teaspoon of the powder in 1 cup of boiled water, cool it, and strain it through a cloth; using an eyecup purchased in a pharmacy, bathe the eyes two or three times a day.

Herbs to Break Up Tumors and Normalize Circulation

FORMULA 68 (GUGGUL RAJ)

Guggul
Triphala (harada, amla, behada)
Pippli
Omum seeds
Chitrak

Guggul is specific for circulatory problems, especially high cholesterol and high triglycerides. In addition, guggul is used for arteriosclerosis, arthritic and rheumatic problems, numbness, and impaired circulation. The active biochemical constituents are called guggulsterones, which contain diterpenes, sterols, esters, and fatty alcohols. All of these seem to have a synergistic effect in lowering cholesterol and triglyceride levels in the blood.

Guggul is one of the most valued herbs in Ayurvedic medicine. It has been used for thousands of years for a variety of conditions, including rheumatoid arthritis and lipid imbalances. Gugulipid has been found in research to be safer and more effective than many cholesterol-lowering drugs, including niacin. Because of this, it was granted approval in India for marketing as a lipid-reducing drug in June 1986.*

Gugulipid lowers cholesterol by increasing the liver's metabolism. Guggulsterone increases the liver's ability to increase the uptake of LDL cholesterol from the blood by the liver. Guggulsterone also has thyroid-stimulating activity, which contributes to the lipid-lowering activity in general.

Guggul is widely used for a variety of circulatory and metabolic purposes. These include inducing weight loss, increasing energy, as a heart

---

*Satyavati, GV. "Gugulipid: A Promising Hypolipidaemic Agent from Gum Guggul (*Commiphora wightii*)." *Econ Med Plant Res* 5: 47–82, 1991.

tonic, improving flexibility and youthful mobility, strengthening the bones to prevent osteoporosis, and treating nervous tissues, cancers and tumors, arthritis and rheumatic complaints, and all circulatory disorders.

Guggul is traditionally combined with triphala to accent its ability to detoxify the channels of the body and to reduce cholesterol and high blood lipids for weight loss.

Fu Zheng Tonic Immune Therapy

Fu zheng is a therapeutic approach to protective the "righteous *qi*" of the body, which represents all those aspects that we would not want to compromise when our system's immune system is under attack. *Fu zheng* formulas like the one below are typically taken to maintain the immune system under all circumstances or when one must undergo chemo- or radiotherapy.

FORMULA 75 (REISHI MUSHROOM COMPLEX)

Reishi mycelial biomass
Shiitake mycelial biomass
Siberian ginseng extract
Schizandra
Astragalus
Atractylodes
Grifola
Ligustrum
Poria cocos
Reishi mushroom extract
Polygala
Ginger root
Green citrus peel

Reishi Mushroom Complex combines *fu zheng* herbs in a special formulation useful for cancer patients undergoing conventional Western medical treatment, for individuals with a depleted immune system, and for protecting one from sickness.

Herbs to Strengthen the Nerves and Help Maintain Calm and Centeredness

FORMULA 8 (NERVE TONIC FOR STRESS)

Valerian
Valerian root extract
Zizyphus seeds
Calcium carbonate
Magnesium citrate (8% of the U.S. recommended daily allowance [RDA] for magnesium)
American ginseng
Black cohosh
Chamomile
Ginger
Hawthorn berries
Hops
Skullcap
Wood betony
Siberian ginseng extract and Siberian ginseng
Licorice

Formula 8 has a mild, neutral, and soothing energy and is a tonic for the nerves. It relieves feelings of stress and tension, insomnia, excessive irritability, anxiety, poor concentration, and the mild pain. It is an ideal formula to use during times of high stress or in the workplace. It will induce a sense of calm centeredness without drowsiness. It can also be taken a half hour before retiring for a sound night's sleep.

Herbs to Clear the Lymphatic System and Metastasis

POKEROOT

Pokeroot (*Phytolacca dicandra;* Chinese *shang lu*) is cooling, bitter, an alterative, anodyne, antibiotic, antiinflammatory, antirheumatic, antiscorbutic, antisyphilitic, antitumor, cathartic, emetic, parasiticide, and toxic. It is considered a specific for all glandular derangements, including breast and other cancers. Because of its strong cathartic and emetic effects, certainly in its fresh state and in too large dose, it can be a gastrointestinal irritant. However, in my opinion, pokeroot is one of the two or three most important native herbs for treating cancer. It can be used with a broad-spectrum blood-purifying formula, such as the Hoxsey formula. The dosage for the tincture is no more than 5–10 drops every 3 hours.

For information on The Hoxsey Formula and Harry S. Hoxsey see Cancer Salves: A Botanical Approach to Treatment by Dr. Ingrid Natman published by Seventh Ray Press, Distributed by North Atlantic books.

Generally, it is best to make a syrup of fresh pokeroot, which tends to lessen gastric irritation. This is made simply by adding fresh green pokeroot tincture to a base syrup or honey. The dose is five to ten drops every three hours. In 1869, Dr. Eli Jones wrote about a formula he used to cure breast cancer. It consisted of equal parts of tinctures of pokeroot (only the fresh green root should be used), gentian root, and dandelion root. These were all added to a simple syrup (they could be mixed with a base of honey and glycerin). He said this was "especially useful for cancer in old people or patients past midlife. It keeps the stomach and bowels in a healthy condition [and] keeps up the appetite and strength."* The dosage for the syrup is no more than 1 teaspoon after each meal.

THUJA

Thuja (Thuja occidentalis) is particularly indicated for cancers of viral origin, including colorectal cancer, uterine cancer, breast cancer, and lung cancer. It enhances the immune system by stimulating T-lymphocytes and increasing interleukin-2 production. This makes it particularly useful for increasing tolerance of chemo- and radiotherapy. Take no more than 10 drops of the tincture three times daily.

See Appendix 3 for formula names.

External Treatment

The internal treatment of cancer is involved with the process of internal purification and normalizing the chemistry of the body to create an unfavorable environment for cancer cells to thrive and thus leading to

---

*Jones, M.D. Eli G., Cancer, Its Causes and Symptoms (first published around 1911; reprinted in India by Jain Publishers, New Delhi, India) in 1994.

their dissolution. The external treatment of cancer, however, actually seeks out and destroys cancer cells with escharotic salves.

Escharotic pastes and salves are caustic compounds that are applied externally on the skin. These are directly applied over the affected area and will erode the tissue to eventually destroy and remove the underlying humor.

The direct application of herbs and herbal juices to tumors has been practiced in many different traditions and cultures far back into antiquity. It is known that the Native Americans commonly applied poultices of roasted onions and bloodroot as well as other substances, which eroded the skin to draw out cancers, tumors, and other undesirable materials. Straight garlic poultice will also cause blistering and open the skin, but, like onions, it is very painful. These formulas were admired and used by medical doctors during the eighteenth century in Europe.

Other examples of topical application of herbs and their expressed juice are the use of chelidonium or dandelion latex to remove warts and other excrescences. The Chinese have a tradition of breaking open the seed of *Brucea javonica* and taping directly over warts and excrescences to stimulate their dissolution. The treatment of breast cancer, particularly through the use of dandelion latex, was used as a folk remedy by the Chinese.

Japanese macrobiotics* uses a grated poultice of the taro potato *(Colocasia esculenta)*, which grows in tropical, hot countries. The Africans call this plant taro; in India, it is called *albi;* in Japan, it is *sato-imo* ("field potato"); and in the Caribbean, it is *malanga* or *yautia.* It is a staple food of the native Hawaiians, who make a porridge called *poi,* which is a staple of the traditional Hawaiian diet.

In the midnineteenth century, Samuel Thompson, a leader of one of the most popular movements of natural healing based primarily on the use of Native American herbs, reported the successful treatment of breast cancer. This was done by using a paste of thickened decoction of red clover blossoms. It was repeatedly and thickly applied to the woman's breast and covered over with a protective bandage. After a short time, the cancer literally sloughed off through the surface of the skin, leaving a shallow crater. It is presumed that if these cases are at all similar to dozens that I have seen or heard of, the breast healed over without any complications.

---

*Michio, Kushi, and Marc Van Cauwenberghe, M.D. *Macrobiotic Home Remedies* (Japan Publications, 1985).

Meanwhile—and previously, from the middle of the eighteenth-century to the midnineteenth century—one of the ways in Europe of treating cancer was by applying zinc chloride directly to tumors until they died and fell off. This was obviously a painful process. Around the midnineteenth century, Native American herbs became very popular in Europe, and a Dr. J. W. Fell, working at Middlesex Hospital in London, developed a paste made of bloodroot, zinc chloride, flour, and water. This was directly applied to a malignant growth and generally destroyed the tumor within 2 to 4 weeks.

Bloodroot (*Sanguinarea canadensis*) is one of the most beautiful eastern North American woodland herbs and was commonly used by the Native Americans to treat cancer. Since that time, it has been identified as a primary ingredient in most escharotic salves and pastes, as these are called, used for the treatment of cancer. The alkaloid sanguinarine has been indeed found to possess powerful anticancer properties.

The Eclectics medical doctors of the nineteenth century, especially Dr. Eli Jones, specialized in the treatment of cancer with an emphasis on internal treatment and lifestyle changes, but they evidently used escharotic salves and ointments with success. The late Dr. Raymond Christopher created a black ointment drawing salve that contained potent anticancer herbs, such as pokeroot and black walnut bark. Many consider this to be only for drawing out slivers and such embedded in the flesh, but in fact the salve is also used for drawing out cancers and tumors. In recent times, various formulas for the salve have been sold or given away by various clandestine individuals who are mostly motivated by the desire to help provide patients with a less invasive and harmful method for removing cancers from various parts of the body.

One of the most startling facts is that the use of escharotics has been and continues to be an accepted and recognized medical procedure. A medical text entitled *Chemosurgery: Microscopically Controlled Surgery for Skin Cancer* was written by Frederic E. Mohs, M.D. and last published by Charles C. Thomas in Publishers 1978. It uses the same basic escharotic paste used by Dr. Eli Jones, Hoxsey, and others for topical application for the removal of various cancers, moles, warts, and other growths and excrescences. At the time he published his book, Dr. Mohs was clinical professor of surgery at the University of Wisconsin Medical School.

As recently as the late 1960s, Vipont Chemical Co. of Fort Collins, Colorado, was formed by a rodeo cowboy named Howard McCrorey and two friends specifically to research and develop the salve for approval by the U.S. Food and Drug Administration (USFDA). At one point, they informally sent it off to an investigator at the Mayo Clinic to be tested for its efficacy in treating cancer. The investigator sent back two letters stating that he had not tested anything having properties that even came close to the antitumor activity of the salve.

In order to keep the company viable, they performed various contract work. As a result, they brought a toothpaste to market called Viadent which used the ingredients of their salve to maintain dental hygiene and prevent and cure periodontal disease. It was and still is very effective and the company was eventually bought up by Colgate, who is the manufacturer of Viadent.

The Escharotic Black Salve researched by Vipont is the basic one that is usually found. It consists of equal parts powdered bloodroot, galangal, zinc chloride, and distilled water. Other versions of this entail adding white flour to make more of a paste consistency.

Besides its topical use, there is a tradition of its internal use for cancer and all infectious and inflammatory diseases. Vipont conducted an LD_{50} toxicity study* of the salve for internal use. It was reported that the LD_{50} was around 700 milligrams per kilogram of body weight. Since the recommended dose for internal use is no greater than 250 milligrams, toxicity is very low at this level. However, it should never be taken on an empty stomach, as it can be too irritating. The salve can be taken in a 00-size gelatin capsule each day.

Vipont and company has documented the use of the salve for a wide variety of problems, ranging from the removal of warts, moles, and skin cancers to other internal cancers, colds, eye problems (diluted in a saline solution, 1 part salve to 1,000 parts water), staff infections, impotency, skin diseases, gastrointestinal inflammations, and other conditions too numerous to list. Clark Bigham, who reported this story and was on the board of directors of Vipont Chemical, stated that his "inclination is to try it for just about any known condition other than stomach ulcers and autoimmune diseases."

This is not the place to thoroughly explore the formulas and methods for the use of escharotic salves. This information, along with a more complete presentation on the botanical treatment of cancer, will be presented in another book. For those who are interested, there is a

---

*LD_{50} means what is the lethal dose at which 50% of rats ingesting it will die.

2½-hour video presentation on the treatment of cancer and the use of escharotic salves, which is available with a more extensive paper on the subject (see page 339).

Dry Skin Brushing and the Medicated Epsom Salts Bath

The skin is one of the most important organs of elimination. As such, it is an extension of the lungs and kidneys. It is important for the cancer patient to improve surface circulation on the skin and keep the pores of the skin open for the regular discharge of metabolic wastes. Each day before you shower, your skin should be vigorously dry-brushed with a natural-fiber brush or loofah sponge. Then take a warm bath or shower, which should always be followed by a cool rinse at the end to invigorate blood circulation and stimulate surface warmth.

The medicated epsom salts bath should be taken at least twice a week before you retire to bed. It neutralizes toxins, relieves pain, and calms the nerves. Simply dissolve 4 tablespoons of epsom salts in warm water in the bathtub. For the treatment of cancer, the best time to take the bath is just before bedtime. Dr. Eli Jones recommends that this bath be taken as often as twice a week. The skin should be vigorously rubbed with a natural bristle brush to remove all the dead skin and other material. The blood needs the magnesium in epsom salts, which neutralizes toxins. The bath also soothes tired nerves and induces sound sleep.

If you have no bathtub, dissolve 1 ounce of Epsom salts in 1 pint of warm water and bathe the body all over with the mixture.

For acute fevers, the bath can be used once or twice a day. For skin diseases, use sulfate of soda.

For the treatment of cancer, the bath should never be omitted.

Enzyme Therapy

Experimental evidence has shown that cancer cells are highly susceptible to lysis (dissolution) when exposed to proteolytic and lipolytic enzymes. The rapid process of cell division of cancer cells causes them to have weaker cell membranes. This is makes them highly susceptible to destruction with enzymes. With age and any degenerative condition, serum levels of proteolytic enzymes (proteases) are at a much lower concentration than normal. Aging causes a general decrease of enzymes throughout the body, which effects many body functions, including digestion, energy production, DNA, and oxygen and amino acid metabolism.

Proteolytic enzymes, such as papain from papaya and bromelain from pineapple, are used in extract form as meat tenderizers. When the more vulnerable membranes of cancer cells are exposed to these enzymes, they tend to break down, with the tumor consequently dissolving.

As tumors break down—by any means—they tend to place an added toxic burden on the body, which can ultimately injure the kidneys. This is one reason that daily coffee enemas and weekly colonics are recommended, to facilitate the discharge of toxic waste from the destruction of the cancer.

Proteolytic enzymes are most effective when taken rectally. Take 3 enzyme wafers in a single enema once a day for 3 days, then 2 wafers in a single enema two times a day for 3 days, then 1 wafer in a single enema once a day for 5 days. A syringe and enema tip accompanies the Wobe Mugos enema wafers. Place the number of wafers in the syringe and draw from 15 to 200 cubic centimeters of distilled water (at body temperature) into the syringe. Shake the syringe a few times until the wafers dissolve and attach the plastic tube to the syringe. Lubricate the tube syringe and insert it into the rectum. Slowly allow the fluid to enter the rectum. This usually does not stimulate bowel movement. The whole process should be performed in 5 to 6 minutes or the enzyme will be deactivated. The enzyme is rapidly absorbed within a few minutes by the large intestine and enters the bloodstream to the site of its action.

Coffee Enemas

Coffee enemas during the initial stages of treatment are important to maintain regular detoxification from the overburdened liver. Coffee specifically draws toxins from the liver through the mesentery of the small intestine. While a small amount of caffeine may be absorbed, the detoxification is of far greater benefit. It may be possible to use other herbs, such as bayberry bark, raspberry leaf, and catnip, to accomplish a similar purpose, but since this is not yet proven by enough experience, the coffee enema may be the better choice.

Dissolve 3 tablespoons of ground organic coffee in 1 quart of water. Boil the coffee for 3 minutes and then simmer it for another 15 minutes.

Strain it and allow it to cool to body temperature. Place it in an enema bag, which can be purchased from a pharmacy. Be sure the stopper on the enema bag hose is closed. Apply oil to the enema tip and the anus. Prepare a place in the bathroom with towels and blankets as necessary. Hang the bag no higher than 3 feet above the area on the floor where you will be lying. Lie on your back and gently insert the oiled enema tip into your anus. Try elevate you feet slightly, perhaps against the wall near where enema bag is hanging. Allow the coffee to flow gently into your bowel slowly so as not to cause cramping. Gentle pressure on the bag will encourage the flow. At the same time, massage upward on the left side of the abdomen from the descending colon to the transverse colon just under the ribs and then down to the ascending colon on the right side of the abdomen. Retain the coffee for 4 or 5 minutes and then expel it. Patients often expel up to 1 gallon of fluid within 20 to 30 minutes. Initially, this can be done once or twice daily for several days in succession. Then the interval can be spread out to a couple of times a week and finally once a week. It can be used anytime the patient feels bogged down and tired or has pain.

High Colonic Enemas

High colonic enemas are done similarly to coffee enemas, but 2 quarts—instead of 1 quart—of fluid are used. This may be an herb tea appropriate for the condition that is being treated. This should be done once a week. One may also engage a colonic therapist to administer the treatment.

· 1 6 ·

MAGNET THERAPY

Magnet therapy is a method of topically applying magnets of varying size and strength over an area to relieve pain and/or inflammation. While magnets can be used for other conditions and in other ways, this is the most common use and the most dramatic in terms of its results. It is my experience that magnet therapy will successfully treat these conditions with approximately 80% to 85% success. The primary limiting factors are the many ingenious methods one may have to devise to attach them to the affected areas of the body and using the correct strength and, most important, the correct polarity.

First, a little background. The use of magnets for the treatment of disease has its origins far back in antiquity. It is recorded that the use of naturally occurring lodestone (magnetic iron ore) was considered by ancient peoples to have magical and sacred properties. These special magnetic stones were used by both the Egyptians and Greeks, as they have been used by the Chinese for healing of a wide variety of common complaints for thousands of years. With the advent of the industrial and electronic ages, it is possible to manufacture specific metal and ceramic material that can hold the highest magnetic charge. Certain minerals, such as cobalt, can be made into supermagnets.

There is a difference between a permanent magnet, which will retain its magnetic power over years, and an electronic magnet, which is only magnetic while it has electricity running through it. The magnetic force of a permanent magnet is a *DC* or *direct current* charge and tends to be regular and organizing to adjacent living cells and tissues. Electronically generated magnetic energy adjacent to high-power electrical lines and appliances, on the other hand, is *AC* or *alternating current*. Because AC electromagnetic energy is irregular, it tends to have a deranging influence on living tissues.

The earth itself is a life-supporting gigantic DC magnet, which, despite its magnetic power, is estimated to have a magnetic strength of approximately only half a gauss. Considering that gauss as a measurement is regarded as very imprecise at best, relatively speaking, a magnet of under 1,000 gauss is considered to be weak and those of 3,000 to 25,000 gauss are considered to be strong. What determines a magnet's strength is its gauss pulling power plus its size. It is the size of the earth, rather than its half-gauss pulling power, that makes the earth a powerful, life-sustaining magnetic force.

In fact, it is now understood that the magnetic force of the earth is absolute necessity to life and it, along with oxygen, must be appropriately provided if we are to survive long journeys into space. Furthermore, since the magnetic strength of the earth waxes and wanes over millennia, there may be a correlation with the great cataclysmic upheavals that have periodically occurred with the variation of the earth's magnetic power. For this reason, there is some justification to consider DC magnetic energy as another form of nutrient, necessary for life.

So how do magnets heal? Over the years, I have used magnets successfully on hundreds of patients for conditions ranging from sinusitis, bronchitis, and coughs to migraine headaches, back and joint pains, carpal tunnel pains, tennis elbow, digestive pains, colitis, and menstrual cramps to brain cancer, to name only a few. Practically every patient who is to undergo magnet therapy is understandably curious as to how they work. After magnets have been on for a few minutes and their condition is relieved, their curiosity changes to astonishment as painful conditions that have caused them distress and pain for years are suddenly alleviated.

With the popularity of magnets in countries like Japan (whose people are among the most health conscious in the world), where you can find 8 of every 10 Japanese people sleeping on magnetic mattresses and an infinite variety of magnetic healing tools on display in pharmacies and openly sold without prescription, there is little or no research on how magnets work. Theories and conjectures abound, however.

On the most direct level, we can understand that magnets relieve pain by relieving congestion and increasing circulation to and through a specific area of the body. However, it is also likely that disease on the macrolevel is a deficiency or blockage of gross tissues, probably accompanied with a weakening or derangement of the relationship of subatomic particles that comprise those tissues on the submicrolevel. In other words, magnets probably supply a much-needed magnetic strength that helps to maintain the proper relationship of electrons, protons, and neutrons in the atomic molecules of the various tissues of the body.

The millions of people who find daily relief of acute and chronic inflammations and pain through magnet therapy need no further evidence of the therapy's worth.

THE NORTH-ATTRACTING AND SOUTH-ATTRACTING SIDES OF A MAGNET

Magnet therapy is very complementary to the use of herbs and diet. Given the energetic classification of herbs and foods as Yin, Yang, hot, cold, positive, or negative, magnets similarly have a south-attracting polarity that is Yang-positive or reinforcing and a north-attracting polarity that is Yin-negative or dispersing. Both have their unique therapeutic applications.

Other than the fact that most therapeutic magnets that one purchases, such as the Acuband magnets that I prefer to use for most conditions, are marked (the small Acuband magnets are purchased in packs of twelve), conveniently attached to an adhesive tape. Usually, these are south attracting and have the smooth side facing outward. By simply reversing these, one can identify the north-attracting side by its indentation. The north side is more dispersing and is indicated more for the relief of pain and inflammation, making it the most commonly indicated side for therapeutic application. The south-facing side is useful if the condition is more chronic and the patient needs strengthening.

Other than this, the best way to determine the therapeutic north and south side of an unmarked magnet is with the aid of a compass. Simply put a small compass up to a magnet. If one side pulls the marked north end of the needle, it should be marked as the north with a little nail polish or a permanent marker. Every other magnet will align itself with this one, which can be used as the marker. Another method is to suspend a magnet by a string. It will naturally align itself with the north and south poles of the earth.

Being one of the most powerful methods of alternative treatment, magnet therapy is often effective in relieving inflammation and pain more quickly and efficiently than either herbal medicine or acupuncture. Properly used, magnet therapy is so powerful and yet safe that it warrants a full discussion, as in my *Biomagnetic and Herbal Therapy* (Lotus Press, 1997).

HOW TO USE MAGNETS FOR HEALING

How does one use magnets for healing? The main considerations for magnet therapy are (1) determining what areas of the body require treatment; (2) selecting the type, size, and strength of magnets to be used; (3) determining, if relevant, the appropriate north or south polarity of the magnet to apply directly to the body; and (4) finding a way to attach them long enough so they have the desired effect.

Determining Areas of the Body to Be Treated with Magnets

The first and experientially most effective method is to apply magnets directly to the most highly reactive or sensitive areas, called "trigger points." While this is not always easy to determine for many conditions, one should do the best possible, since the difference of even a couple inches off the active trigger point can make a difference in therapeutic effect.

Another method that I find less experientially substiated are to apply either north-attracting or south-attracting magnets at specific acupuncture points both near and distal to the site of the affected area. This can be combined with the use of magnets over the site of vital organs that may be involved with the presenting condition. For instance, if the problem involves a headache, north-attracting magnets can be applied to the temples, forehead, or the base of the occiput. Usually, this alone is enough to relieve most headaches. However, if the headache is unresponsive or tends to be chronic, one might select areas over the liver or stomach, at relevant acupoints along the spine, or along meridians involved.

Choosing the Appropriate Type, Size, and Strength Magnet

Magnets come in various types, sizes and strengths. Magnetic strength is classified as follows:

GAUSS CATEGORY	STRENGTH (IN GAUSS)
Low	300– 700
Medium	1,000– 2,500
High	3,000– 6,000
Super	7,000–12,000

Generally speaking, it is best to begin by applying low-gauss magnets. Use low-strength magnets for the sensitive, the weak, small children, or the very aged. The inexperienced should use only lower-strength magnets on the head or chest.

There are large, bulky, circular or bar magnets that are intended to be applied to the affected area for a prescribed period of time (usually around 30 minutes) two or three times a day. This method is most suitable for high-strength magnets.

Smaller acupoint magnets come with a self-adhesive. These are intended to be applied to specific trigger points, acupoints, or affected areas.

Flexible bipolar magnets are flat and generally much wider and cover a larger area. They are generally of lower gauss strength, but their proponents claim that the bipolar configuration has the effect of further helping to increase blood circulation by dilating blood vessels. In my experience, these bipolar magnets are weaker, which compromises the overall therapeutic effectiveness, but they do have the advantage of being simpler to use for the inexperienced.

Determining the Correct Application of North and South

General Method

Correctly applying the north- or south-facing magnet, especially for higher-strength magnets, is essential to successful treatment. The north-facing side of a magnet is dispersing. It is used for acute pain and inflammation and to disperse stagnations of all kinds. The south-facing side is strengthening. It tends to coalesce the energy and should be used for tonification and for more chronic conditions.

In general, one should begin with the north side first and if results are unsatisfactory, simply reverse the polarity to south. Since there can be acute inflammatory episodes associated with chronic conditions, there are many conditions for which a combined north and south bipolar magnet is more effective than either polarity used alone. Further, there are conditions in which one might place a north-facing magnet over the acutely sensitive area of pain and inflammation and a south-facing magnet over a depleted organ, such as with lower back involving the kidneys and adrenals.

The Tapping Method

One fantastic method that I personally discovered for determining whether a condition requires north- or south-facing magnet therapy is to tap on the magnet once it is applied to the affected area. Incredible as it may seem, I have had patients on whom I have applied an Acuband magnet who, after suffering for over 2 years with such conditions as shoulder pain, tennis elbow, or carpal tunnel pain, received relief within 2 minutes. After lightly tapping on the top of the Acuband magnet approximately fifty times, I ask them to challenge their injury—to actually try to make it hurt. If the correct polarity was used, the pain immediately lessens within 2 minutes; if the incorrect polarity was chosen, it is aggravated.

In general, more recent or acute pains are relieved with the north-attracting side of the magnet and are aggravated by the south-attracting side. Chronic pains caused by weakness or deficiency are often relieved by south-attracting magnets and aggravated by the north-attracting.

DIFFERENT FORMS OF THERAPEUTIC MAGNETS

Therapeutic magnets come in many different sizes and shapes. Overall, for therapy, I prefer to use the Acuband magnets at a minimum of 6,000 gauss to relieve specific pain and inflammation. One must learn to reverse them as needed for the appropriate north or south side as described above. Other than these magnets, there are some other common forms in which magnets are purchased and used.

Flexible Magnets

Flexible magnets come in various shapes and sizes and are taped or fastened with a special clothing accessory to be worn on the lower back, knees, elbows, or wrist, for instance. They can come with either north or south polarity or may be bipolar.

Ceramic Industrial Magnets

Ceramic magnets come in all sizes and shapes. They are extraordinarily strong and can be dangerous to handle, as they can easily pinch one's fingers because they tend to violently slam together. The proper method is to slide them together or apart. Because they are made of a ceramic alloy, they can also shatter. I don't recommend these for use by the layperson. When I use them in my clinic, I wrap them with several layers of adhesive tape, which somewhat prevents them from shattering and also allows them to be marked according to their north or south side.

Magnetic Mattresses

As stated earlier, recent estimates are that eight out of ten Japanese people sleep on a magnetic mattress or magnetic mattress pad. In general, because they are used continuously, these mattresses and pads should be low—under 1,000 gauss—and either bipolar or with the north-facing side toward the reclining body. One oft-quoted study by Kyoichi Nakagawa, M.D., director of Isuzu Hospital in Tokyo, described a condition called magnetic field deficiency syndrome (MFDS)* that causes a variety of symptoms, including stiff shoulders, back, and neck; chest pains; habitual constipation; and general fatigue.

He mailed questionnaires to 11,648 users of magnets 2.5 millimeters thick by 5 millimeters in diameter with an external gauss strength of 590. Only the north magnetic side was in direct contact with the skin. Women represented 57% of respondents and men represented 43%, with ages ranging between 40 and 49 years. There were a variety of conditions represented, including stiff neck and shoulders, lumbago, neuralgia, painful muscles, and rheumatism. No adverse effects were reported; positive effects were noticed from the second to the fourth day of treatment. Even with this short-term study of every low strength magnets, over 90% of the users classified results as very efficacious, efficacious, or fairly efficacious; only 10% classified results as either ineffective or not very effective. Another study of 400 people with pain of the neck, shoulders, back, arms, or hands and legs, conducted by professors Akio Yamada and Shuwichi-Hirose of the Faculty of Medicine of the University of Tokyo, found the effectiveness range to be between 60% and 80% within a treatment period of 7 to 14 days.

Most who sleep on a magnetic mattress experience deeper, more relaxed sleep and a need for less sleep. Only a few may initially experience some heightened restlessness the first few nights. This may be caused by an increased level of detoxification as circulation is increased. The condition will usually even out after a few days.

Magnetic Insoles

Circulation of the feet and legs is considered vital to the health of the entire body. Magnetic insoles aids in the circulation in these vital areas.

---

*Nakagawa, Kyoichi, M.D. "Magnetic Field Deficiency Syndrome and Magnetic Treatment." *Japan Medical Journal* #2745, 12/4/76.

They can be considered for helping to maintain the health of the feet and treating such problems as neuropathy in these areas.

Magnetic Balls

Magnetic balls are special balls that are attached to a holder and vigorously rolled over an area of pain. The effect is temporarily or permanently relieved pain over the affected area, which wins many converts to the health-giving properties of magnetics.

Acupods

Acupods are exclusively manufactured by Norso Biomagnetics.* They represent an innovation in therapeutic magnet design: the magnet is encased in a small round plastic case to take advantage of the fact that when a magnet is rolled, tapped, or vibrated, it sends electrons deeper into the tissues of the body and more quickly relieves pain.

Magnetized Water

Magnet therapists believe that water exposed to a north, south, or bipolar magnetic field for a period of time is somehow altered to have a systematic therapeutic value when taken internally. For this reason, one may find various specially manufactured magnetic containers in Japan that are used to store drinking water.

Magnetic Jewelry

Magnetic jewelry includes magnetic bracelets, necklaces, and earrings, which are used for a variety of purposes ranging from addiction treatment to appetite control to treatment of heart palpitations.

CONTRAINDICATIONS FOR MAGNET THERAPY

For obvious reasons, magnets should not be used on individuals with pacemakers, metal pins, or metal parts in the body. They should also be

---

*Norso Biomagnetics, 4105 Starboard Court, Raleigh, NC 27613; phone: (800) 480-8601.

avoided during pregnancy. Strong magnets can be very dangerous when they are placed near each other. Care and proper handling is essential to prevent injury of fingers or other delicate bodily parts. Strong magnets are usually a ceramic ferrite alloy that can easily shatter, so the proper method of attaching and separating them should be to slide them together and apart. Finally, magnets will demagnetize computer hard disks, other computer floppy disks, credit cards, CDs and CD-ROMs, and magnetic tapes, so care should be taken to keep these away from all magnetic products.

PLANETHERBS ONLINE!

Planetherbs is Dr. Michael Tierra's web site and the web site for the East West Herbal Correspondence Course. This web site features the following:

- Information on the East-West Herbal Correspondence Course, including the 12-Lesson Home Study Course and the 36-Lesson Professional Herbalist Course
- Various audio- and videotapes by Dr. Michael Tierra on herbal medicine, including the twenty-four-set course
- The *Way of Herbs* video
- A revolving number of special herbal articles by Dr. Tierra and associates
- An online forum where one can comment or ask questions regarding herbs, health, and healing
- A cyberstore where one can safely purchase online a number of hard-to-find specialty products, including Planetary Formulas, products, magnets, Nikken magnets (along with information on distributorship opportunities), Barefoot Doctor tools, Chinese herbs, Ayurvedic herbs, soy extract, and much more
- Video on the use of escharotic pastes and the botanical treatment of cancer. This highly informative unedited 2½-hour video tape presentation given at the 1997 American Herbalists' Guild symposium in Cincinnati, Ohio, describes various healing approaches, including the application of escharotic pastes for the removal of external and internal cancers. On this video are two women who had the courage to successfully treat themselves for breast cancer. One segment is a dramatic home video presentation by one patient who videotaped herself with her recently extracted tumor. This comes with a descriptive booklet on the botanical treatment of cancer. Order online from East-West Store at

    http://supplies.planetherbs.com/

- You'll also find this site to be a source for special links to other herbal sites and sites of related interest. The online supplies service's "shopping basket" employs the latest SSL (secure sockets layer) encryption methods to enable you to safely order books and herbal supplies online.

Use the following URLs (universal resource locators):

> http://www.planetherbs.com/
> http://supplies.planetherbs.com/mall/
> http://forums.planetherbs.com/

APPENDIX 1

Traveler's First Aid

Condition to Treat	Herbal Preparation to Carry	Method of Application
SUNBURN	aloe vera gel (may be purchased or squeezed fresh from the leaf)	Apply thin layer over affected area, reapply frequently.
BLEEDING	tincture of amaranth or powder of tienchi	Apply directly to wound, and internally as needed.
INFECTED WOUNDS	salve of equal parts goldenseal, myrrh and calendula	Apply to affected area.
SORE MUSCLES	liniment of equal parts eucalyptus, bay and rosemary, with one-quarter part lobelia	Apply to affected area.
BITES, SNAKE AND INSECT	tincture of echinacea	Apply to bite; also take internally one teaspoon every two hours for venomous bites.
REPELLING INSECTS	oil of pennyroyal and citronella	Apply to exposed areas, avoid contact with mucous membranes.
POISON OAK AND IVY	tincture made with equal parts witch hazel, mugwort, comfrey root, plantain and white oak bark	Apply to affected area.
DYSENTERY AND DIARRHEA	capsules of blackberry bark and capsules of equal parts goldenseal and chaparral	Take two of each every four hours.

Condition to Treat	Herbal Preparation to Carry	Method of Application
CONSTIPATION	capsules of equal parts cascara, licorice and psyllium seed	Take two capsules every four hours.
IRRITATIONS	powder of equal parts comfrey root, slippery elm and marshmallow	For external use, add a little water and apply to affected area. For internal irritations, fill gelatin capsules and take two every two hours.
HYPERACIDITY	pieces of calamus root	Chew a small piece.
COLDNESS	capsules of composition powder, angelica, cayenne or prickly ash bark	Take two capsules as needed, not to exceed eight per day.
TO INDUCE VOMITING	Ipecac	Take as directed.
MENSTRUAL CRAMPS AND MUSCLE CRAMPS	capsules of dong quai, cramp bark or black haw	Take two as needed, not to exceed eight per day.
HEADACHE	tincture of rosemary	Fifteen to thirty drops as needed, internally.
INSOMNIA	tincture of equal parts valerian and kava kava	Take one teaspoon as needed.
FATIGUE	capsules of equal parts ginseng and astragalus	Take two capsules as needed, not to exceed eight per day.
RED EYES	goldenseal tea preserved with tincture of benzoin	Make fresh before each trip, apply a few drops as needed.
COLDS AND FLU	oil of garlic and capsules of cayenne	Take a teaspoon of garlic oil and two capsules of cayenne every four hours.
POOR DIGESTION	tincture of agrimony or gentian	Take one or two teaspoons before meals.

How to carry: Put tinctures, liniments and oils in small plastic containers with flip-up dropper spouts. Carry capsules in plastic, multicompartment containers like those used by fishermen to separate small items. Salves, gels and powders can be carried in small, tightly capped jars.

How much to carry: Bring at least one ounce of the tinctures and oils; at least two ounces of the salves, liniments and gels; and at least eight of each capsule for each remedy you think you may need.

Other things to bring: Bandages, empty gelatin capsules, cloth and a small scissors.

APPENDIX 2

Sources for Herbs and Herb Products

Threshold Enterprises
23 Janis Way
Scotts Valley, CA 95066
Phone: (408) 438-1700
Fax: (408) 438-7410

Manufacturer and wholesale distributor of Michael Tierra's Planetary Formula herbal products. Those interested in the wholesale distribution of these products should contact this company.

ORGANIC WESTERN HERBS

Frontier Herbs and Nature's Herbs
P.O. Box 118, Department 34, Q
Norway, IA 52318
Phone: (800) 365-4372

Trinity Herb Company
P.O. Box 199
Bodega Bay, CA 94222
Phone: (707) 874-3418

CHINESE HERBS

Min Tong Chinese Herbs Company
5221 Central, suite 105
Richmond, CA 94804
Phone: (800) 538-1333

This company offers high-quality Chinese herbs in concentrated dry extract form, which is most convenient to use.

Great China Herb Company
857 Washington Street
San Francisco, CA 94108
Phone: (415) 982-2195

This is the oldest herb store in San Francisco's Chinatown and a source of quality Chinese herbs.

HERBAL NURSERY

Companion Plants
7447 N. Coolville Road
Athens, OH 45701
Phone: (614) 593-3092

Elixir Botanicals
General Delivery
Brixey, MO 65618
Phone: (417) 261-2393

Horizon Herbs
P.O. Box 69
Williams, OR 97544
Phone: (541) 846-6704
Fax: (541) 846-6233

Oregon Exotics
1065 Messinger Road
Grants Pass, OR 97527
Phone: (541) 846-7578

Richter's Nursery
Phone: (905) 640-6677
Fax: (905) 640-6641

This is one of the world's finest sources of herb plants and seeds. They ship herb seeds and plants worldwide. Visit and order from them online (www. richters.com). They are located in Ontario, Canada. Ask for a catalogue.

APPENDIX 3

Educational Resources

WHERE TO STUDY HERBS: SCHOOLS, COLLEGES, AND COURSES

For a listing of schools and courses, write or call the American Herbalists Guild (AHG), P.O. Box 70, Roosevelt, UT 84066; (435) 722-8434.

East/West School of Herbalism
Michael Tierra, O.M.D., L.Ac., founder of the AHG
P.O. Box 712
Santa Cruz, CA 95061
Phone: (408) 336-5010 or (800) 717-5010
Fax: (408) 336-4548

A correspondence course with yearly weeklong seminars, integrating the study of Western, Chinese, and Ayurvedic herbal medicine. The East/West Course is also an official registered professional herb course in the United Kingdom. Contact David and Sarah Holland, Hartswood Marsh Green, Hartfield, E. Sussex, United Kingdom TN7 4ET, or call 011-44-134-282-2312 or fax 011-44-134-282-6347.

ASSOCIATIONS

American Association of Acupuncture and Oriental Medicine (AAAOM)
433 Front Street
Catasauqua, PA 18032-2526
Phone: (610) 266-1433
Fax: (610) 264-2768

The AAAOM is a national professional association for practitioners of acupuncture and Oriental medicine. Contact them for a list of schools of traditional Chinese medicine (TCM).

American Association of Naturopathic Physicians (AANP)
601 Valley Street, suite 105
Seattle, WA 98109
Phone: (206) 298-0126
Referral line: (206) 298-0125
Fax: (206) 298-0129

The AANP is the unifying professional association for naturopathic medicine.

American Botanical Council
Mark Blumenthal
P.O. Box 201660
Austin, TX 78720-1660
Phone: (512) 331-8868
Fax: (512) 331-1924

Publishes *HerbalGram* in association with the Herb Research Foundation, as an educational project.

American Herb Association
Kathi Keville
P.O. Box 1673
Nevada City, CA 95959

Publishes a quarterly newsletter on the latest developments on herbal medicine.

The American Herbalists Guild
P.O. Box 70
Roosevelt, UT 84066
Phone: (435) 722-8434
Fax: (435) 722-8452
e-mail: ahgoffice@earthlink.net or http://www.healthy.net/herbalists

Represents the interests of student and professional clinical herbalists of North America. Professional membership is through peer review. Anyone may join as an associate and receive its quarterly newsletter, information on herb schools, and a discount on the cost of the guild's annual herbal symposiums. It is also a source for obtaining authoritative information on the therapeutic use of herbs.

American Holistic Medical Association
4101 Lake Boone Trail, suite 201
Raleigh, NC 27607
Phone: (919) 787-5146
Fax: (919) 787-4916

Herb Growing & Marketing Network
P.O. Box 245
Silver Spring, PA 17575-0245
Phone: (717) 393-3295
Fax: (717) 393-9261

Herb Research Foundation (HRF)
1007 Pearl Street, suite 200
Boulder, CO 80302
Phone: (303) 449-2265 or (800) 748-2617
Fax: (303) 449-7849
e-mail: rmccaleb@herbs.org

HRF is an internationally recognized center for herbal research and education.

National Institute of Medical Herbalists (NIMH)
56 Longbrook Street
Exeter, Devon, United Kingdom EX4 6AH
Phone: 011-44-39-242-6022
Fax: 011-44-39-249-8963

Membership and certification organization for medical herbalists in the United
Kingdom.

National Institutes of Health (NIH), Office of Complimentary and
    Alternative Medicine (OCAM)
9000 Rockville Pike, building 31
Bethesda, MD 20829
Phone: (301) 402-2466 or (301) 402-4334

Ontario Herbalists Association
11 Winthrop Place
Stoney Creek, Ontario, Canada L8G 3M3
Phone: (905) 536-1509
Fax: (905) 536-1567

United Plant Savers (UPS)
P.O. Box 420
East Barre, VT 05649
Phone: (802) 479-9825
Fax: (802) 476-3722

UPS is devoted to replanting endangered and threatened medicinal plant species for nonharvestable purposes.

JOURNALS AND NEWSLETTERS

The Business of Herbs
Northwind Farm Publications
P. Oliver, Route 2, Box 246
Shevlin, MN 56676
Phone: (219) 657-2478
Fax: (218) 657-2447

Bimonthly trade journal for herb businesses

The Herb Companion
Interweave Press
201 East Fourth Street
Loveland, CO 80537
Phone: (970) 669-7677 or (800) 272-2193
Fax: (970) 667-8317
e-mail: hc@1wp.ccmail.compuserve.com

Bimonthly full-color magazine "celebrating the useful plants"

HerbalGram
One of the most respected and beautiful herbal magazines, attempting to bring science and herbalist together; See the listing for the American Botanical Council

The Herbalist
Quarterly newsletter for members of the AHG; see listing for the American Herbalist Guild

International Journal of Oriental Medicine
Oriental Healing Arts Institute
1945 Palo Verde Avenue, suite 208
Long Beach, CA 90815
Phone: (310) 431-3545

Medical Herbalism
Paul Bergner, editor
P.O. Box 20512
Boulder, CO 80308
Phone: (303) 541-9552

An outstanding newsletter for the clinical herbalist

Robyn's Recommended Reading
Robyn Klein, editor (herbalist and member of AHG)
1627 West Main, suite 116
Bozeman, MT 59715
e-mail: rklein@sunrise.alpinet.net

Townsend Letter for Doctors
911 Tyler Street
Port Townsend, WA 98368

A forum for alternative medical practitioners

PLANETARY FORMULA NAMES MENTIONED IN THE TEXT

Formula number 2 is Diurite
Formula number 8 is Stress Free
Formula number 12 is HepatoPure
Formula number 14 is River of Life
Formula number 15 is Complete Pau D'Arco
Formula number 23 is Triphala
Formula number 68 is Guggul Raj

For online information and ordering of these and Michael Tierra's other Planetary Formulas, enter http://supplies.

APPENDIX 4

Weights and Measures

1 pound = 453 grams
1 ounce = 28.3 grams
16 ounces (dry) = 1 pound
1 quart = 2 pints
1 pint = 2 cups
1 cup = 8 ounces (fluid)
1 teaspoon = 60 drops
1 tablespoon = 3 teaspoons
1 fluid ounce = 2 tablespoons
1 cup = 16 tablespoons

Capsules and Powders

15.4 grains = 1 gram
1 gram = 1000 milligrams (mg)
contents 1 "00" capsule = about 650 mg = 10 grains
(well packed)*
contents 1 "0" capsule = about 500 mg = 8 grains
(well packed)
Two gelatin capsules = one teaspoon of the tincture
Two tablespoons tincture = one-half cup of tea

---

*1 teaspoon of powder will fill about two "00" capsules. Thus one ounce of powdered herb will fill 40 to 50 "00" capsules or 50 to 70 "0" capsules, depending on the type of herb, fineness of powder, and tightness of packing.

BIBLIOGRAPHY

BOOKS BY MICHAEL TIERRA, L.Ac., O.M.D.

Planetary Herbology (Lotus Press, 1988)

The Natural Remedy Bible, with John Lust (New York: Pocket Books, 1990)

Biomagnetic and Herbal Therapy (Lotus Press, 1997)

The Herbal Tarot, with Candis Cantin (US Games, 1992)

The Spirit of Herbs: A Guide to the Herbal Tarot, with Candis Cantin (1993) by U.S. Games

American Herbalism: Essays on Herbs & Herbalism, by members of the American Herbalist Guild; edited by Michael Tierra, O.M.D. (Crossing Press, 1992, out of print)

The East/West Herb Course (East/West Herbal Correspondence Course, Box 712, Santa Cruz, CA 95060)

Chinese-Planetary Herbal Diagnosis, with Lesley Tierra

The Way of Chinese Herbs (Pocket Books, 1998)

BOOKS BY LESLEY TIERRA

The Herbs of Life (Crossing Press, 1992)

Healing with Chinese Herbs (Crossing Press, 1997)

A Children's Herbal (Forthcoming)

HISTORY OF HERBAL MEDICINE

Griggs, Barbara. *Green Pharmacy: The History and Evolution of Western Herbal Medicine*, revised edition (Rochester, VT: Healing Arts Press, 1997)
> Don't miss reading this book. It is the best book on the subject by far and is highly informative and entertaining.

Griggs, Barbara. *The Food Factor: Why We Are What We Eat* (Viking Press, 1986)
> If you can find this book, it is almost as good as *Green Pharmacy*. It essentially is the history of the various nutrition movements through the ages. I think the title of the book is misleading, but the book is fascinating reading.

Vogel, Virgil J. *American Indian Medicine* (Ballantine Books, 1970)
> The most authoritative single book on the vast herbal healing traditions of the Native Americans

Brooke, Elisabeth. *The Women Healers: A Portrait of Herbalists, Physicians, and Midwives* (Rochester, VT: Healing Arts Press, 1995)
A fascinating book on the little-known but extremely important tradition of women herbalists and healers from ancient times
Conrow and Hecksel. *Herbal Pathfinders: Voices of the Herb Renaissance* (Woodbridge Press, 1983)

MISCELLANEOUS AND USEFUL BOOKS ON HERBS

Brown, Deni. *The Encyclopedia of Herbs and Their Uses.* (Dorling Kindersley, under the auspices of the Herb Society of America, 1995)
Over 1,000 plants and 1,500 photographs oriented for the gardener, but provides very good information on plants' medicinal uses; a beautiful book
Weiss, Rudolf Fritz, M.D. *Herbal Medicine* (Gothenburg, Sweden: AB Arcanum, 1988; Beaconsfield, England: Beaconsfield Publishers Ltd; distributed in the United States by Medicina Biologia, 4839 N.E. 32nd Avenue, Portland, OR 97211)
An excellent book written by a German medical doctor who used herbs extensively in his medical practice
Ritchardson, Jack, N.D. *The Little Herb Encyclopedia,* 3rd edition. (Woodland Health Books, P.O. Box 160, Pleasant Grove, UT 84062)
The Macdonald Encyclopedia of Medicinal Plants (Macdonald & Co., 66-73 Shoe Lane, London, United Kingdom EC4P 4AB)
Foster, Steven, and James Duke. *Peterson Field Guides Eastern/Central Medicinal Plants* (Boston, Houghton Mifflin, 1990)
Pederson, Mark. *Nutritional Herbology* (Wendell W. Whitman Co., 302 E. Winona Ave., Warsaw, IN 46580, 1-800-241-2401; 1994)
Murray, Michael T., N.D. *The Healing Power of Herbs* (Prima Publishing, P.O. Box 1260BK, Rocklin, CA 95677; 1992, 1995)
A book with a lot of useful information but tending to be overly scientific, as it recommends standardized constituents
Mabey, Richard. *The New Age Herbalist* (Collier Books, Macmillan, 1988)
Mills, Simon Y. *Out of the Earth: The Essential Book of Herbal Medicine* (Viking Arcana, 1991)
Priest and Priest. *Herbal Medication: A Clinical and Dispensary Handbook* (Fowler)
Thomson, William A. R., M.D., editor. *Medicines from the Earth,* revised, with a foreword by Richard Evans Schultes. (Alfred Van Der Marck Editions, 1978; distributed by Harper & Row, San Francisco)
Lust, John. *The Herb Book* (New York: Bantam Books, 1974)
Scott, Julian, Ph.D. *Natural Medicine for Children* (Avon Books, 1990)

HERBAL CLASSICS

Culpepper, Nicholas. *Culpepper's Complete Herbal* (W. Foulsham and Co.)
Grieve, Maude. *A Modern Herbal*, 2 volumes (Dover Press)
    A classic book, originally published in the early 1930s, with a lot of great
    herbal lore
Strehlow, Dr. Wighard and Gottfried Hertzka, M.D. *Hildegard of Bingen's Medicine*
    (Santa Fe, NM: Bear and Company, 1988)
Millspaugh, Charles F. *American Medicinal Plants* (Dover Press)
Shook, Dr. Edward E. *Elementary and Advanced Treatise in Herbology* (Trinity Center
    Press and CSA Press)
    First published in the early twentieth century. If you can get past the author's
    tendency to rant and rave, this is still one of the more important books on
    Western clinical herbal medicine.
Christopher, Dr. John R. *The School of Natural Healing* (Christopher Publications,
    P.O. Box 412, Springville, UT 84663)
Wren, F.L.S., R. C., *Potter's New Cyclopaedia of Botanical Drugs and Preparations*,
    revised. (Saffron Walden, C. W. Daniel Company Limited, 1988)

HERBALS BY AND FOR WOMEN

Crawford, Amanda McQuade, M.N.I.M.H., American Herbalists' Guild *Herbal
    Remedies for Women* (Prima Publishing, 1997)
    An important book by one of the best women herbalists for women and for
    men who are supporters and helpers of women
Gladstar, Rosemary. *Herbal Healing for Women* (New York: Fireside, Simon &
    Schuster, 1993)
    Rosemary is one of the most important and revered herbalists of our time; her
    book is simple and empowering.

BOOKS BY SUSAN S. WEED

Breast Cancer? Breast Health! The Wise Woman Way (Woodstock, NY: Ash Tree
    Publishing, 1992)
Menopausal Years (Woodstock, NY: Ash Tree Publishing, 1992)

OTHER HERBALS

Pengelly, Andrew, Medical Herbalist. *The Constituents of Medicinal Plants: An Intro-
    duction to the Chemistry & Therapeutics of Herbal Medicines* (Sunflower Herbals,
    "Athlone," Dorset Road, Muswellbrook, NSW 2333, Australia

This is a very useful book for the serious student who is interested in better understanding herbal biochemistry.

BOOKS BY DAVID HOFFMANN, FOUNDING MEMBER OF THE AMERICAN HERBALISTS' GUILD AND GRADUATE OF THE BRITISH SCHOOL OF MEDICAL HERBAL MEDICINE

The Holistic Herbal (Element Press, 1992)
    A modern herbal classic
The Elements of Herbalism (Element Inc., 42 Broadway, Rockport, MA 01966; 1991)
The Herbal Handbook: A User's Guide to Medical Herbalism (Healing Arts Press, 1987)
An Elder's Herbal
Successful Stress Control by David Hoffman (Thorsons Publishing Group, Rochester, Vermont, 1986)
Therapeutic Herbalism
Welsh Herbal Medicine (Abercastle Publications, 1988, Wales)

BOOKS BY CHRISTOPHER HOBBS, L.Ac., FOUNDING MEMBER OF THE AMERICAN HERBALISTS' GUILD

Medicinal Mushrooms: An Exploration of Tradition, Healing, & Culture
Echinacea, The Immune Herb
Foundations of Health: on Digestion
Ginkgo, Elixir of Youth
Milk Thistle, The Liver Herb
Natural Liver Therapy
Usnea, The Herbal Antibiotic
Valerian, The Relaxing and Sleep Herb
Vitex, The Women's Herb
St. John's-wort
The Ginsengs: A User's Guide
    An excellent and growing collection of authoritative books by one of the most prolific authors on herbal medicine in our time. All of Hobbs' books are published by Botanica Press, 201 E. 4th Street, Loveland, CO 80537; (800) 272-2193.

BOOKS BY MICHAEL MOORE, MEMBER OF THE AMERICAN HERBALISTS' GUILD

Medicinal Plants of the Desert and Canyon West
Medicinal Plants of the Pacific West

Medicinal Plants of the Mountain West
    All of the above are published by Museum of New Mexico Press

Los Remedios: Traditional Herbal Remedies of the Southwest 1977, by Author
Herbal Repertory in Clinical Practice
    Michael Moore is the dean of mid–twentieth century herbalists.

BOOKS BY TERRY WILLARD, MEMBER OF THE AMERICAN HERBALISTS'
GUILD

Reishi Mushroom: Herb of Spiritual Potency and Medical Wonder Sylvan Press, Issa-
    quah, WA, (1990)
The Wild Rose Scientific Herbal (Wild Rose College of Natural Healing Ltd., 1220
    Kensington Road N.W., Calgary, Alberta, Canada T2N, 3P5)
Edible and Medicinal Plants of the Rocky Mountains and Neighbouring Territories (Wild
    Rose College of Natural Healing Ltd.)
Textbook of Modern Herbology (C. W. Progressive Publishing, 515 42nd Avenue
    S.E., Calgary, Alberta, Canada T2G 1Y7)

BOOKS BY PAUL BERGNER, MEMBER OF THE AMERICAN HERBALISTS' GUILD

The Healing Power of Ginseng & the Tonic Herbs (Prima Publishing, 1996)
The Healing Power of Garlic (Prima Publishing, 1996)
The Healing Power of Minerals, Special Nutrients, and Trace Elements (Prima Publish-
    ing, 1997)

BOOKS BY KENNETH JONES

Pau d'Arco: Immune Power from the Rain Forest (1995)
Reishi: Ancient Herb for Modern Times
Shiitake: The Healing Mushroom
    These are all excellent researched, well-written, and definitive books, pub-
    lished by Healing Arts Press, Rochester, Vermont, on important herbs.

BOOKS BY STEVEN FOSTER

The Herbal Renaissance: Growing, Using & Understanding Herbs in the Modern World,
    revised edition of *Herbal Bounty*
    The finest book on herbal cultivation by one of the masters; well written and
    with some of the most beautiful herbal photographs and line drawings (by
    Mimi Dowden) that you will ever see

Herbal Emissaries: Bringing Chinese Herbs to the West, a Guide to Gardening, Herbal Wisdom, and Well-being, with Yue Chongxi (Rochester, VT: Healing Arts Press)

Herbs for Your Health: A Handy Guide for Knowing and Using 50 Common Herbs (Interweave Press, 1996)

Forest Pharmacy: Medicinal Plants in American Forests (Durham, NC: Forrest History Society)

BOOKS BY JAMES GREEN, MEMBER OF THE AMERICAN HERBALISTS' GUILD

The Male Herbal: Health Care for Men and Boys (Freedom, CA: Crossing Press, 1991)

The Herbal Medicine Makers' Handbook [Simplers Botanical, Box 39, Forestville, CA 95436, (707) 887-2012]

An excellent short book on making herbal preparations

BOOKS BY VARRO E. TYLER, PH.D., S.C.D.

The Honest Herbal (George F. Stickley Company)

The New Honest Herbal (George F. Stickly Company)

Herbs of Choice: The Therapeutic Use of Phytomedicinals (Pharmaceutical Products Press)

Dr. Tyler's perspective on the use of herbs is strictly scientific and pedantic. He is the country's most respected pharmacognocist. His opinions often clash with the practical clinical experience of herbalists, for which he is justly criticized. However, his work is worthy of consideration.

ECLECTIC PUBLICATIONS

Unless otherwise indicated, all Eclectic publications are reprinted by Eclectic Medical Publications, 11231 SE Market Street, Portland, OR 97216, (503) 252-5617.

Ellingwood, Finley, M.D. *American Materia Medica, Therapeutics, and Pharmacognosy*

King, John Felter, M.D., and John Uri Lloyd. *King's American Dispensatory*

Lloyd, John Uri. *Dose Book of Specific Medications* (from the original edition, 1915)

Scudder, John Milton. *Specific Medications and Specific Diagnosis*

ESCOP (European Scienfitic Cooperative on Phytotherapy). *Herbal Monographs on the Medicinal Uses of Plant Drugs* (European Scientific Cooperative on Phytotherapy)

AYURVEDIC, TRADITIONAL EAST INDIAN MEDICINE

Lad, Dr. Vasant. *Ayurveda: The Science of Self Healing* (Lotus Press, 1984)

Lad, Dr. Vasant, and Frawley, Dr. David. *The Yoga of Herbs* (Lotus Press, 1986)

Frawley, David, O.M.D. *Ayurvedic Healing* (Lotus Press, 1989)

Heyn, Birgit. *Ayurvedic Medicine* (Thorsons, 1987)

Nadkarni, Dr. K. M. *Indian Materia Medica,* two volumes (Bombay: Popular Praka-
    shan, 1976)

DIET AND NUTRITION

Ballentine, Rudolph, M.D. *Diet and Nutrition: A Holistic Approach* (Himalayan Inter-
    national Institute, Honesdale, PA, 1978)

Fallon, Sally. *Nourishing Traditions* [ProMotion Publishing, 3368F Governor Drive,
    suite 144, San Diego, CA. 92122, (800) 231-1776]

Turner, Kristina. *The Self Healing Cookbook* (Earthtones Press, P.O. Box 2341B,
    Grass Valley, CA 95945; 1987)

Flaws, Bob. *The Book of Jook* (Blue Poppy Press)

MACROBIOTICS

Kushi, Michio. *The Book of Macrobiotics* (Japan Publications)

Colbin, Annemarie. *Food and Healing,* revised (New York: Ballantine Books, 1996)

CHINESE MEDICINE

Holmes, Peter. *Jade Remedies: A Chinese Herbal Reference for the West,* 2 volumes
    (Boulder, CO: Snow Lotus Press, 1996)

L'Orange, Darlena. *Herbal Healing Secrets of the Orient* (Englewood Cliffs, NJ:
    Prentice-Hall)
    An outstanding and practical book for Westerners on the practical use of
    Chinese herbs

Beinfield, Harriet, L.Ac., and Efrem Korngold, L.Ac., O.M.D. *Between Heaven and
    Earth: A Guide to Chinese Medicine*
    An outstanding introduction to the principles of traditional Chinese medicine
    with many practical uses for everyday life

Kaptchuk, Ted J., O.M.D. *The Web That Has No Weaver* (Congden and Weed,
    1983)

Bensky and Gamble. *Chinese Herbal Medicine Materia Medica* (Eastland Press)

Bensky and Barolet. *Formulas and Strategies* (Eastland Press)

Yeung, Him-Che, Ph.D. *Handbook of Chinese Herbs* and companion book *Chinese
    Herbal Formulas* [Institute of Chinese Medicine, 602 San Gabriel Boulevard,
    Rosemead, CA 91770, (818) 280-8811]

A Barefoot Doctor's Manual (Cloudburst Press)

BOOKS BY DANIEL P. REID

Chinese Herbal Medicine (Shambhala, 1987)
The Complete Book of Chinese Health and Healing (Shambhala, 1994)

THE BOTANICAL TREATMENT OF CANCER

Boik, John. *Cancer and Natural Medicine: A Textbook of Basic Science and Clinical Research* [Oregon Medical Press, 315 10th Avenue North, Princeton, MN 55371; phone and fax, (612) 389-0768]

Minyi, Chang, et al. *Anticancer Medicinal Herbs* (Hunan Science and Technology Publishing House, 1992)

Hsu, Hong-Yen. *Treating Cancer with Chinese Herbs* (Oriental Healing Arts Institute, 1982)

Dai-Zhao, Zhang. *The Treatment of Cancer by Integrated Chinese-Western Medicine*, translated by Zhang Ting-Liang and Bob Flaws (Blue Poppy Press)

Keane, Maureen, M.S., and Daniella Chace, M.S. *What to Eat If You Have Cancer* and *The What to Eat If You Have Cancer Cookbook* (Contemporary Books, Two Prudential Plaza, Chicago, IL 60601-6790; 1996)
These are the best two books available on traditional cancer nutrition—A must for individuals treating cancer or who have cancer

CANCER SALVES

Naiman, Dr. Ingrid. *Cancer Salves: A Botanical Approach to Treatment* (Seventh Ray Press; distributed to the public by North Atlantic Books; distributed to the trade by Publishers Group West)
This book is available over the internet at www.cancersalves.com or www.northatlanticbooks.com (ISBN: 1-55643-270-4).

BOOKS ON MAGNET HEALING

Tierra, Michael, L.Ac., O.M.D. *Biomagnetic and Herbal Therapy* (Lotus Press, 1997)

Davis, Albert Roy, Ph.D. *The Anatomy of Biomagnetism*
This is an important work describing the pioneer research in the use of bio-magnetics by one of the late leaders of the field in North America. It is available from Schafer's Health Centre, Box 251, Unity, Sask., Canada S0K 4L0

Bengali, Dr. Neville S. *Magnet Therapy Theory and Practice* (Jain Publishers, 10 Chuna Mandi Street, Paharganj, New Delhi 110055, India)
This is a very authoritative and informative book, but the reader should be

aware of a semantic difference that causes the author to reverse the description of the qualities of north and south magnetic poles.

Washnis, George J., and Richard Z. Hricak. *Discovery of Magnetic Health* (Rockville, MD: Nova)

Philpott, M.D., and Sharon Taplin. *Biomagnetic Handbook* [Enviro-Tech Products, 17171 SE 29 Street, Choctaw, OK 73020, (405) 390-3499]

INDEX